HUMAN
MOVEMENT

AN INTRODUCTORY TEXT FOR PHYSIOTHERAPY STUDENTS

HUMAN MOVEMENT

AN INTRODUCTORY TEXT FOR PHYSIOTHERAPY STUDENTS

P. M. Galley B. Phty, M.Ed.St.

Lecturer, Department of Physiotherapy, University of Queensland

A. L. Forster Hon. B. Phty, F.C.S.P.

Former Head of Department of Physiotherapy, University of Queensland

SECOND EDITION

Churchill Livingstone ▦

MELBOURNE EDINBURGH LONDON AND NEW YORK 1987

CHURCHILL LIVINGSTONE
Medical Division of Longman Group UK Limited

Distributed in Australia by Longman Cheshire Pty
Limited, Longman House, Kings Gardens, 95 Coventry
Street, South Melbourne 3205, and by associated
companies, branches and representatives throughout the
world.

First edition 1982
Second edition 1987
  Reprinted 1988
  Reprinted 1990
  Reprinted 1991
  Reprinted 1992
  Reprinted 1993 (twice)
  Reprinted 1994

ISBN 0 443 03390 0

British Library Cataloguing in Publication Data
A catalogue record for this book is available from the
British Library.

Library of Congress Cataloging in Publication Data
Galley, P. M.
  Human movement,
  Includes bibliographies and index.
  1. Human mechanics.   2. Exercise therapy.
1. Forster, A.L.   II. Title.   [DNLM: 1. Movement.
2. Physical Therapy. WE 103 G167h]
QP303.G26   1986   612'.76   85-26897

Produced by Longman Singapore Publishers (Pte) Ltd
Printed in Singapore

Preface to the Second Edition

In this new edition many chapters have been enlarged and updated. The bibliography has been extended. Several new chapters have been added including some which briefly discuss the reaction of the patient to disability, the rehabilitation team and the role of the physiotherapist in the planning and treatment of patients. It is hoped that this book will help the student appreciate the links between basic theoretical knowledge and its application to certain treatment procedures.

Queensland, 1987

P. M. G.
A. L. F.

Preface to the First Edition

The purpose of this book is to provide a text for physiotherapy students and for those returning to the profession. It is also hoped it will be of interest to clinicians.

The book aims to provide readers with some basic knowledge related to human movement which can be used in their treatment of patients.

The authors hope it will stimulate readers and promote a desire to read more widely, exploring many of the factors underlying physiotherapy practice. An effort has been made to define many of the terms commonly used by physiotherapists.

For brevity and clarity the patient is referred to as 'he' and the physiotherapist as 'she' throughout the text.

Queensland, 1982

P. M. G.
A. L. F.

Acknowledgements

We acknowledge with gratitude the many suggestions and helpful criticism of the first edition of the book given to us by practising physiotherapists and by the students of the Department of Physiotherapy, University of Queensland.

We also acknowledge the help once again given to us by Dr B. Lasich of the Department of Physics, University of Queensland, on the chapter on The Basic Principles of Mechanics.

Our very special thanks to our two typists; in particular, to Miss Joan Chapman who has so willingly and patiently typed many of the drafts as well as most of the final manuscript, and also to Mrs A. Weston.

The new line drawings are the work of Ms J. Chernside and Mr D. Sheehy of the Graphic Design Section of the Department of Audio-visual Services, University of Queensland.

Contents

1
Introduction

All people move constantly although few realise how complex their movements may be and even fewer stop to analyse how these movements come about. Yet it is through their movements that people have the ability and the means to interact with their environment, express their feelings and relate meaningfully to one another.

Kinesiology is the study of movement. For the physiotherapist and others who are involved in the treatment of the disabled, 'how man moves' is an important question. It is just not enough to register that a movement has occurred but rather how the movement was produced, if it was normal, and if not, what was the cause of the abnormality and what must be done to correct or improve it. Only by such an analysis can the physiotherapist plan an appropriate programme to help restore normal function, prevent deterioration and to use to advantage what remaining movement the patient has, so that all possible independence is gained.

The study of human movement

Because of its complexity, the study of human movement in all its forms may be conducted from many points of view – all of which at some time may concern the physiotherapist.

Five major theoretical approaches, considered to be of more immediate concern to the physiotherapist, are identified. They are:
1. Anatomical – which describes the structure

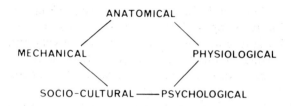

Fig. 1.1   The study of human movement.

of the body and its parts and their potential for movement.
2. Physiological — which studies the processes involved in the initiation, continuation and control of movement.
3. Psychological — which examines the sensations, perceptions and motivations that stimulate movement and the neurological mechanisms which control them.
4. Mechanical — which considers the force, time and distance relationships involved in body movement.
5. Socio-cultural — which considers the meanings given to various movements in different human settings.

Although these different approaches are often taught as separate subjects, it is advisable that relevant areas be linked up wherever possible so a wider appreciation of movement and its control is achieved by the student (Fig. 1.1).

Also based on these early studies will be studies of the cause, effects, course and overall management of the most common conditions treated by physiotherapy, many of which will involve disorders of movement.

Knowledge of human movement through direct experience

Few people consciously explore their full potential for movement. Therefore, in addition to the more formal approaches to the study of movement, is the self-knowledge that can be gained by the student as he or she moves and as the movements of others are carefully observed in daily life.

Much can be learned about a movement skill, even by a lay person through doing the movement and/or watching others perform. For the future physiotherapist, these are basic skills which must be deliberately acquired and developed to a high degree. It is suggested that the student becomes more aware of:

1. His or her own body — its structure — the shape of the whole and its parts, and how it changes in space with movement.
2. What the body feels like when it moves, in contrast to when it is still. What are the kinaesthetic sensations perceived? What movements give a feeling of pleasure or discomfort?
3. The internal sensations as individual muscle groups work to move the body parts from one position to another. What is the qualitative difference between a stretched, contracted and relaxed muscle? How long does it take before a muscle group becomes fatigued?
4. The growth of personal skill in moving.
5. How to use his or her own body effectively in order to prevent unnecessary strain.

As careful observation of others is basic to good clinical practice, every opportunity should be taken to observe the movements of as many people as possible, comparing and contrasting them in terms of age, sex, ethnic group, social and occupational status. Through doing this systematically, the student may begin to develop a concept of what is the 'normal' movement that could be expected from any particular person, as well as exploring the full range of human movement possibilities of which pathological movement is one extreme.

These studies need to be extended to consider those factors which are necessary for normal individuals to function adequately in society. Therefore an attempt should be made to define those skills which are necessary in performing the common tasks of daily living and to analyse what movements are involved. The specialised tasks of different work situations can be approached in the same way. How these skills may be improved is also an important consideration.

This broader appreciation of what is 'normal'

should provide the student with useful guidelines for later clinical work, particularly when evaluating a disabled person's difficulties and the effectiveness of the various treatment methods applied.

Knowledge of testing and exercise procedures

With the building up of knowledge of human movement and needs will come the learning of skills involved in testing and analysing abnormal movement, as well as in the selection and teaching of therapeutic exercise. A wide repertoire of exercises to give a number of options and the ability to select and teach them is necessary if treatment of patients is to be relevant, accurate, interesting and stimulating, while at the same time encouraging active independent participation in the programme.

Understanding human movement and its clinical application

Knowledge derived from the various sources outlined in this chapter, can be applied by the physiotherapist during each stage of the clinical problem-solving process.

Through the senses of hearing, sight and touch, much information is collected about the patient and his problems. The skills of interviewing — listening with understanding; looking and seeing; palpating sensitively and testing contribute towards this pool of information as well as aiding in the development of visual and auditory memory.

Knowledge so gained is then recorded quickly, accurately and concisely. It is interpreted in the light of the knowledge acquired primarily through the formal study of movement, its abnormalities and their cause. Thus problems are identified. Goals are then formulated, keeping in mind what would be considered the norm for the patient's reference group, as well as his personal needs and desires.

Treatment follows in which therapeutic exercise often plays a major role. Here self-knowledge related to the therapist's own potential for movement will be found most helpful if treatment is to be applied sensitively and imaginatively. Finally, the patient's progress is regularly evaluated and goals altered when necessary.

Thus, through systematically approaching each situation in this way, clinical judgement can be developed and clinical practice should become effective.

REFERENCES AND FURTHER READING

1. Brooke, J. D. & Whiting, H. T. A. (1973) *Human Movement — a field of study*. London: Henry Kimpton.
2. Higgins, J. R. (1977) *Human Movement — an integrated approach*. St Louis: C. V. Mosby.
3. Mainland, D. *Anatomy*. London: Hamish Hamilton Medical.
4. Muybridge, E. (1955) *The Human Figure in Motion*. New York: Dover Publications.
5. Penrod, J. (1974) *Movement for the Performing Artist*. Palo Alto, California: National Press Books.

2

Early growth and development

Human growth and development involves the whole spectrum of life and living from conception through to old age and death. Growth and development, though closely related, refer to different processes which change with time. Normally both these processes work in harmony.[42,43]

It is useful to study the various aspects of growth and development at different phases in the life span. In reality, one phase merges into the next without a definite line of demarcation, although there are some obvious exceptions notably birth and menarche. These phases are:

1. Prenatal — from conception to birth
2. Neonatal — from birth to 4 weeks of age
3. Infancy — until the child is able to exist independent of its caregiver, in that he is capable of feeding himself, walking and talking
4. Childhood — until puberty
5. Adolescence — until the adult social role is achieved
6. Adulthood — in which biological and social maturity are reached
7. Old age.

Both experience and organic changes contribute to the overall progression through all these phases.

In this chapter, the major emphasis will be on the development of movement but it must be stressed that this is only one aspect of the total developmental process. Other aspects include personality, intellectual, language, social, emotional and moral development.

GROWTH

Growth involves a series of anatomical and physiological changes which alter the body's size and composition. It is a continuous process although the rate of growth is far more obvious during the first years of life than at any other time. The interaction between an individual's genetic endowment and the environmental influences to which he is exposed is a major issue in development.

An individual's genetic heritage will determine the type of body he should possess as a mature human being.

Environmental factors can alter this potential, as is demonstrated by children who suffer severe early brain damage.

Different parts of the body grow at variable rates. The brain, whose growth and maturation is most closely related to the development of human behaviour, grows more rapidly during the prenatal period than at any other time during the life span. Tissues involved in reproductive function grow most rapidly at puberty. The bony epiphyses close at different ages.

Periods of rapid growth of body systems are called growth spurts. After a period of time, the fast rate of growing is lessened. When this occurs, the growth spurt is said to have ceased.

Growth, as a general phenomenon, does not cease once maturity is reached. If this were so there would be no healing of bone after a fracture or no repair of wounds to skin and muscle. In nearly every tissue and organ, there is a recurring cycle of growth, death and replacement.[44] An obvious everyday example is the growth of hair and nails.

A major exception to this cycle of events involves the neurons. Once their numbers have been established during the early part of the life span they cannot be replaced when they are destroyed.[44,47]

After maturity is reached in the early twenties, the body begins to age. With aging comes a decline in the number of cells in the body. This is called the period of negative growth.[44]

Cell loss first occurs in the central nervous system. Even people in their early twenties will demonstrate such changes when the special senses, memory and co-ordinated movements may begin to show deficits which are indicative of aging.

Both organic changes and experience contribute towards the performance of any behaviour. So although organic factors reach their peak in the early twenties and then decline, the level of experience still continues to rise throughout life. This has important implications for skill development.[53]

As the individual approaches old age, physical decline becomes most apparent. For example, control of the upright posture is reduced and elderly people are much more susceptible to falls.[21,34] Yet in the actual performance of a well learned task, those neurons still remaining function effectively, serving the individual well. Old people still retain the ability to learn new tasks, striking evidence of the versatility of the human nervous system.

Though the body loses much of its earlier capacity to move and in old age becomes biomechanically less efficient, experience accumulated over the years can make up much of this deficit. This factor is most important for those physiotherapists working with aged people to realise.

Measurement of growth

There have been many studies reported which examine changes in the dimensions of the body such as height, weight and body composition. The position of the growing individual's centre of gravity is altered as the body proportions change[35,41] (Fig. 2.1).

Muscle strength, which is partly though not completely related to the size and composition of the muscle concerned, has been examined in children of various ages.[33,56] Results have shown a predictable trend. As the child approaches adulthood, strength increases and

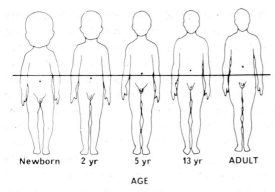

Newborn   2 yr   5 yr   13 yr   ADULT

AGE

Fig. 2.1 Body proportions at different ages. Note the relative height of the centre of gravity from birth to maturity. *After Palmer, C.E. 'Studies of the centre of gravity in the human body'. Child Development, vol 15, no. 2–3, June — September 1944, p. 134.*

the sex differences become even greater during adolescence. These sex differences remain throughout the life span.[14]

Other studies have plotted the decline of strength in the old, relating these strength measures to changes in the composition of the aging tissue.

Biochemical and cellular changes have been found in relation to aging and endurance.[30]

Growth of the brain

Human development depends on the gradual elaboration of the structure and function of the brain. In other words it depends on brain maturation and this becomes more complete with time.

The structure of the brain and the sequence it follows as it matures is principally determined by the genetic code. There are fixed ages at which certain changes are programmed to occur in the human species. This phenomenon can be observed in the baby, when certain primitive reflexes disappear within fairly narrow time limits during the first year of life. Therefore when comparing the performance of very young infants, it is important to know their post-conceptual ages. This information becomes less useful as the child gets older, as environmental factors come to exert an increasing influence on his performance.

Stages in brain growth

A brief outline based on work by Dobbing[15] is given below.

1. During the first weeks of intra-uterine life, the gross shape of the brain is determined. By ten weeks conceptual age, the brain though very small, can already be differentiated into a forebrain, midbrain, hindbrain, cerebral hemispheres and cerebellum.[25]

2. By 18 weeks, the adult number of neuronal cells has been achieved in most areas of the brain, although there are exceptions such as the cerebellum.

3. At about mid-pregnancy, there commences a very rapid period of growth called the brain growth spurt which lasts from mid-pregnancy until the child is in his fourth postnatal year. After this time the brain grows at a relatively much slower rate as adult proportions are approached.

4. The early part of the brain growth spurt involves a rapid multiplication of glial cells. This process eases off only when the child has reached his second year. There are still not the adult number of glial cells present in the brain.

5. In the early months after birth, there is an increased growth and branching of neuronal dendrites, which in turn form synapses with other cells. This branching adds to the complexity of the brain's structure.[37]

6. The latter part of the brain growth spurt represents a period of rapid myelination. After the major brain growth spurt is over, at about four years of age, myelination still continues, though now at a much slower rate as the child progresses to adulthood.

7. Different parts of the brain grow at different rates.

The cerebellum has a dramatic growth spurt. Notice in Figure 2.2 that the growth spurt of the cerebellum occurs during the period of growth spurt of the whole brain but its cells begin to multiply at a later date than those in the forebrain and the brainstem. They also grow very much faster and in a shorter period of time. At 15 months postnatal age, the cerebellum has already reached its adult number

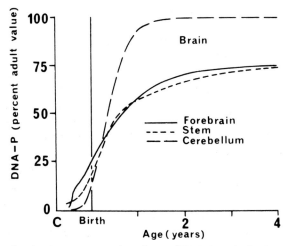

Fig. 2.2 Comparative values for total DNA-P equivalent to total numbers of cells in three brain regions. Values shown in this figure for forebrain, cerebellum and stem have been calculated as a percentage of adult value. *Reproduced with kind permission from Dobbing, J. and Sands, J. (1973) 'Quantitative growth and development of human brain.' Archives of Disease in Childhood, vol 48, p. 766.*

of cells, whereas the rest of the brain still only has about 65 per cent of its adult number.

The effects of the environment on brain growth

The brain possesses the quality of plasticity. It can be moulded by events. This fact holds promise particularly for young handicapped children.

Brain structures which are undergoing growth spurts are particularly sensitive to environmental factors.[15,16,47] This sensitivity allows the developing infant to benefit from experiences in an intensified form. Should these experiences be of a detrimental kind, or should the appropriate experience be withheld from him, the result can be much more extensive than it would have been at a less vulnerable time.

Some factors which have been shown to have such an effect include viral infections, chemical agents, malnutrition[16] and radiation,[32] particularly during the period of neuronal growth in the first 18 weeks after conception.

It is also possible, that more subtle features of the postnatal environment, such as an unstimulating nursery environment or emotional deprivation may have a direct effect on the basic structure and function of the brain. Failure to thrive has been demonstrated in children who have undergone such conditions.[18] Whether this actually has direct effects on the structure of their brains is unknown. Deprived children do demonstrate lower intellectual ability, as well as retarded growth, but how permanent this is, is not clear.

Research with animals, on the other hand, has shown that actual changes do occur in brain structure as well as alterations in function which are apparently related to the type of stimulation received during infancy. For example, rats exposed to stimulating environments as youngsters have been shown to develop larger and biochemically and histologically different brains to those rats brought up in a dull environment.[52] Kittens reared in different visual environments have been shown through the use of sophisticated neurophysiological techniques to have permanent changes in the functioning of their brain cells depending on whether they experienced horizontally or vertically striped early visual environments.[4]

Obviously these findings cannot be extrapolated directly to human beings. All the same they do demonstrate that subtle environmental features can have a very direct effect of the brains of living organisms and as a consequence influence their behaviour.

DEVELOPMENT

Development refers to the continuous process of unfolding and elaboration of behaviour which results from the interaction between the human organism and the environment over a lifetime.[25] Learning is implicated in development although it is not the same.[11]

In broad terms the developmental process continues throughout life although much of the literature indicates that 'development'

Table 2.1 Summary of development in the first year. *Reproduced with kind permission from Holt, K. S. (1977) Developmental Paediatrics. London: Butterworths, pp. 70–71.*

Age (months)	Gross motor	Vision and manipulation	Hearing and vocalization	Social
1	Gradual development of head control. Movements coarse and jerky.	Begins to fixate on nearby familiar objects. Watches mother's face.	Cries when hungry or uncomfortable. Freezes or quietens to sounds.	Sleeps and feeds. Evokes much affection and accepts this passively.
2	Dominance of primary reflexes on posture and movements.	Following with eyes. Visually takes 'hold' of objects.		Quiets in response to cooing and rocking.
3	Head lag, when pulled from supine to sitting, disappearing.	Holds objects placed in hands momentarily.	Response to sounds varies, e.g. dislikes loud harsh sounds, may excite to familiar sounds.	Regards nearby face. Smiles in response. Reacts to familiar pleasant situations e.g. feeding, bathing.
4	In prone head and chest raised. Later, support taken on forearms.	Visually associated reaching develops.	Cry pattern more mature. Vocalizes in response to overtures.	Likes handling. Feeding now a social activity.
5	Feet to mouth, plays with toes. Rolls front to back, and usually later back to front.	Recognizes everyday objects, e.g. cup. Watches hands.		
6	Held upright takes weight in legs.	Mature visual following and convergence. Eyes used together, no squint.	Turns to sounds. Wider range of vocalization. Chuckles.	Spontaneously responsive and smiling.
7	In sitting head steady and back straight.	Transfers objects, e.g. cubes, hand to hand.	Beginning to imitate rhythms of sounds.	
8	Reciprocates with legs. Protective support reflexes of limbs appearing.	Looks for dropped objects.	Practises vocalization.	Beginning to be aware of strangers and to modify responsiveness.
9	Stable in sitting position. Sideways and forward support with arms.	Moves cover in order to see object. Index finger use appearing.	Babbles, uses voice purposefully. Vocal imitation.	Responds to adults; plays imitative games.
10	Attempts to move – creep, crawl, squirm, shuffle. Pulls to stand.	Visually very alert. Pincer grip for small objects.	Mature localization of sounds.	Reacts to encouragement and discouragement.
11	Plays standing holding on. Cruises around furniture.	Glances around, makes quick visual appraisals. Beginning to look at pictures and may point with index finger.	Beginning to understand words and single simple commands. Beginning to vocalize recognizable words.	Shows affection. Plays pat-a-cake; waves bye-bye.
12	May take first steps.			

appears to have been reserved for that period of life from conception to maturity. To date, research into developmental trends occurring after maturity is reached, has been largely ignored, although in the movement field there are some exceptions.[31,38]

As the development of basic motor abilities is a feature of the early years, this section will concentrate on that period of the life span.

Principles of development

There are a number of basic principles which underlie the changes observed during the early years of life. These can be readily appreciated by examining the developmental changes occurring during the infant's first year. A summary of this period is given in Table 2.1.

The following list of developmental principles is adapted from Illingworth.[27]

1. Development is a continuous process. There is continuity of development as the infant at each stage prepares for the next. He practises newly learned skills which in their turn will form the basis for his next developmental step forwards. Much is going on at any one time in the different areas of development. This is well illustrated in Table 2.1 which compares development in the first year laterally and longitudinally.

2. Development depends primarily on the maturation of the nervous system. Maturation here refers to the gradual elaboration of the structure and function of the nervous system as it approaches its complete adult form.[48]

3. The sequence of development is much the same for all children but the rate will vary from child to child. The age at which a few children first show the ability in question is called the 'initial age'. The age at which the majority of children can perform the task is called the 'limit age'. Tables 2.2 and 2.3 illustrate the 'initial' and 'limit' ages for some early childhood abilities.[25] Detailed studies of

Table 2.2 Initial ages for various childhood abilities. *Reproduced with kind permission from Holt, K. S. (1977) Developmental Paediatrics. London: Butterworths, p. 250.*

Age	Ability, observation of which indicates a minimum developmental age level	Age	Ability, observation of which indicates a minimum developmental age level
1 month	Regards object in line of vision and follows for short distances. Immobilizes to nearby sound and social approach. Prone, raises head just clear of table.	1 year	Gives a toy; releases cube into cup. Co-operates with dressing. Walks one hand held. Responds to 'No' and 'Give it'.
4 months	Very slight head lag when pulled to sitting. Almost complete head stability in sitting. Prompt visual regard. Holds ring, reaches for it with free hand and takes it to mouth.	1½ years	Sits down on chair. Builds tower of 4–5 cubes. Spontaneous scribble. Looks at picture book and may name or point to one picture. Carries doll or teddy and hugs it. Obeys simple directions.
6 months	Immediate reach for object and retention in radial palmar grasp. Transfers object (cube) from hand to hand. Sits momentarily on a firm surface. Takes feet to mouth. Discriminates strangers.	2 years	Towers 6–7 cubes. Imitates vertical stroke and circle. Names pictures (2 or 3). Kicks ball. Follows directions. Walks up and down stairs.
9 months	Index finger approach to small objects. Early pincer grasp. Shakes bell. Pulls objects towards himself with string. Pulls to standing. Pat-a-cakes (claps hands) and waves 'Bye bye'. Imitates sounds and uses 'Mama', 'Dada' with meaning.	3 years	With book turns pages singly and names pictures. With crayon early tripod grip, copies circle and names drawing. Asks questions: may answer one or two. Knows name and sex. Repeats up to 3 digits. Matches 3 colours.

Table 2.3 Limit ages for various childhood abilities. *Reproduced with kind permission from Holt, K. S. (1977) Developmental Paediatrics. London: Butterworths, p. 251.*

Age in months	Ability which should be shown by stated age (if absent or doubtful further examination is indicated)
1	Some indication of attention.
2	Attention to objects. Some response to nearby voices and everyday noises.
3	Head held erect.
4	Hands not fisted. Shows ordinary interest in people and playthings.
5	Reaches for object.
6	ATNR not present or producible. Visual fixation and following established. Turns to sounds.
7	Holds objects in hands.
9	Gives attention to gestures.
10	Sits independently on firm surfaces. Uses tuneful babble to self and others. Bears most of weight on legs. Chews lumpy food.
12	Attends to words.
15	Releases held object.
18	Walks alone. No casting, mouthing, drooling.
21	Kicks when standing. Says single words with meaning.
27	Puts 2–3 words together into a phrase.
3 years	Can stand on one leg. Talks in sentences.
4 years	Uses fully intelligible speech.

sequential development which are available, include those of Gesell[19] and Sheridan.[42]

4. The direction of development is in the head to feet (cephalocaudal) direction. The infant gains head control before he can sit. He can use his hands with some finesse before he can stand and walk.

5. Development involves differentiation of behaviour. There is a gradual change of behaviour from relatively repetitive and stereotyped forms to more elaborate ones. At birth a baby's movements are limited but by the time of his first birthday he can roll, sit, stand, walk and play with toys.

6. Generalised mass activity gives way to specific individual responses. A young baby responds with a crude grasp reflex to stimulation of his palm (Fig. 2.3a). This involves all his fingers and his thumb moving at once. By his first birthday he can pick up a bead using a delicate pincer-like movement of his index finger and thumb, (Fig. 2.3c).

PRENATAL DEVELOPMENT OF MOVEMENT

Sensori-motor behaviour begins a long time before birth. Initially the muscle fibres develop separately from the nervous system. At about 7½ weeks these muscle fibres begin to come

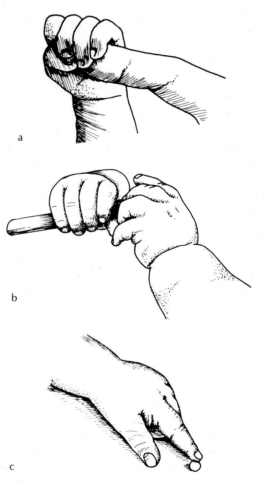

Fig. 2.3 Stages in the early development of hand function. a. Neonatal grasp. b. At 6 months, infant manipulates objects passing them from hand to hand. c. At 9 months infant pokes at small objects with his index finger.

under the influence of the nervous system, through the formation of the earliest crude reflex arcs.[47,57] Once this occurs each muscle fibre is placed in a position to be able to respond to the many influences which will come to act on the nervous system as the individual matures.

All the earliest movements *in utero*, are the result of reflex activity. Reflex activity also dominates the baby's movements for the first three months after he is born.

Reflexes which produce a response to tactile stimuli are the first to develop prenatally. Initially stimulation to the mouth region only will produce a response. This is at 7½ weeks.[26] At 10 weeks the palms of the hands become sensitive followed soon after by the soles of the feet. Sensitivity to touch develops in the limbs in a disto-proximal direction whereas motor ability develops in the opposite direction.[28] By the time the baby is born, widespread sensitivity to touch is present.

Proprioceptive reflexes, such as those responding to muscle stretch, develop later in the prenatal period. The muscle spindles begin to differentiate at 12 weeks and only at 24 to 31 weeks become structurally and functionally mature. At birth they are functioning well.[40,57]

Proprioceptors in the capsules of the synovial joints of the limbs and vertebral column have to await postnatal weight-bearing experiences before they approach maturity.[57]

The early developmental sequence of some of these neuromuscular mechanisms is presented in Table 2.4.

THE DEVELOPMENT OF MOVEMENTS RELATED TO FEEDING

The movements related to feeding are some of the earliest to become most fully developed. This occurs rapidly during the prenatal period because these movements need to be refined by the time the baby is born, in order to assure his survival. Other movements associated with survival include those associated with breathing. A summary of these events follows, based on material from Humphrey,[26] Jacobs,[28] Timiras,[47] Twitchell[50] and Wyke.[57]

The earliest movements that have been observed in the fetus occur in response to light touch around the mouth region at 7½ weeks of age. The motor response at this stage is a crude mass movement of the head, neck and trunk away from the stimulus. One week later, when more reflex arcs have been formed, more areas of the body join in this mass response. Only when the structures involved have undergone a period of further maturation will these movements become more differentiated.

By 13–14 weeks, the fetus can now turn with his head and lip movements towards the stimulus rather than withdrawing from it. When he does turn away, he can now turn his face without trunk movement. Already, the movements in response to the same stimulus around the mouth are becoming more refined. Both movements of turning towards the stimulus and turning away from it will be necessary when he is born; the former if he is to be able to feed and the latter if he is to prevent himself from suffocating when he is placed in prone.

Swallowing and tongue movements are present at 13–14 weeks and sucking movements soon follow. They are still very primitive but by the time the baby is born at 40 weeks these movements which are associated with the movement sequence of feeding, are qualitatively far in advance of any others.

Sucking, in the newborn, seems to be the only purposeful movement in the infant's repertoire. Therefore it is not surprising that research workers interested in early learning have attempted to condition these particular movement responses.[29,45] The fact that sucking can be conditioned in the neonate suggests that the cerebral cortex may be beginning to assume some control over motor behaviour at this time.[40]

Stimulation on the baby's cheek or the corner of his mouth will produce an automatic turning of his head and movement of his mouth towards the stimulus. This is called the

Table 2.4 Developmental emergence of neuromuscular behaviour. *Reproduced with kind permission from Wyke, B. (1975) The Neurological Basis of Movement – a developmental review. In Holt, K. S. (Ed) Movement and Child Development. London: William Heinemann Medical Books Ltd, p. 21.*

Developmental period	Weeks of age from conception	Neuromuscular developmental phenomena
EMBRYONIC	5–6	Excitable muscle fibre differentiation. Innervation from alpha motoneurones.
	6–7	Motoneurone activation of motor units (through fine unmyelinated axons).
	7–8	Afferent neurones establish fine unmyelinated peripheral and central connexions (trigeminal system first).
	8	Oro-facial cutaneous mass reflexes elicitable. Ampullary cristae active.
FETAL	9–10	Mass 'spontaneous' movements of whole musculature. Moro reflex elicitable (from vestibular receptors).
	12	Muscle spindles differentiate. Movements of eyeballs. Generalized cervical reflexes. Palmar and plantar reflexes elicitable.
	14	Spinal grey nuclei differentiate. Fusimotor neurones active. Localized movements of lips, tongue (swallowing), head, trunk, limbs.
	16	Respiratory muscle movements (intercostals before diaphragm). First myelin lamellae in CNS (in cervical intersegmental tracts and vestibular nerves).
	24	Myelin lamellae in spinal dorsal columns and medial longitudinal bundle. Commencing myelinization of cranial motor nerves, followed by afferents (vestibular first); and of reticulospinal, tectospinal and vestibulo-spinal tracts. Myelin lamellae in spinal nerves (motor before afferent).
	28	Facial mimetic muscle reflexes. Cervical reflexes regionally co-ordinated (Magnus and de Kleyn reflexes). Myelin lamellae in spinocerebellar and spinothalamic tracts.
	32	Vestibular reflex effects on eye and limb muscles.
	36	Myelin lamellae in cortical projection tracts, and in optic nerves.
BIRTH	36–37	
NEONATAL	38	Reflex walking, crawling and swimming movements elicitable.
	40	Ocular pursuit movements present. Voluntary control begins.
INFANCY	42	Reflex head extension in prone position.
	50	Visuo-motor reflex effects on neck, trunk and limb muscles. Positive supporting reflexes in arms.
	60	Head held up in supported sitting position.
	64	Sits unsupported. Exploratory creeping.
	68	Stands with support. Cerebral dominance emerging.
	70	Exploratory crawling. Positive supporting reflexes in legs.
	80	Walks with support.
	100	Stands and walks unaided.

rooting response. The infant 'roots around' for his mother's nipple so he can feed.

The fact that the sensitivity of the mouth region is far in advance of other areas is also important in early learning. The baby will take his hands to his mouth as well as any toys, food or other objects he may be given. As he mouths a toy, for example, the sensations this activity produces, provides his cortex with information about the texture of the toy as well as the consequences of his movements upon it. Information about what the toy looks like, as well as any sound it makes will also be passing to the cerebral cortex at the same time. In time the baby will gradually piece together, or integrate, all the information about the toy coming to his brain from these various sources, to form a concept about the toy. He will also be building a perception or awareness of his own body.

The formation of early concepts, on the basis of such experience, is the beginning of early cognitive development.

As the baby's manipulative ability becomes more refined, the mouthing of objects will become less.[27] The hands now become the dominant source of tactile information for the brain to use.

Although the feeding movements described earlier have obvious survival value, they are also important because they form the basis of the movements involved in speech. Speech development must await the development of language, which is a very high level cortical function.

THE PERCEPTUAL ABILITIES OF VERY YOUNG INFANTS

Research has shown that the very young infant is probably much more aware of his surroundings than was previously thought.[6,39,46] Although his motor abilities are primitive during the early months after birth, his perceptual abilities are apparently more advanced. Some examples are given here.

A number of studies have shown that young babies prefer patterns of human faces rather than any other representation. Even babies a few minutes after birth have been shown to demonstrate this preference.[20] Three week old babies have been able to distinguish between their mother and another object — a fuzzy monkey.[7] In this study, the babies moved differently depending on whether their mother or an object was in front of them. Babies aged 2–11 weeks apparently respond quite differently to looming shadows depending on whether these shadows are on a 'hit or miss' path as they move towards the baby.[2] Even babies aged 1–14 days of age have been shown to move in synchrony with adult speech.[8,9] Adults themselves do this too when listening to another speaker.

These studies and many others like them, raise questions as to whether the development of higher levels of brain functioning may be much more advanced than previously supposed. They also point to the importance of movement in the very early period of development particularly in the subtle areas of interpersonal communication.[49] There is much about early movement that is still to be discovered.

THE DEVELOPMENT OF GROSS MOTOR ABILITIES

The motor ability of a newborn baby is very limited. Yet one year later he will probably be ready to take his first independent steps and 18 months later he will be running. With increasing mobility many more opportunities for learning present themselves to the child.

This dramatic change in motor behaviour is dependent on the infant's increasing ability to automatically maintain a stable background posture against the influence of gravity. The development of an adequate postural reflex mechanism[5] is one of the major tasks for young human beings to accomplish.

The motor behaviour of the newborn and young infant has been described in great detail by many authors.[3,19,23,27,36,42,51]

The newborn baby adopts a flexed attitude irrespective of the position in which he is placed (Fig. 2.4a).

Over the first year his ability to extend against gravity must be developed in order to stand erect. Then control over flexion must be achieved. Extension takes precedence.

A brief summary of the major features involved in early motor development in supine, prone and the upright position is presented in Table 2.5. Patterns of movement that can be developed in each position vary. For example the infant's hands are not free in prone but they are free in supine from the start and eventually become free in the upright sitting position. Therefore reaching and grasping activities will obviously be practised in the latter positions after they emerge. Eventually the infant comes to change from one position to another with ease as his movements develop.

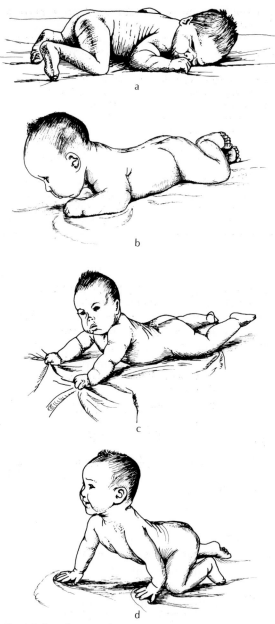

Fig. 2.4 Development in prone. a. 2 weeks old. b. 3 months. c. 5–6 months. d. 9 months.

Early reflex activity

From birth to about two to three months of age, the baby's movements in response to a wide variety of stimuli are predominantly reflex. This is thought to be due to the current immaturity of the cerebral cortex and its related pathways to and from other parts of the nervous system. It is via these pathways that the cerebral cortex comes to exert control over the motor neurons to any one muscle or group of muscles. As this control increases, the early reflex activity becomes modified.

Most of the reflexes present at birth, involve the lower levels of the central nervous system, such as the spinal cord, hindbrain and midbrain, for their integration. Some of these which have postural functions are listed in Table 2.6. As well as the feeding reflexes mentioned previously, other reflexes and integrated motor activities of the neonate, include protective reflexes such as the withdrawal reflex, locomotor movements such as the primitive walking reflex, palmar and plantar grasping and the Moro response.[47]

Postural reflexes such as the tonic labyrinthine and tonic neck reflexes and the more advanced neck righting reaction can be elicited in the newborn.[5,25]

The importance of the position of the neck and the presence of tonic neck reflexes in controlling muscle tone throughout the body cannot be overestimated. For, although the tonic neck reflexes have faded by six months of age their presence can still be detected in normal adults.[22]

At six months of age other more advanced postural reactions, the equilibrium reactions, are beginning to emerge. By this time muscle tone has settled into a more normal state, due to the fading of the tonic neck reflexes.

The tonic reflexes affect the positioning of the body, by creating particular arrangements of the body parts and then holding that attitude. Righting and equilibrium reactions also affect body positioning but in a changing, more dynamic, way.

The neck righting reaction is the only righting response present at birth. When the head is turned the body follows. This is a dynamic response, compared to the static position of the limbs adopted, if an asymmetrical tonic neck reflex were elicited.

Righting reactions are those automatic movements of the body which help in the establishment of the head and body

Table 2.5 Features of early motor development in supine, prone and upright postures. *Reproduced with kind permission from Holt, K. S. (1977) Developmental Paediatrics. London: Butterworths, p. 189.*

Posture	Requirements for progress	Advantages	Disadvantages
Supine	Head flexion & stability Symmetry Ability to support trunk upright	Hands free early facilitating early play & hand-eye co-ordination	A static posture apart from babies who shuffle
Prone	Head extension & stability Control of symmetrical tonic neck reflex Symmetry	Leads to early mobility by hauling or crawling	Hands occupied
Upright	Stability of head & trunk against gravity Balance and fine control of distribution of body weight	Socially acceptable and effective mobility Hands free	Time taken to acquire anti-gravity postural control

Table 2.6 Principal postural reflexes. *Reproduced with permission from Ganong, W. F. (1979) Review of Medical Physiology, 9th edition. Copyright(c) 1979 by Lange Medical Publications, Los Altos, California, p. 139.*

Reflex	Stimulus	Response	Receptor	Integrated In
Stretch reflexes	Stretch	Contraction of muscle	Muscle spindles	Spinal cord, medulla
Positive supporting (magnet) reaction	Contact with sole or palm	Foot extended to support body	Proprioceptors in distal flexors	Spinal cord
Negative supporting reaction	Stretch	Release of positive supporting reaction	Proprioceptors in extensors	Spinal cord
Tonic labyrinthine reflexes	Gravity	Extensor rigidity	Otolithic organs	Medulla
Tonic neck reflexes	Head turned: (1) To side (2) Up (3) Down	Change in pattern of rigidity (1) Extension of limbs on side to which head is turned (2) Hind legs flex (3) Forelegs flex	Neck proprioceptors	Medulla
Labyrinthine righting reflexes	Gravity	Head kept level	Otolithic organs	Midbrain
Neck righting reflexes	Stretch of neck muscles	Righting of thorax and shoulders, then pelvis	Muscle spindles	Midbrain
Body on head righting reflexes	Pressure on side of body	Righting of head	Exteroceptors	Midbrain
Body on body righting reflexes	Pressure on side of body	Righting of body even when head held sideways	Exteroceptors	Midbrain
Optical righting reflexes	Visual cues	Righting of head	Eyes	Cerebral cortex
Placing reactions	Various visual, exteroceptive, and proprioceptive cues	Foot placed on supporting surface in position to support body	Various	Cerebral cortex
Hopping reactions	Lateral displacement while standing	Hops, maintaining limbs in position to support body	Muscle spindles	Cerebral cortex

relationship in space as well as in the relationship of the head and body to one another.

Development of head and trunk control

At birth, the baby has no head control. When held in ventral suspension the head drops forwards. When pulled up to sitting from supine lying, his head lags behind (Fig. 2.5a). The development of head control is an important first step in achieving the upright posture.

It is also important because it allows the baby to begin to use his eyes and ears more effectively, directing them independent of gravity, with considerable implications for the development of perceptual ability and cognition.

The development of the labyrinthine righting reaction is involved in the early attainment of head control. This important reaction begins to emerge at 4–6 weeks of age and is retained throughout life.

By 12 weeks when the baby is lying in prone he can lift and hold his head. At this stage he takes his weight on his forearms. If he is pulled into sitting from supine at the same age, his head lag is only slight (Fig. 2.5b). By 20 weeks this head lag has disappeared.

By 28 weeks he spontaneously lifts his head from supine in anticipation of being lifted, evidence that his ability to alternate control between his flexor and extensor muscle groups is well on the way to being perfected in the head and neck region. The same process will occur later for other regions of the body.

Although he has attained head control at 20 weeks he still needs to be supported when he is in a sitting position. By 29 weeks he can sit using his own hands placed forward to prop himself.

A key factor in this developmental step is the emergence of protective reactions of his arms where they extend spontaneously to act as a prop. Protective extension reactions of the arms also occur when the baby is tipped forwards and later sideways and backwards.

The baby can recover his balance in sitting if

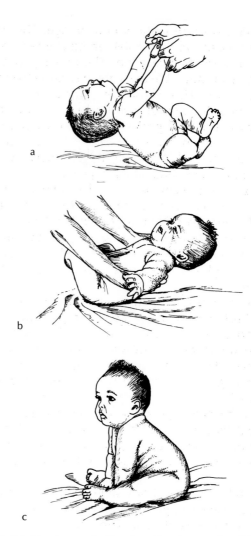

Fig. 2.5 Development of head and trunk control. a. Baby of 6 weeks when pulled to sitting still has a head lag. b. Baby at 20 weeks where head lag has disappeared. c. Baby at 28 weeks can sit alone using his own hands placed in front of him to prop himself.

he is toppled forward at 36 weeks, but not until 44 weeks can be recover himself if he falls sideways. At 38 weeks, rotation of the trunk in sitting becomes possible. The infant can now turn round to pick up a toy placed behind him.

During this first year the infant gradually perfects extension activities in the prone position, (Fig. 2.4).

The development of rotational movements of the body takes a major step forward with the emergence of the body-on-body righting reaction at six to eight months of age. This in effect breaks up the earlier 'en bloc' effects of the neck righting reaction. The upper part of the trunk is now able to rotate in relation to the lower part. This allows the infant to start rotating around his own vertical axis so that the ability to roll from prone to supine (24 weeks), and from supine to prone (28 weeks) emerges at this time. At 28 weeks he can now bear weight on one hand when in prone.

Vision eventually becomes the dominant influence in maintaining the normal relationship of the head to body throughout life. With the emergence of the optical righting reaction the earlier 'head', 'body-on-head' and 'body-on-body' righting reactions become partially inhibited.

Vision does not play as great a role in the establishment of stable positional postures as it does in the achievement of mobility. Developmental studies with blind babies have shown that gross motor abilities primarily involving stability are achieved within normal limits.[1]

As the righting reactions are becoming fully established at about six months, the highly complex equilibrium reactions emerge. Gradually, the righting reactions become modified.

Equilibrium reactions operate to keep the body's centre of gravity over its base. They are varied patterns of automatic movement which allow the body to compensate for changes in its position in space and its relationship to the supporting surface.

'They manifest themselves in either very slight changes of tone throughout the whole body musculature or in visible automatic countermovements to restore the disturbed balance.'[5] After three to four years of age and from then on, the righting and equilibrium reactions are closely integrated — the righting mechanism becoming part of all the equilibrium reactions.

Equilibrium reactions require that the cerebral cortex, basal ganglia and cerebellum have reached an adequate level of maturity before they can occur. The first equilibrium reactions develop in prone and supine lying at about six and seven months. Later they appear in other positions after the position itself has already been accomplished by the infant.[17] The developmental history of standing and walking illustrates this point.

At 24 weeks the infant takes a large part of his weight through his lower limbs when held in the standing position. By 36 weeks he is standing holding on to furniture and at 40 weeks can pull himself into the standing position. At 44 weeks he can lift one foot while standing holding on, and by one year of age he walks while held by one hand. By 13 months he stands alone and by 15 months walks alone. Only now when the infant is achieving independence in walking, based on a position – standing – do we see the equilibrium reactions in standing emerging.

His dynamic ability develops rapidly. He is running at 18 months and by two years can go up and down stairs.

Perfecting these postural mechanisms continues over the next few years.[41] This would account for some of the obvious differences in the patterns of movement observed in children at different ages, as they attempt the same activity; for example, running, (Fig. 2.6) catching or throwing a ball.[55] From now on, the development of new skills will have as their background an efficient postural mechanism on which to build.

THE DEVELOPMENT OF PREHENSION

The ability to reach out and grasp an object with the hand is a major human achievement which develops rapidly during the first year of life after birth. In order to do this the infant must:

1. Become visually aware of the object he wants to grasp
2. Be able to direct his arm and hand to the object with accuracy
3. Be able to grasp the object
4. Be able to release the object when he has finished playing with it.

In the normal infant the senses of vision and touch come to be integrated with the move-

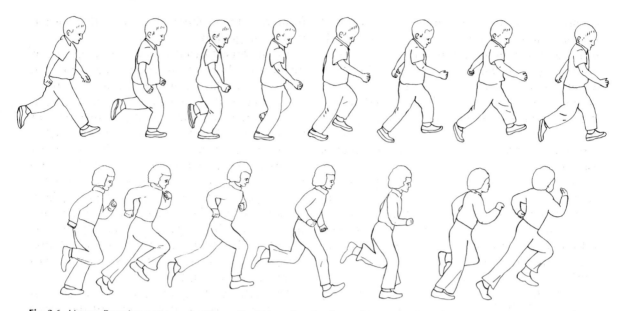

Fig. 2.6 *Upper.* Running pattern of a 27 month old boy showing bounding, vertical emphasis and limited range of motion. *Lower.* More advanced form of an 8 year old girl with strong horizontal emphasis and more extensive movement. *Reproduced with kind permission from Wickstrom R. L. (1975) Developmental Kinesiology; maturation of basic motor patterns. In Wilmore, J. H. & Keogh, J. F. (Eds) Exercise and Sport Sciences Reviews vol. 3, p. 171.*

ments of the arm and hand. Vision is dominant. Blind children show a conspicuous delay in the development of reaching behaviour.[1]

At birth, reflex activity dominates and all the factors previously mentioned for the development of reaching and grasping are not yet integrated. Reflex activity affects the upper limbs in some of the following ways:

1. Stretch applied to any of the flexor muscles leads to an increase of flexion of the fingers and wrist. This tightening is called the traction response.[50]
2. Tactile stimulation lightly applied to the palm of the baby's hand will also lead to the baby's fingers reflexly flexing and curling around the stimulating object,[36] (Fig. 2.3a).
3. Movements of the upper limb as a whole are very limited and not well organised. The asymmetrical tonic neck reflex has some influence.

During the first two months, the baby's visual capacity improves rapidly. He develops the ability to focus his eyes on objects at various distances, rather than having his focus-

sing capacity locked into the narrow range present at birth. At the same time he is rapidly developing head control which will help to direct his eyes where he wills more readily.

Reaching activities which have been widely studied by White and his associates[54] forms the basis of the following summary.

At two months the infant begins to swipe at objects hanging in his cot, although his hands are still fisted at this stage, indicating that reflex activity is still present. The grasp reflex is weakening.

By 12 weeks he can hold on to objects placed in his hand, using the ulnar side of his palm. As his grasp develops there will be a shift of this contact area in a radial and distal direction so that by 36 weeks, objects can now be held between his thumb and index finger in a pincer type grip. Small objects can be retained in this way.[13]

The ability to release an object develops later than the ability to grasp. At 40 weeks of age the infant begins to demonstrate his ability to let go.[25]

Grasps used by older children beginning to use implements, such as pencils and paintbrushes, also show developmental trends.[25] Children initially holding a pencil use a cylindrical grasp with the point of the pencil projecting from the ulnar border of the hand towards the paper. Later the pencil is held between the thumb and fingers, particularly the first two. At about three years of age the adult-like dynamic tripod grip formed between the thumb, index finger and middle finger is adopted.

The development of a mature grasp and the ability to manipulate objects in the hand requires tactile sensitivity.[50] The development of reaching normally requires vision, although with blind children auditory stimuli can be used as a substitute.[1]

At about two to three months, the baby's eyes can focus on objects which are potentially within reach, including his hands. As his arms move, he sees what happens to his hands. Through these experiences, he begins to integrate information coming to his brain from his eyes, with kinaesthetic information arriving from his upper limbs. This is called visual-motor integration.

When three to four months of age, he can deliberately bring both hands together in the midline. He plays with his hands, one hand manipulating the other, as he watches. Both hands touch each other as they move and are moved. Now the baby can relate the tactile experiences of both hands with the movements he experiences. As he is watching, he links in his visual experiences as well. All this sensorimotor integration is a necessary prerequisite to visually directed reaching, which first makes its appearance at about five months. The child can now reach out and grasp what he sees, and at this stage he tries to grasp everything that he sees.

Through reaching activities the infant becomes more aware of himself and the space he occupies. He can now deliberately begin to act on and in his environment and develop his cognitive skills.

REFERENCES AND FURTHER READING

1. Adelson, E. & Fraiberg, S. (1974) Gross motor development in infants blind from birth. *Child Development*, Vol. 45, pp. 114–126.
2. Ball, W. & Tronick, E. (1971) Infant responses to impending collision: optical and real. *Science*, Vol. 171, pp. 818–820.
3. Beintema, D. J. (1968) *A Neurological study of Newborn Infants. Clinics in Developmental Medicine. No. 28.* London: Heinemann.
4. Blakemore, C. & Cooper, G. F. (1970) Development of the brain depends on the visual environment. *Nature*, Vol. 228, pp. 477–478.
5. Bobath, K. (1980) *A Neurophysiological Basis for the Treatment of Cerebral Palsy – Clinics in Developmental Medicine. No. 75.* London: William Heinemann Medical.
6. Bower, T. G. R. (1977) *A Primer of Infant Development.* San Francisco: W. H. Freeman and Co.
7. Brazelton, T. B., Koslowski, B. & Main, M. (1974) The origins of reciprocity: The early mother-infant interaction. In *The Effect of the Infant on its Caregiver*, Lewis, M. & Rosenblum, L. A. (Eds.) Ch 3. pp. 49–76. New York: John Wiley and Sons.
8. Condon, W. S. (1977) A primary phase in the organisation of infant responding behaviour. In *Studies in Mother-Infant Interaction*, Schaffer, H. R. (Ed.) Ch. 7, pp. 153–176. London: Academic Press.
9. Condon, W. S. & Sander, L. W. (1974) Neonate movement is synchronized with adult speech: interactional participation and language acquisition. *Science*, Vol. 183, pp. 99–101.
10. Connolly, K. J. (Ed.) (1970) *Mechanisms of Motor Skill Development.* London: Academic Press.
11. Connolly, K. J. (1972) Learning and the concept of critical periods in infancy. *Developmental Medicine and Child Neurology*, Vol. 14, pp. 705–714.
12. Connolly, K. J. (1977) The nature of motor skill development. *Journal of Human Movement Studies*, Vol. 3, pp. 128–143.
13. Connolly, K. J. & Elliott, J. M. (1972) Evolution and ontogeny of hand function. In *Ethological Studies of Child Behaviour*, Blurton Jones, N. (Ed.) London: Cambridge Uni. Press.
14. Cuddigan, J. H. P. (1973) Quadriceps femoris strength. *Rheumatology and Rehabilitation*, Vol. 12, pp. 77–83.
15. Dobbing, J. (1974) The later development of the brain and its vulnerability. In *Scientific Foundations of Paediatrics*, Davis, J. A. & Dobbing, J. (Eds.) Ch. 32, pp. 565–577. London: Heinemann.
16. Dobbing, J. & Smart, J. L. (1974) Vulnerability of developing brain and behaviour. *British Medical Bulletin*, Vol. 30, No. 2, pp. 164–168.
17. Fiorentino, M. R. (1973) *Reflex Testing Methods for Evaluating C.N.S. Development.* Springfield: Charles C. Thomas.
18. Gardner, L. I. (1972) Deprivation dwarfism. *Scientific American*, Vol. 227, no. 1, pp. 76–82.
19. Gesell, A. (1940) *The First Five Years of Life.* New York: Harper and Brothers.
20. Goren, C. C., Sarty, M. & Wu, P. Y. K. (1975) Visual following and pattern discrimination of face like

stimuli by newborn infants. *Paediatrics*, Vol. 56, No. 4, pp. 544–549.

21. Hasselkus, B. R. & Shambes, G. M. (1975) Aging and postural sway in women. *Journal of Gerontology*, Vol. 30, No. 6, pp. 661–667.

22. Hellebrandt, F. A., Schade, M. & Carns, M. L. (1962) Methods of evoking the tonic neck reflexes in normal human subjects. *American Journal of Physical Medicine*, Vol. 41, No. 3, pp. 90–139.

23. Holle, B. (1976) *Motor Development in Children*. Oxford: Blackwell Scientific Publications.

24. Holt, K. S. (Ed.) (1975) *Movement and Child Development. Clinics in Developmental Medicine, No. 55*. London: Heinemann.

25. Holt, K. S. (1977) *Developmental Paediatrics*. London: Butterworths.

26. Humphrey, T. (1969) Postnatal repetition of human pre-natal activity sequences with some suggestions of their neuro-anatomical basis. In *Brain and Early Behaviour*, Robinson, R. J. (Ed.) pp. 43–71. London: Academic Press.

27. Illingworth, R. S. (1979) *The Normal Child*, 7th edn. Edinburgh: Churchill Livingstone.

28. Jacobs, M. J. (1967) Development of normal motor behaviour. *American Journal of Physical Medicine*, Vol. 46, No. 1, pp. 41–51.

29. Koupernik, C., Mackeith, R. & Francis-Williams, J. Neurological correlates of motor and perceptual development. In *Perceptual and Learning Disabilities in Children*, Vol. 2, Cruickshank, W. M. & Hallahan, D. P. (Eds.) Chap. 2, pp. 105–135. Syracuse: Syracuse Uni. Press.

30. Larsson, L. & Karlsson, J. (1978) Isometric and dynamic endurance as a function of age and skeletal muscle characteristics. *Acta Physiol. Scand.* Vol. 104, pp. 129–136.

31. Leme, S. A. & Shambes, G. A. (1978) Immature throwing patterns in normal adult women. *Journal of Human Movement Studies*, Vol. 4, pp. 85–93.

32. Miller, R. W. & Blot, W. J. (1972) Small head size after in-utero exposure to atomic radiation. *The Lancet*, Vol. 2, pp. 784–787.

33. Molnar, G. E. & Alexander, J. (1974) Development of quantitative standards of muscle strength in children. *Archives of Physical Medicine and Rehabilitation*, Vol. 55, pp. 490–493.

34. Overstall, P. W., Exton-Smith, A. N., Imms, F. J. & Johnson, A. L. (1977) Falls in the elderly related to postural imbalance. *British Medical Journal*, Vol. 1, pp. 261–264.

35. Palmer, C. E. (1944) Studies of the centre of gravity in the human body. *Child Development*, Vol. 15, Nos. 2–3, June-Sept., p. 99.

36. Prechtl, E. H. (1977) The neurological examination of the full term newborn infant. *Clinics in Developmental Medicine, No. 63*. London: Heinemann.

37. Purpura, D. (1976) Discussants comments. In *Intervention Strategies for high risk infants and young children*, Tjossem, T. D. (Ed.) pp. 75–83. Baltimore: Uni. Park Press.

38. Roberton, M. A. (1978) Longitudinal evidence for developmental stages in the forceful overarm throw. *Journal of Human Movement Studies*, Vol. 4, pp. 167–175.

39. Schaffer, H. R. (Ed.) (1977) *Studies in Mother-Infant Interaction*. London: Academic Press.

40. Schulte, F. J. (1974) The neurological development of the neonate. In *Scientific Foundations of Paediatrics*, Davis, J. A. & Dobbing, J. (Eds.) Ch. 34, pp. 587–615. London: Heinemann.

41. Shambes, G. M. (1976) Static postural control in children. *American Journal of Physical Medicine*, Vol. 55, No. 5, pp. 221–252.

42. Sheridan, M. D. (1973) *Children's Developmental Progress*. NFER Publishing Company Ltd.

43. Sheridan, M. D. (1978) The fashioning of a human life style. *Child: care, health and development*, Vol. 4, pp. 425–429.

44. Sinclair, D. C. (1969) *Human Growth after Birth*, 2nd edn. London: Oxford Uni. Press.

45. Siqueland, E. R. & Delucia, C. A. (1969) Visual reinforcement of nonnutritive sucking in human infants. *Science*, Vol. 165, pp. 1144–1146.

46. Stone, L. J. (Ed.) (1974) *The Competent Infant*. London: Tavistock Publications.

47. Timiras, P. S. (1972) *Developmental Physiology and Aging*. New York: MacMillan.

48. Touwen, B. C. L. (1974) The neurological development of the infant. In *Scientific Foundations of Paediatrics*, Davis, J. A. & Dobbing, J. (Eds.) Ch. 35, pp. 615–625. London: Heinemann.

49. Trevarthan, C. (1974) Conversations with a two month old. *New Scientist*, 2nd May, pp. 230–235.

50. Twitchell, T. E. (1965) Normal motor development. *Journal of the American Physical Therapy Association*. Vol. 45, pp. 419–423.

51. Van Blankenstein, M., Welbergen, U. R. & de Haas, J. H. (1962) *Le développement du nourisson*. Paris: Presses Universitaires de France.

52. Walsh, R. N., Cummins, R. A. & Budtz-Olsen, O. R. (1973) Environmentally induced changes in the dimensions of the Rat cerebrum: A Replication and Extension. *Developmental Psychobiology*, Vol. 6, No. 1, pp. 3–7.

53. Welford, A. T. (1958) *Aging and Human Skill*. London: Oxford Uni. Press.

54. White, B. L., Castle, P. & Held, P. (1964) Observations on the development of visually-directed reaching. *Child Development*, Vol. 35, pp. 349–364.

55. Wickstrom, R. L. (1975) Developmental kinesiology: Maturation of basic motor patterns. In *Exercise and Sport Sciences Reviews (vol. 3)* Wilmore, J. H. & Keogh, J. F. (Eds.) pp. 163–192. New York: Academic Press.

56. Williams, H., Tomberlin, J. A. & Robertson, K. J. (1965) Muscle force curves of school children. *Journal of the American Physical Therapy Association*, Vol. 45, pp. 539–549.

57. Wyke, B. (1975) The Neurological Basis of Movement – A developmental review. In *Movement and Child Development*, Holt, K. S. (Ed.) Ch. 4, pp. 19–33. London: Heinemann.

3

The musculoskeletal basis for movement

The framework of the body consists of bones articulating at the joints. It is at the joints that motion can take place.

The bones form a hard core for the various body segments which move around the joints. Soft tissue structures, such as muscles, connective tissues, blood vessels, nerves and skin complete each segment's mass.

There are considered to be eight principal body segments (Fig. 3.1).[2,26] These are:

1. Axial skeleton
    (i) head-neck
    (ii) trunk
2. Upper extremity
    (iii) arm
    (iv) forearm
    (v) hand
3. Lower extremity
    (vi) thigh
    (vii) leg
    (viii) foot.

Muscles, via their attachments to the bony core of the segments, provide the motor force to move them.

Description of movement

All movements are conventionally described as being initiated from the anatomical position. For ease of description they are related to planes and axes.

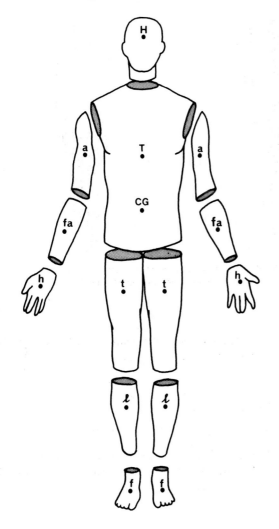

Fig. 3.1 The principal body segments where: H = head and neck; T = trunk; a = arm; fa = forearm; h = hand; t = thigh; l = leg; f = foot. The dots in the segments of the upper and lower limbs represent the centres of gravity for those segments. Note that they are placed near the heavier end. CG = the centre of gravity of the entire body.

There are three cardinal planes of the body which:

1. Divide the body into equal parts
2. Lie at right angles to each other
3. Intersect at the centre of gravity of the body.

They are:

1. The cardinal sagittal plane, which is a vertical plane dividing the body into equal right and left halves (Fig. 3.2 a). Any plane parallel to this is called a sagittal plane. Movement in a sagittal plane takes place about a frontal axis.
2. The cardinal frontal (coronal) plane, which is a vertical plane dividing the body into equal front and back halves (Fig. 3.2b). Any plane parallel to this is called a frontal plane. Movement in a frontal plane takes place about a sagittal axis.
3. The cardinal transverse (horizontal) plane, which divides the body into equal upper and lower halves (Fig. 3.2c). Any plane parallel to this is called a transverse plane. Movement in a transverse plane takes place about a vertical axis.

The following general definitions of movement are used descriptively for some of the more major movements.

1. Movements in a sagittal plane about a frontal axis. These are best observed from the side.
   a. Flexion, in which the angle between the surfaces of two adjacent segments decreases as the joint is bent.
   b. Extension, in which the angle between the segments increases. It is the opposite movement to flexion. An exception to this is flexion and extension of the thumb which takes place in a frontal plane.
   c. Dorsiflexion, where the foot is pulled up towards the leg.
   d. Plantar flexion, in which the foot moves downwards from the leg.

2. Movements in a frontal plane about a sagittal axis. These movements are best observed either standing in front or behind the person moving.
   a. Abduction, in which the segment moves away from the midline of the body.
   b. Adduction, in which the segment moves towards the midline of the body. A special case is movements of the digits. In the foot the midline is taken as the second digit; in the hand it is the third digit. Abduction and adduction of the thumb takes place in the sagittal plane.

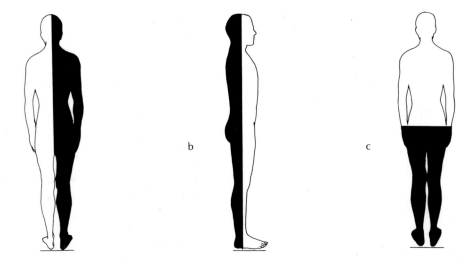

Fig. 3.2 The three cardinal planes. a. The sagittal, which divides the body into equal right and left halves. b. The frontal, which divides the body into equal front and back halves. c. The transverse, which divides the body into equal upper and lower halves.

    c. Ulnar deviation, in which the hand moves in the direction of the little finger at the wrist.

    d. Radial deviation, in which the hand moves in the direction of the thumb at the wrist.

    e. Lateral flexion, of the trunk or head and neck to the left or right.

3. Movements in a horizontal plane about a vertical axis.

    a. Medial (internal) rotation, in which the anterior surface of the segment turns inwards – towards the midline.

    b. Lateral (external) rotation, in which the anterior surface of the segment turns outward – away from the midline.

    c. Rotation to the left or right of the vertebral column.

    d. Supination, in which the hand is in the anatomical position with reference to the forearm.

    e. Pronation, in which the palm of the hand is turned away from the anatomical position so it now faces posteriorly.

4. Circumduction, in which a combination of the movements, flexion, abduction, extension and adduction is performed in sequence, so the segment traces out a conical shape in space.

Causes of motion

Joint motion may be caused by:

1. Internal forces – muscle contraction
2. External forces – gravity and/or manual and mechanical forces.

JOINTS

A joint is the junction between two bones. Joints may be broadly classified as being:

1. Synovial or freely movable
2. Cartilagenous or slightly movable
3. Fibrous or fixed.

    Only the behaviour of synovial joints will be discussed in this section as they are more directly involved in human movement.

Joint function

The function of a joint basically depends upon the shape of the contours of the contacting surfaces and how well they fit together. By convention, the larger convex surface is termed the 'male' surface, whereas the smaller concave surface is called the 'female' surface.

Movements of these surfaces relative to each other may be typed as:

1. Spinning
2. Rolling
3. Sliding.[36]

This is shown in Figure 3.3.

In most actual movements that one observes in real life, these 'fundamental' movements are combined (Fig. 3.4).

Stability of a joint is dependent on:

1. The shape of the articular surfaces and their congruency
2. The ligaments
3. Muscle tension in surrounding musculature
4. Fascial structures
5. Atmospheric pressure.[35]

All synovial joints have only one position where the surfaces fit together precisely and where there is maximal contact between the

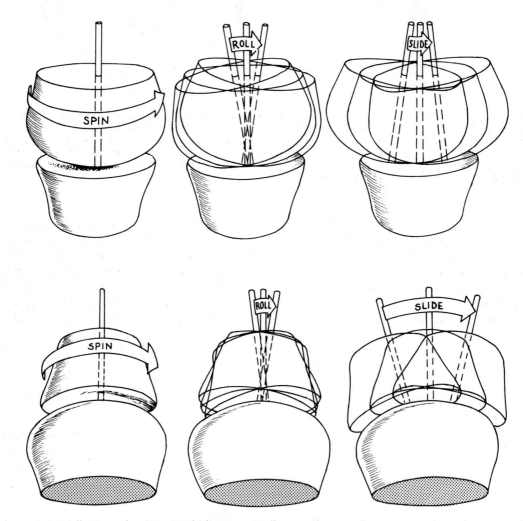

Fig. 3.3 An analysis of the types of movement which occur (usually in combination) between articular surfaces when a. a male surface moves over a stationary female surface and b. a female surface moves over a stationary male surface. *Reproduced with kind permission from Warwick, R. & Williams, P. L. (1973) Gray's Anatomy, 35th Edn. Edinburgh: Churchill Livingstone, p. 405.*

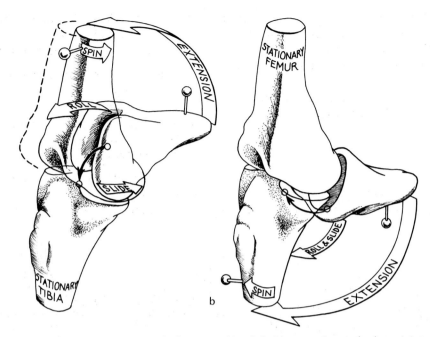

Fig. 3.4 An analysis of the articular movements which are combined during extension at the knee joint. a. With a stationary tibia, i.e. a moving male surface. (The broken line in a. represents the hypothetical position of the femur had slide not occurred). b. With a stationary femur, i.e. a moving female surface. Notice that in each case elements of slide, roll and spin occur together. In a. the roll and slide are in opposite directions, whereas in b. they are in the same direction. *Reproduced with kind permission from Warwick, R. & Williams, P. L. (1973) Gray's Anatomy, 35th edn. Edinburgh: Churchill Livingstone, p. 406.*

'male' and 'female' surfaces. This is called the close-packed position (Fig. 3.5a).

In the close-packed position, the articular surfaces are pressed firmly together and the bones cannot be separated by force. The two bones united by the joint now behave as one segment, no movement being possible between them. In the close-packed position, the ligaments are taut and twisted, because as the close-packed position is approached the fibrous capsule and the ligaments undergo a final spiral twist to screw home the articular surfaces. The close-packed position is the final limiting position of the joint (Table 3.1).

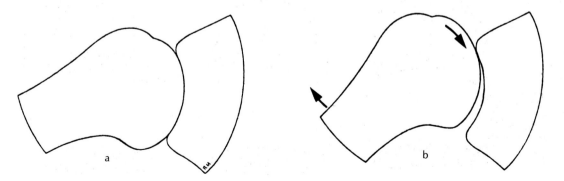

Fig. 3.5 Congruence of articular surfaces. a. The close packed position of the joint, with close-fitting or full congruence, of the surfaces. b. In loose-packed positions of a joint, the surfaces are not congruent (this has been over-emphasized for clarity). *Reproduced with kind permission from Warwick, R. & Williams, P. L. (1973) Gray's Anatomy, 35th edn. Edinburgh: Churchill Livingstone, p. 407.*

Table 3.1 Close-packed position of important joints. *Reproduced with permission from MacConaill, M. A. & Basmajian, J. V. (1977) Muscles and Movements – a basis for Human Kinesiology, 2nd edition. New York: Robert E. Kreiger Publishing Company, p. 60.*

Joint	Close-packed position
Shoulder	Abduction + lateral rotation
Ulno-humeral	Extension
Radiohumeral	Semiflexion + semipronation
Wrist	Dorsiflexion
Metacarpophalangeal (2–5)	Full flexion
Interphalangeal	Extension
1st carpometacarpal	Full opposition
Hip	Extension + medial rotation
Knee	Full extension
Ankle	Dorsiflexion
All toe-joints	Dorsiflexion
All other foot joints	Full supination

Note: Semipronation is the position of maximal congruence (fit) of radioulnar joints and of the greatest tension of the interosseous ligament.

Further forces acting to produce more movement are resisted by reflex contraction of the appropriate musculature. This operates to protect the joint.[24]

A joint not in the close-packed position, is said to be in a loose-packed position (Fig. 3.5b). In these loose-packed positions, the articular surfaces do not fit each other well and allow the fundamental movements of

Table 3.2 Least-packed position of important joints. *Reproduced with permission from MacConaill, M. A. & Basmajian, J. V. (1977) Muscles and Movements – a basis for Human Kinesiology, 2nd edition. New York: Robert E. Kreiger Publishing Company, p. 60.*

Joint	Least-packed position
Shoulder	Semiabduction
Ulnohumeral	Semiflexion
Radiohumeral	Extension + supination
Wrist	Semiflexion
Metacarpophalangeal (2–5)	Semiflexion + ulnar deviation
Interphalangeal	Semiflexion
First carpometacarpal	Neutral position of thumb
Hip	Semiflexion
Knee	Semiflexion
Ankle	Neutral position
Foot joints	Semipronation

spin, roll and slide to occur. The laxity of the capsular structures allows distractive forces to separate the articular surfaces.[24]

Every joint has a least-packed position, in which the capsule is most relaxed but not the musculature (Table 3.2). The joint most readily assumes this position to accommodate the maximal amount of fluid in its cavity after injury or in some disease processes such as osteoarthritis.[24]

Classification of synovial joints

Synovial joints are of most interest in human movement studies. They can be classified into seven sub-categories, all of which allow movements of body segments around at least one axis, except those classified as gliding joints, which are non axial.

Joints may be described as being:

1. Uniaxial (hinge joint; pivot joint) where motion takes place only about one axis. Body segments move in only one plane which is perpendicular to this axis. Uniaxial joints are said to possess one degree of freedom, for example, the elbow and atlanto-axial joints.

2. Biaxial (condyloid joint; ellipsoid joint) where motion takes place about two axes which are perpendicular to each other. Movement is now possible in two planes. Biaxial joints possess two degrees of freedom, for example, the metacarpophalangeal joints.

3. Multiaxial (ball and socket joint; saddle joint) where motion occurs around three major axes which pass through the centre of the joint. Movement is now possible in the three major planes: frontal, sagittal and transverse. Movement is also possible in oblique planes because such joints possess many secondary axes which also pass through the centre of the joint. A multiaxial joint, for example the hip joint, has three degrees of freedom, which is the maximum that any joint may possess.

4. Non axial (gliding joint) where only translatory motion can take place as compared to the rotary motion possible in the previous

subcategories, for example, the intercarpal and intertarsal joints.

Joint chains[12,26,35,37]

Broadly speaking, the joints unite the various body segments. Just as the concept of body segment is useful when describing mass distribution, so the use of the concept of body links, borrowed from engineering, is most helpful when describing body motion.

A body link is the distance between joint axes – a link unites joint axes (Fig. 3.6).

When a number of links are united in series they form what is called a kinematic or joint chain. A kinematic chain is a combination of several successively arranged joints constituting a complex motor system. Such chains may be open or closed. In an open kinematic chain the distal segment terminates free in space, whereas in a closed kinematic chain the distal segment is fixed. Open chains are more common in the body.

In the limbs, the 'links' and 'segments' generally correspond. Such a statement cannot yet be confidently made with respect to the torso.[26]

Use of the link and kinematic chain concepts

By using the concept of links, a link diagram can be drawn of the body in various positions (Fig. 3.7).[12,26] Using these diagrams, calculations are made which provide a more detailed description of the position than can be obtained from simple observational methods alone.

Limb motion can be described in terms of kinematic chains because the segments and links correspond in the limbs. Therefore, by adding the degrees of freedom at each of the joints in an open chain such as the upper limb, the degrees of freedom of each segment can be determined. Obviously, the more distal the segment, the greater the degrees of freedom it possesses. For example, each of the distal phalanges in the hand has 17 degrees of freedom relative to the trunk (Fig. 3.8).[12,35]

Such a linkage system allows the degrees of freedom of the many joints in the chain to be pooled, giving the segments, particularly those more distal, greater potential for achieving a variety of movements than any one joint could possibly have on its own.

When movements are required at many joints in order to place a distal segment in a position to carry out a task, most of the degrees of freedom available may be required. Such may be the case when reaching forward to pick up a small object from a shelf set at eye level. Other tasks may only require that just a few of the available degrees of freedom are used.

Should a joint in the chain become restricted, through injury, disuse or disease, the versatility of the distal segments will be

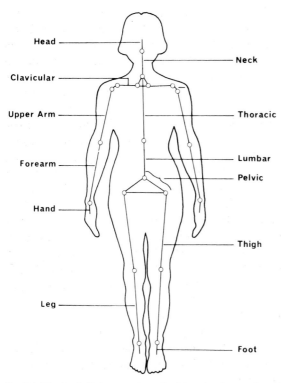

Fig. 3.6 The body linkage system. *Redrawn and reproduced with permission from Reynolds, H. M. (1978) The Inertial Properties of the Body and its Segments, Chapter IV. In Anthropometric Source Book Volume 1: Anthropometry for designers NASA Reference Publication 1024, p. IV–9.*

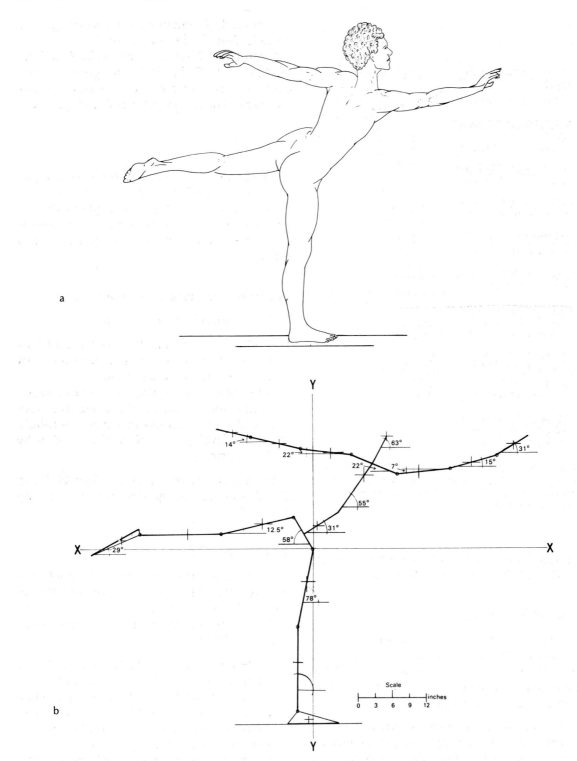

Fig. 3.7 a. Photographic tracing and b. corresponding link diagram drawn from it. *Reproduced with kind permission from O'Connell, A. L. & Gardner, E. B. (1972) Understanding the Scientific Bases of Human Movement. Baltimore: The Williams and Wilkins Company, pp. 114–115.*

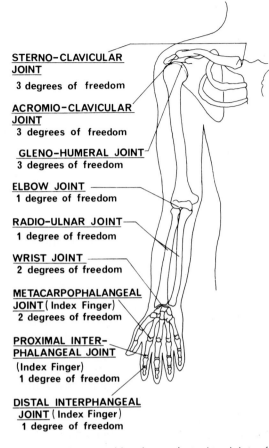

STERNO-CLAVICULAR
JOINT
3 degrees of freedom

ACROMIO-CLAVICULAR
JOINT
3 degrees of freedom

GLENO-HUMERAL JOINT
3 degrees of freedom

ELBOW JOINT
1 degree of freedom

RADIO-ULNAR JOINT
1 degree of freedom

WRIST JOINT
2 degrees of freedom

METACARPOPHALANGEAL
JOINT (Index Finger)
2 degrees of freedom

PROXIMAL INTER-
PHALANGEAL JOINT
(Index Finger)
1 degree of freedom

DISTAL INTERPHANGEAL
JOINT (Index Finger)
1 degree of freedom

Fig. 3.8 The degrees of freedom at the various joints of the upper limb. Added together this makes for seventeen degrees of freedom for each of the distal phalanges relative to the trunk.

reduced by a factor which is equivalent to the number of degrees of freedom lost.

Range of joint motion

The range of joint motion is the maximum amount of displacement possible at any one joint. Joints are said to be more or less stable, depending on their resistance to displacement, which in turn depends on:

1. The shape of the articular surfaces
2. The restraining effects of the ligaments and muscles crossing the joint as well as overlying skin and other soft tissue
3. The bulk of tissue in the adjacent segments.

A method of measuring and recording joint range is described in Appendix 1.

A standard reference source is the American Academy of Orthopaedic Surgeons (1966) *Joint motion, method of measuring and recording.* Edinburgh: Churchill Livingstone.

MUSCLES

Muscles can be divided into three major types – skeletal, cardiac and smooth. Skeletal muscle which contributes significantly to movements at the joints and to the maintenance of posture, will be the subject of this section.

Structural characteristics of skeletal muscle

A skeletal muscle is made up of:

1. Contractile components – the muscle fibres which are involved in the generation of active tension by the muscle.
2. Non-contractile elastic connective tissue components – tendons, intra-muscular septa and muscle coverings which contribute to the development of passive tension by the muscle.

All muscles have a rich capillary bed and blood flow can be greatly increased during activity.[4]

Muscle fibres[9,18,36]

Muscle fibres are the long multi-nucleated muscle cells, which may or may not extend the whole length of the muscle.

Within the cell membrane, or sarcolemma, are to be found:

1. Many myofibrils running longitudinally and parallel to each other embedded in a protein intracellular substance, the sarcoplasm. The myofibrils blend with the sarcolemma at each end of the muscle cell.
2. Two tubular systems. These are:
   a. The transverse tubules, which run from the outside into the centre of the muscle fibre. They are involved in the trans-

mission of an electrical impulse into the central parts of the muscle fibres to set up a sequence of events resulting in a muscle contraction.

b. The sarcoplasmic reticulum, which forms a net around the myofibril and is involved in the storage and release of calcium ions. On excitation of the muscle, calcium is released to contribute towards muscle contraction. Relaxation occurs when the calcium ions are pumped back into the sarcoplasmic reticulum.

3. Mitochondria, which are involved in the production of adenosine triphosphate that provides energy for contraction processes to take place. The mitochondria increase in number and size during endurance training, particularly in muscles involved in sustained postural activity.

The myofibril and muscle contraction[6,9,16,17]

Each myofibril is composed of repeating units called sarcomeres, which can be considered as the basic contractile units of the muscle fibre. Sarcomeres are enclosed between two bands which adhere to the sarcolemma called the Z lines (Fig. 3.9).

Within each sarcomere are to be found two sets of protein filaments:

1. Thick filaments made up of myosin molecules. Each myosin molecule has a heavy 'head' which projects from the side of the

filament (Fig. 3.15). These 'heads' appear to be involved in forming 'crossbridges' with the thin actin filaments, resulting in a muscle contraction.

2. Thin filaments made up of the proteins actin, troponin and tropomyosin.

Figure 3.9 illustrates that where the two sets of filaments overlap, each myosin filament is surrounded by six actin filaments between which crossbridges may be formed. The relative alignment of these filaments gives skeletal muscle its banded appearance when seen in a longitudinal section. The myosin filaments are lined up to form the darker A bands. In the middle of each thick filament there is a bulge. Slender cross connections pass from filament to filament at this point to hold the thick filaments apart. These form the M line. The actin filaments form the light I bands.

In the centre of the A band, when the muscle is relaxed, there is a less dense area, the H zone. It becomes obliterated when the muscle is fully contracted, as the actin and myosin filaments then are fully overlapping each other. Electron-microscopy research into the behaviour of these bands led to the emergence of the sliding filament theory of muscle contraction.

The sliding filament theory of muscle contraction[16,17]

When a muscle contracts, the filaments themselves do not change their length but slide past each other. This sliding action is thought to be brought about by direct contact between the 'heads' of the myosin molecules and the actin filaments. The 'heads' attach to the actin filaments at binding sites and supposedly move the thin filaments a short distance towards each other. The myosin 'heads' are then released from the binding sites and are again free to make new connections at other binding sites along the actin filaments. This further propels the thin filaments towards each other within each sarcomere. The cycle of binding, moving and breakage, is repeated a number of times.

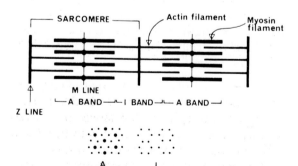

Fig. 3.9 Two sarcomeres. A represents a cross section through that part of the A band where the actin and myosin filaments overlap. I represents a cross section through the I band.

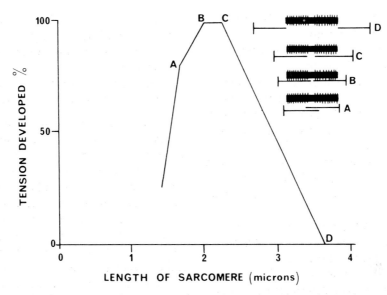

Fig. 3.10 Length tension diagram for a single sarcomere. Note the tension relationship to the overlap occurring between the actin and myosin filaments at A, B, C and D. *After Gordon et al (1966) – reproduced with kind permission from Guyton, A. C. (1976) Textbook of Medical Physiology, 5th edn. Philadelphia: W. B. Saunders Co. p. 137.*

The active tension that the muscle can produce depends on the number of such bridges formed as a result of stimulus to the muscle. Active tension will not be possible or will be markedly reduced if a muscle is either stretched to a point where there is no overlap of filaments or shortened to a point where the actin filaments from both sides overlap each other, thereby reducing the number of binding sites available. Such is the microstructural basis of the length–tension observations illustrated in Figure 3.10.

The motor unit[3,8,14,20,25,27,28,32,37]

Muscles are under the control of the nervous system. An alpha motor neuron and the muscle fibres it innervates is called a motor unit (Fig. 3.11). The motor unit is the basic functional unit of a muscle.

Motor unit size depends on the number of muscle fibres supplied by a single motor neuron. All muscle fibres in any one motor unit are of the same type. They cannot be mixed.

The muscle fibres of any one motor unit are

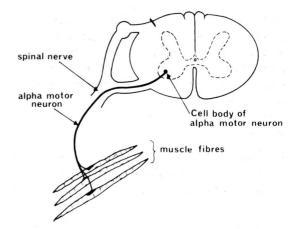

Fig. 3.11 A motor unit. In this case it is a skeleto-motor unit because it involves an alpha motor neuron and the extrafusal muscle fibres it serves.

often widely spread throughout the muscle but when the alpha motor neuron is excited all the muscle fibres supplied by it contract. Any one muscle has many motor units.

The dominant size of these motor units varies from muscle to muscle depending on the functional demands usually placed on the muscle. Muscles involved in activities needing precision, for example those of the eye and hand, have very few muscle fibres per motor unit, whereas muscles involved in gross forceful activities, such as those in the lower limbs, have a larger number of muscle fibres supplied by any one alpha motor neuron.

The manner in which a muscle contracts is determined by the number and types of motor units activated and the rate at which they are stimulated to contract. The cell bodies of the smallest motor units are the most excitable of the motor neuron pool of the spinal cord, whereas those of the larger motor units need a high level of stimulus before they will respond. As the small units can be turned on more readily, this allows for muscle force production to be finely tuned at low levels through small adjustments in the number of muscle fibres active at any one time.

Electromyography is used to study the activation of motor units.

Types of muscle fibre[5,6,7,13,18,27,32]

There are two basic types of muscle fibre, although histological examination of muscle stained to highlight the presence of oxidative enzymes would suggest that more categories could be used. These are:

1. Type I or slow twitch fibres, also called 'tonic' because they are involved in maintained activity. Slow twitch fibres are found in the smaller motor units. They have a high capacity for aerobic metabolism and are fatigue resistant. Another term for Type I fibres is slow-oxidative (SO) fibres.
2. Type II or fast twitch fibres, also called 'phasic' because they are involved in sharp bursts of activity as occur when changing from one position to another. Type II fibres are found in the larger motor units and rely on anaerobic metabolism. Another term for Type II fibres is fast-glycolytic (FG) fibres.

There is another type of Type II motor unit with fibres showing intermediate characteristics between Type I and Type II fibres. These are called fast-oxidative-glycolytic (FOG) fibres. Sometimes Type I and Type II fibres are

called 'red' and 'white' respectively. These colour terms should not be used interchangeably with slow or fast twitch, as the correlation between colour and contraction speed is not perfect.[7]

Whether muscle fibres behave as Type I or Type II depends on their innervation. Cross-innervation experiments, where nerves from fast fibres are transposed to slow, and vice versa, have shown that Type II – fast – muscles can assume the characteristics of Type I – slow – muscles, and to a lesser extent, the reverse. This is a good example of the dominance of the nervous system in regulating muscle activity.

Human muscles tend to contain a mixture of both Type I and Type II muscle fibres, the proportion in any particular muscle being an indication of its potential for performing specific tasks.

Muscles with predominantly Type I fibres are more efficient in maintaining isometric tension and are best suited for holding positions over a long period of time. They have high aerobic activity and are resistant to fatigue. Postural muscles such as soleus come into this category. Muscles containing mainly Type II fibres are said to be more efficient during dynamic muscle activity which requires the generation of a high force and high velocity action over a short period. Gastrocnemius is such a muscle.

Muscle twitch and tetanus[13,20,27]

When a single electrical pulse of an adequate intensity is applied to a muscle via the motor nerve, there is a latent period in which there is no activity after which it will respond with a quick contraction followed by a relaxation phase. This is called a muscle twitch. Muscles differ in the time taken to reach a full contraction and achieve a full relaxation depending on which type of muscle fibre is dominant in the gross muscle structure (Fig. 3.12).

When two identical stimuli are given to a muscle with a suitable time interval separating them, the peak force produced for each muscle twitch will be identical. If the stimuli

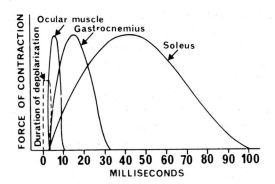

Fig. 3.12 Contraction-relaxation curves for fast twitch muscles, for example gastrocnemius, and slow twitch muscles, for example soleus. Note the very short duration of the ocular muscles. *Reproduced with kind permission from Guyton, A. C. (1976) Textbook of Medical Physiology, 5th edn. Philadelphia: W. B. Saunders Co. p. 142.*

are then moved closer together in time so the first twitch is not fully completed before the second stimulus is applied, the second twitch reaches a higher force maximum than the first. With even more rapid stimulation, the degree of summation of successive contractions becomes progressively greater until a frequency of stimulation is finally reached when successive contractions fuse together so they cannot be distinguished from each other. Further increases in stimulus frequency do not produce any increase in muscle tension at this stage. This is called tetanus (Fig. 3.13). The tension produced by a muscle in this state may be four to five times greater than that exerted by a single muscle twitch.

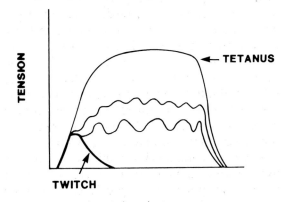

Fig. 3.13 Isometric twitch and tetanus.

Recruitment order of motor units[14,25,27,28,37]

Not all activities require the same amount of muscle tension to be produced. Some require a minimal tension level to be sustained over a long period, whereas others require an immediate all-out effort. Even within the same activity sequence there is a need for grading force production as the action proceeds. Whatever the case, a certain number of motor units will need to be recruited into action.

The order of recruitment of motor units is determined by their size – the size principle. The smallest motor units are recruited first because of the high excitability of their cell bodies in the spinal cord. If a stronger contraction is required, more motor units become progressively recruited until when a maximal voluntary contraction is required the largest units also become involved.

Gradation of muscle force can be made in smaller steps when only a 'weak' muscle contraction is all that is required. As the intensity of the muscle contraction increases the steps become progressively greater because larger motor units are included.

The sequence is reversed when the force level falls. Here the largest motor units cease their activity first followed later by progressively smaller units.

Obviously a maximal muscle contraction will not be needed for many activities so the number of motor units recruited will vary according to the circumstances but the sequence of recruitment will still follow the size principle.

The gross structure of muscles[30,36]

The muscle fibres are grouped into bundles called fasciculi. The size of these bundles varies – muscles performing fine movements having small fasciculi, whereas muscles performing more gross movements have a larger number of muscle fibres in each fasciculus. The fasciculi are not to be confused with the motor units previously described.

The arrangement of the fasciculi determines the basic shape of the muscle, which in turn has some bearing on the amount of tension produced and the speed of muscle contraction. Parallel fibres are usually seen in muscles which are more fast acting, for example sartorius, whereas a pennate-type shape is associated more with a design for strength, for example, gluteus maximus (Fig. 3.14).

Each fasciculus is surrounded by a connective tissue sheath called the perimysium. All fasciculi are then collected together and covered by a strong epimysium, to form the whole muscle belly.

Figure 3.15 summarises most of the levels of organization in the skeletal muscle which have been discussed so far.

The non-contractile coverings of the muscle merge at both ends of the contractile section of the muscle to become part of a round-shaped tendon or a flat fibrous sheet, an aponeurosis, which in turn attaches to bone. These connective tissue elements possess a degree of elasticity which needs to be considered in the total tension that can be generated in a muscle.

Elasticity refers to a material's resistance to being deformed when a force is applied to it. After the deforming force is released the material returns to its original position.

Tendons form part of the series elastic

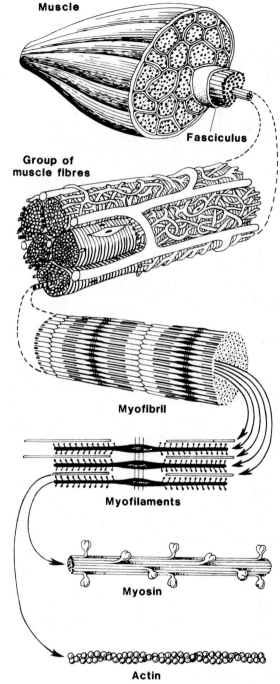

Fig. 3.15 Diagram showing the various levels of organisation within a skeletal muscle, from whole muscle, through fasciculi, fibres, myofibrils, myofilaments, down to molecular dimensions. *Reproduced with kind permission from Warwick, R. & Williams, P. L. (1973) Gray's Anatomy, 35th edn. Edinburgh: Churchill Livingstone, p. 481.*

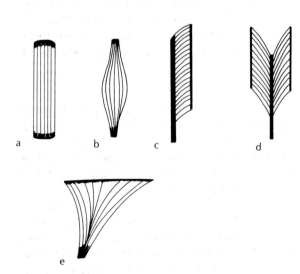

Fig. 3.14 Gross shapes of muscles. a. Strap b. Fusiform (Latin fusus – spindle) c. Unipennate d. Bipennate e. Triangular.

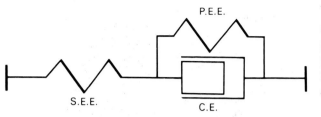

Fig. 3.16 An analogue model of muscle. C.E. = contractile element (the cross-bridge system). S.E.E. = series elastic element, part of which resides in the tendinous extremities of the muscle, and part in the necks of the myosin molecules. P.E.E. = parallel elastic element, the connective tissue surrounding the muscle fibres. *Reproduced with kind permission from Buller, A. J. (1973) Posture and Movement. Physiotherapy, vol 59, no. 11, p. 347.*

element of a muscle. The connective tissue surrounding the muscle fibres is called the parallel elastic element because it is in parallel with the contractile material (Fig. 3.16).

Muscle attachments

A muscle exerts a force at all its attachments when it contracts. One of the bones to which the muscle attaches remains relatively steady anchoring one end of the muscle. Thus the force of the contracting muscle can be used efficiently to move the bony lever to which the other end of the muscle is attached.

In the traditional anatomical description of muscles of the extremities, the proximal attachment which is usually the more stationary, is called the origin and the more distal attachment, the insertion. There are many instances when the distal attachment is the more stationary of the two. Thus this system of naming can lead to confusion; so in movement analysis, it is perhaps best to refer to the muscle attachments as being either fixed or moving.

Roles of muscles

Muscles rarely act alone. Usually several different muscles collaborate one with another to achieve the movement required, through an interplay of individually increasing and decreasing tensions produced within them.

This is under the control of the nervous system. Depending on the movement being performed each muscle has its own role to play in producing that movement. For another movement, that same muscle may play quite a different role.

A muscle can act as:

1. A prime mover, or agonist, where the muscle is the major muscle involved in initiating, carrying out and maintaining a particular movement. Other muscles in the same group may play a significant though lesser role in producing a similar movement to the prime mover. These muscles may be called assistant movers.

2. An antagonist, where the muscle wholly opposes the prime mover. Antagonists relax reciprocally during the contraction of the prime mover, through the process of reciprocal inhibition. An exception occurs when hinge joints are moved in a whip-like fashion. In this case the antagonist contracts briskly at the end of the movement as a protective device.

3. A stabiliser or fixator which contracts to position a bone, to keep it as a controlled steady base from which a prime mover can act. Thus stabilisers act to provide the fixed attachment of another muscle.

4. A synergist, where the muscle teams up with another muscle in the production of a movement which neither could perform alone. Both muscles in the team are called synergists.

There are two types of synergist, helping and true.[30] An example of the former is found when flexor carpi radialis and extensor carpi radialis longus, usually antagonists in the movements of flexion and extension of the wrist, team up as synergists to produce radial deviation.

An example of true synergists is as follows – gripping an object effectively, using the long finger flexors, means that the unwanted action of these same muscles at the wrist needs to be eliminated. Contraction of the wrist extensors synergically does this.

Types of muscle contraction

The contractile components of the muscle tend to shorten when they are activated by efferent impulses. This shortening produces a force which tends to stretch the elastic tendon which lies in series with the contractile material. In this way active muscle tension is produced.

This attempt of the activated muscle to develop tension and shorten is called a muscle contraction. Whether the muscle actually does shorten or remains at the same length or is forcibly stretched depends on the external resistance offered. The term muscle action can be used to describe any type of tension development in the muscle when it is activated.[31]

Muscle contractions can be classified on the basis of the relationship of the internal force developed by the muscle itself and the external force applied to the muscle. There are two major divisions:

1. Dynamic
2. Isometric.

1. A dynamic muscle contraction is one in which the muscle actively alters its length. There are two types which are readily identifiable in everyday activities.

a. Shortening (concentric) contraction, in which the internal force generated is greater than the external force applied, so the muscle actively shortens.
b. Lengthening (eccentric) contraction, in which the external force applied is greater than the internal force generated. During this type of contraction, the muscle is allowed to lengthen while still maintaining tension. It acts as a braking force.

Muscles produce less heat when they are actively lengthening than when actively shortening.

Work is done by muscles when they actively shorten to move an external load. This is termed positive work. When muscles are actively lengthening, work is being done on them by an external force, for example gravity, to produce the movement. This is called negative work.[1]

Dynamic muscle contractions can also be isotonic and isokinetic in nature.[22,31]

a. Isotonic muscle contractions involve the production of a constant force as the muscle actively alters its length. In real-life situations this is not the case as the effective force developed alters because of leverage effects around the joints.
b. Isokinetic muscle contractions are those in which the rate of shortening or lengthening of the muscle is constant.

During a dynamic muscle contraction it changes its length through a certain range.[15] It is called full range when the muscle length changes from the position in which it is fully stretched within the body to where it is fully contracted if working concentrically, and vice versa if acting eccentrically. Full range muscle excursion can be further subdivided into:

a. Outer range – where the muscle changes its length from full stretch to the mid-point of full range if working concentrically, and vice versa if acting eccentrically.
b. Inner range – where the muscle changes its length from the mid-point of full range to the fully contracted position if working concentrically, and vice versa if acting eccentrically.
c. Middle range – where the muscle changes its length from the mid-point of outer range to the mid-point of inner range if working concentrically, and vice versa if acting eccentrically. This descriptive terminology should not be confused with range of joint motion.

2. An isometric contraction is one in which the internal force developed by the muscle is such that the total muscle neither shortens nor lengthens. The muscle attempts to contract against a resistance without producing any motion, the internal force generated being equal to the external force applied. When a muscle acts isometrically, no mechanical work is done as a load is not moved.

Table 3.3 Types of muscle contraction: a summary

Type of contraction	Function	External force on muscle	External work by muscle	Energy cost (O_2) demand	Maximal force produced
Shortening (concentric)	Acceleration	Less	Positive	More than lengthening contraction	Lowest
Isometric	Fixation	Same	None		Intermediate
Lengthening (eccentric)	Deceleration	More	Negative	Less than shortening contraction	Highest

Although at the gross level the total muscle does not alter its length, there is a redistribution of lengths within the muscle for there is:

a. Slight shortening of each sarcomere, due to the filaments sliding past each other
b. Slight stretching of the tendon, due to its elastic properties.

Most forms of daily activity will involve a combination of varying proportions of concentric, eccentric and isometric types of contraction. A summary of some of the characteristics of the different types of muscle contraction used in everyday activities is given in Table 3.3.

Muscle length and tension production

The length of a muscle when it is stimulated to contract, influences the amount of tension it can produce at that length. This can be displayed graphically in a length-tension curve (Fig. 3.17). These curves differ for various

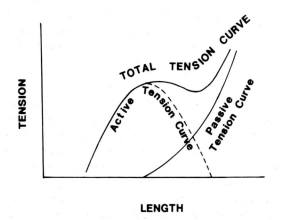

LENGTH

Fig. 3.17 Length–tension curve for a skeletal muscle.

muscles depending on their gross shape and connective tissue content.[27]

Length–tension curves have mainly been obtained using muscles that have been removed from the body. The length that an unattached unstimulated muscle adopts is called its equilibrium length and tension is zero.[9] Very little work has been done on muscles *in vivo*.

A 'total' tension curve is obtained by measuring the tension produced by the muscle when it is tetanised at different lengths. The curve for passive tension is obtained by measuring the tension produced at different lengths as the muscle is simply stretched beyond its equilibrium length.

An increase of passive tension occurs slowly at first and then more rapidly as stretching proceeds. When the muscle is about three times its equilibrium length rupture occurs.[9]

In the living body, most muscles which cross only one joint are not normally stretched enough to cause passive tension to rise sufficiently high enough for it to play a significant role in overall force production, but this is not so for muscles which cross two or more joints, where tension can become so great as to limit range of joint motion.

Generally speaking, the amount of passive tension produced by muscles lying more distally in the extremities is much higher than those more proximally placed. Likewise, the passive tension produced by the muscles of the lower extremities is higher than that of the upper extremities.[19]

The difference between the total and passive tension curves gives an estimate of the active or developed tension curve (Fig. 3.17).

In the living body, unstimulated muscle is normally under slight passive tension due to stretch on the parallel elastic element. This resting length is approximately 20 per cent greater than the equilibrium length.[38]

Active tension decreases when the muscle is either lengthened or shortened relative to its resting length and becomes zero, either at twice the resting length or as the muscle approaches its maximally shortened position. This observation can be readily explained by the sliding filament theory of muscle contraction, for either there is no overlap of the filaments, as when the muscle is excessively stretched, or there is too much overlap so effective 'crossbridges' cannot be established[11] as illustrated in Figure 3.10.

Many muscles of the body develop maximal active tension at the resting length and are often naturally positioned at this length for tasks requiring a strong muscle contraction. In normal movement, the posture of the body is automatically adjusted so as to keep muscles at a favourable length.[29]

Re-education of a muscle is best undertaken at its optimal length in order to achieve a maximal amount of active tension. For a muscle crossing only one joint, this means its most elongated position in the normal body, but this does not necessarily hold true for muscles crossing two or more joints.

Active and passive insufficiency[12,22]

Muscles placed so that they cross only one joint are normally capable of shortening and lengthening to such an extent that they can permit full range of motion of that joint. This is not necessarily the case for muscles crossing two or more joints.

A muscle crossing two or more joints and producing simultaneous movement at all the joints it crosses, soon reaches a shortened length at which it can no longer generate a useful force (active tension). At this point the muscle is said to be actively insufficient, as, for example, if the hamstrings are used to simultaneously flex the knee while extending the hip.

In contrast, a muscle crossing two or more joints but unable to stretch across these joints

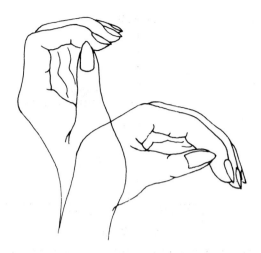

Fig. 3.18 The tenodesis action.

sufficiently to allow for their full displacements is said to be passively insufficient. Reaching towards the floor while keeping one's knees fully extended may be limited by the passive insufficiency of the hamstrings, as they are stretched across both the hip and knee joints.

Increasing passive tension in a muscle crossing two or more joints may produce movements at these joints. This is called tenodesis. For example, when the wrist is flexed and the fingers are relaxed, the fingers will automatically extend as full wrist flexion is reached. Likewise, if the wrist is extended, the fingers will tend to flex (Fig. 3.18).

Velocity of contraction and tension[21,27,31,37]

The amount of tension a muscle can produce is also influenced by its velocity of contraction. If a muscle of a predetermined length is made to contract maximally at different velocities, force measurements can be made and a force–velocity curve constructed (Fig. 3.19).

More is known about the force–velocity behaviour of concentric than eccentric muscle contractions at high velocities because of difficulties in devising equipment to do work on muscle – negative work – with safety and accuracy.

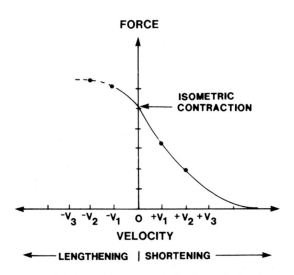

FORCE

ISOMETRIC CONTRACTION

$-v_3 \quad -v_2 \quad -v_1 \quad 0 \quad +v_1 \quad +v_2 \quad +v_3$

VELOCITY

← LENGTHENING | SHORTENING →

Fig. 3.19 Relation of force to velocity for an isolated muscle preparation under maximal stimulation. From left to right on the abscissa are rapid eccentric (lengthening) contraction, slow eccentric contraction, isometric contraction (zero velocity), slow concentric (shortening) contraction, rapid concentric contraction.

The following observations can be made from the force–velocity curve:

1. Isometric (zero velocity) and eccentric muscle contractions develop greater tension than concentric contractions of any velocity.
2. As the velocity of a concentric muscle contraction increases less tension is developed.
3. Eccentric contractions develop more tension than isometric and concentric contractions.
4. The faster the eccentric contraction the greater the tension that can be produced, but at very high velocities more needs to be discovered.

The velocity at which a muscle contracts influences its power output. Power is a measure of the force which the muscle can produce and the velocity at which the muscle shortens.

Clinically it is important to consider the velocity at which muscles are tested and exercised as well as considering the load involved. Erroneous measures of increased tension production capacity of a muscle (strength) could occur if the speed of testing is not kept constant from test to test.

REFERENCES AND FURTHER READING

1. Astrand, P. O. & Rodahl, K. (1977) *Textbook of Work Physiology*, 2nd edn. New York: McGraw Hill.
2. Barham, J. N. (1978) *Mechanical Kinesiology*. St Louis: C. V. Mosby.
3. Basmajian, J.V. & De Luca, C. J. (1985). *Muscles Alive*, 5th edn. Baltimore: Williams & Wilkins.
4. Bowden, R. E. (1968) The structure and function of striated muscle. *Physiotherapy*, Vol. 54, No. 6, pp. 190–196.
5. Burke, R. E. & Edgerton, V. R. (1975) Motor unit properties and selective involvement in movement. In *Exercise and Sport Sciences Review*, Wilmore, J. H. & Keogh, J. F. (Eds) Vol. 3. New York: Academic Press.
6. Buller, A. J. (1973) Posture and movement. *Physiotherapy*, Vol. 59, No. 11, pp. 344–349.
7. Buller, A. J. (1975) The Physiology of Skeletal Muscle. In Hunt, C. C. (Ed.) *Physiology Series One: Volume 3 – Neurophysiology*. London: Butterworths.
8. English, A. W. & Wolf, S. L. (1982) The Motor Unit. *Physical Therapy*, Vol. 62, No. 12, pp. 1763–1772.
9. Ganong, W. F. (1979) *Review of Medical Physiology*, 9th edn. Los Altos: Lange Medical.
10. Gardiner, M. D. (1963) *The Principles of Exercise Therapy*, 3rd edn. London: Bell & Hyman.
11. Gordon, A. M., Huxley, A. F. & Julian, F. J. (1966) The variation in isometric tension with sarcomere length in vertebrate muscle fibres. *Journal of Physiology*, Vol. 184, pp. 170–192.
12. Gowitzke, B. A. & Milner, M. (1980) *Understanding the Scientific Bases of Human Movement*, 2nd edn. Baltimore: Williams & Wilkins.
13. Guyton, A. C. (1981) *Textbook of Medical Physiology*, 6th edn. Philadelphia: W. B. Saunders.
14. Henneman, E., Somjen, G. & Carpenter, D. (1965) Excitability and Inhibitability of motoneurons of different sizes. *Journal of Neurobiology*, Vol. 28, pp. 19–41.
15. Hollis, M. (1981), *Practical Exercise Therapy*, 2nd edn. Oxford: Blackwell Scientific.
16. Huxley, A. F. (1974) Muscular contraction. *Journal of Physiology*, Vol. 243, pp. 1–43.
17. Huxley, H. E. (1965) The mechanism of muscular contraction. *Scientific American*, Vol. 213, No. 6, pp. 18–27.
18. Ianuzzo, C. D. (1976) The cellular composition of human skeletal muscle. In Knuttgen, H. G. (Ed.) *Neuromuscular Mechanisms for Therapeutic and Conditioning Exercise*. Baltimore: University Park Press.
19. Inman, V. T. & Ralston, H. J. (1968) The mechanics of voluntary muscle. In Klopsteg, P. H. & Wilson, P. D. (Eds) *Human Limbs and Their Substitutes*. New York: Hafner Publishing.
20. Keynes, R. D. & Aidley, D. J. (1981) *Nerve and Muscle*. Cambridge: Cambridge University Press.
21. Knuttgen, H. G. (1976) Development of muscular strength and endurance. In Knuttgen, H. G. (Ed.) *Neuromuscular Mechanisms for Therapeutic and Conditioning Exercise*. Baltimore: University Park Press.
22. Lehmkuhl, L. D. & Smith, L. K. (1983) *Brunnstrom's*

Clinical Kinesiology, 4th edn. Philadelphia: F. A. Davis Co.

23. Le Veau, B. (1977) *Williams and Lissner: Biomechanics of Human Motion*. Philadelphia: W. B. Saunders.

24. MacConaill, M. A. & Basmajian, J. V. (1977) *Muscles and Movements*, 2nd edn. New York: Robert E. Krieger Publishing.

25. Maton, B. (1980) Fast and slow motor units. Their recruitment for tonic and phasic contractions in man. *European Journal of Applied Physiology*, Vol. 43, pp. 45–55.

26. McConville, J. T. & Laubach, L. L. (1978) Anthropometry. In *Anthropometric Source Book Volume I: Anthropometry for Designers*, N.A.S.A. Reference Publication 1024 Chapter III. National Aeronautics and Space Administration, Scientific and Technical Information Office.

27. McMahon, T. A. (1984) *Muscles, Reflexes and Locomotion*. Princeton: Princeton University Press.

28. Milner-Brown, H. S., Stein, R. B. & Yemm, R. (1973). The orderly recruitment of human motor units during voluntary isometric contractions. *Journal of Physiology*, Vol 230, pp. 359–370.

29. Ralston, H. J. (1953) Mechanics of voluntary muscle. *American Journal of Physical Medicine*, Vol. 32, pp. 166–184.

30. Rasch, P. J. & Burke, R. K. (1978) *Kinesiology and Applied Anatomy*, 6th edn. Philadelphia: Lea and Febiger.

31. Rodgers, M. M. & Cavanagh, P. R. (1984) Glossary of Biomechanical Terms, Concepts and Units. *Physical Therapy*, Vol 64, No 12, pp. 1886–1902.

32. Rose, S. J. & Rothstein, J. M. (1982) Muscle Mutability. Part 1.–General Concepts and Adaptations to Altered Patterns of Use. *Physical Therapy*, Vol. 62, No. 12, pp. 1773–1787.

33. Rothstein, J. M. (1982) Muscle Biology – Clinical considerations. *Physical Therapy*, Vol. 62, No. 12, pp 1823–1830.

34. Singh, M. & Karpovich, P. V. (1966) Isotonic and isometric forces of forearm flexors and extensors. *Journal of Applied Physiology*, Vol. 21, No. 4, pp. 1435–1437.

35. Steindler, A. (1955) *Kinesiology of the Human Body*. Springfield, Illinois: Thomas.

36. Williams, P. L. & Warwick, R. (Eds) (1980) *Gray's Anatomy*, 36th Edn. Edinburgh: Churchill Livingstone.

37. Winter, D. A. (1979) *Biomechanics of Human Movement*. New York: John Wiley & Sons.

38. Woodbury, J. W., Gordon, A. M. & Conrad, J. T. (1965) Muscle. In Ruch, T. C., Patton, H. D., Woodbury, J. W. & Towe, A. L. *Neurophysiology*, 2nd edn. Philadelphia: W. B. Saunders.

4

The neurological basis of human movement

The purpose of this chapter is to introduce some basic neurological concepts related to the control of skeletal muscle activity.

BASIC STRUCTURE AND FUNCTION OF THE NERVOUS SYSTEM

Gross structure of the nervous system

The spinal cord and the brain form the central nervous system.

The brain may be considered as an elaborate extension of the spinal cord which has become increasingly complex in higher animals.

The spinal nerves and cranial nerves form the peripheral nervous system.

Afferent or sensory nerve fibres carry information from various sensory receptors into the central nervous system. This information is integrated at all levels of the central nervous system to produce appropriate motor responses in both skeletal and smooth muscles and glands. Information is relayed to these effectors via the efferent motor fibres.

In spinal nerves, afferent fibres pass into the spinal cord via the dorsal nerve root and efferent fibres leave via the ventral nerve root.

The neuron

The basic structural elements of the nervous system are neurons or nerve cells and glial cells. The function of the latter is uncertain.

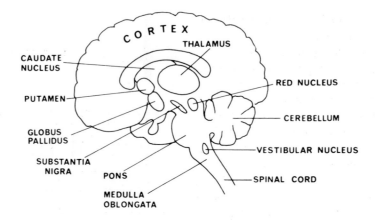

Fig. 4.1 Major regions of the brain.

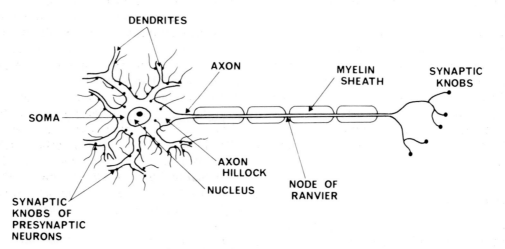

Fig. 4.2 A typical motor neuron. Impulses are passed along the single axon towards the next cell. The axon eventually branches and terminates in a number of synaptic knobs or terminal boutons, which release a chemical transmitter substance when suitably excited.

Neurons are highly specialised excitable cells which receive messages from other nerve cells or specific sensory receptors (Fig. 4.2).

Neurons vary widely in their size, shape and amount of branching. For example, the axon of a motor neuron can sometimes be very long as is the case from the lower segments of the spinal cord to the muscles of the foot. Likewise the process of a sensory neuron running from a receptor in the foot to its cell body in the dorsal root ganglion may be lengthy.

Electrical activity in nerve cells

A semi-permeable cell membrane separates the intracellular fluid compartment from the interstitial fluid surrounding the nerve cell. These two fluid compartments have different ionic concentrations. Na^+ and Cl^- ions are more concentrated in the interstitial fluid, whereas K^+ ions are more concentrated in the intracellular fluid.

Because the cell membrane is semi-permeable, certain ions such as Na^+, K^+ and Cl^- can move across it. It is much more permeable to K+ than to either Na+ or Cl−.

Inside the cell are large protein molecules which are negatively charged. These cannot move across the cell membrane. Therefore there is a tendency for the outside of the membrane to be charged positively in relation to the inside of the cell membrane, which is charged negatively. This produces a potential difference across the cell membrane.

The resting membrane potential, which in neurons is usually −70 millivolts, is maintained by energy processes which 'pump' Na+ out of the cell and K+ back into it. This sodium-potassium 'pump' is important in keeping the charge on what amounts to a condensor, correct.

Any alteration in relative ionic concentrations on both sides of the cell membrane may change the potential difference across it. Sometimes this may decrease the resting membrane potential which leads to excitation of the neuron. At other times this may increase the resting membrane potential, which leads to inhibition of the neuron to firing.

Action potential

When for any reason the resting membrane potential is reduced, it may reach a threshold level for firing. This occurs after a 15 mV depolarisation in nerve cells. Reduction in the potential difference across the cell membrane is called depolarisation. There is a discharge when the nerve cell fires which creates an action potential (Fig. 4.3).

During the action potential, the polarity across the resting membrane is abolished and for a few milliseconds is even reversed before repolarisation occurs and the resting membrane potential of −70 mV is re-established after a short period of hyperpolarisation. With hyperpolarisation there is an even greater potential difference across the cell membrane than occurs with the resting membrane potential.

When the period of reversed potential occurs, the outside of the membrane becomes negatively charged relative to the inside of the

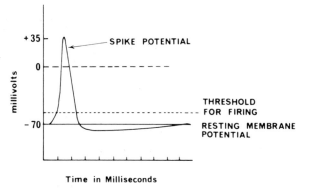

Fig. 4.3 An action potential.

cell. Positive charges now flow into the areas of negativity, thereby decreasing the potential difference across the cell membrane ahead of the action potential to the threshold level for firing. The nervous impulse is thereby propagated along the nerve fibre due to the circular current flow so caused.

Depolarisation in myelinated axons jumps from one Node of Ranvier to the next, thereby short-circuiting that part of the axon which lies in between. This is called saltatory conduction and explains why conduction by myelinated fibres is more than 100 m/sec compared to only 1 m/sec in the non-myelinated fibres.

'All or none' law

If a stimulus is applied to a neuron which is at or above the threshold level for firing, the action potential generated will be constant in amplitude and form, irrespective of the strength of the stimulus.

The action potential is said to obey the 'all or none' law.

Synapses

Synapses are regions of specialised contact between cells where cell to cell communication takes place. A gap, called the synaptic cleft, is always present between the cells. Transmission across this gap takes time, causing a delay called synaptic delay. Therefore neuronal circuits, involving many synapses,

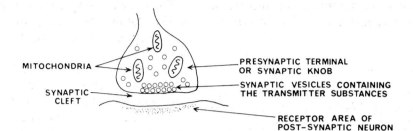

Fig. 4.4 An inter-neuronal synapse.

take longer to traverse than those with fewer synapses.

At synapses impulses are transmitted, usually via a chemical mediator, from the axon or some other portion of the pre-synaptic cell to the soma, dendrites or other portion of the post-synaptic cell (Fig. 4.4). Muscle fibres are the post-synaptic cells at the neuro-muscular junction.

Chemical transmitter substances are released from the synaptic vesicles when an action potential passes into the terminal endings of the pre-synaptic axon. For example, an action potential arriving at the neuro-muscular junction, leads to a release of acetylcholine which passes across the synaptic gap to the muscle membrane, bringing about changes which lead to a muscle contraction.

Another excitatory transmitter substance is dopamine, whereas the amino acid, glycine, acts as an inhibitory chemical mediator.

Greater understanding of transmitter substances and their modes of action will lead to a better understanding of the nervous system and its function.

Convergence and divergence

The cell body and dendrites of a post-synaptic neuron are often densely covered by a multitude of synaptic knobs from many other pre-synaptic cells (Fig. 4.2). When many cells influence one neuron this is called convergence.

It has been calculated that there may be as many as 5000 synaptic knobs applied to a single motor neuron. Some of these synaptic knobs may secrete a transmitter substance such as acetylcholine which decreases the resting membrane potential of the post-synaptic neuron. Other synaptic knobs from different pre-synaptic cells may secrete substances which raise the resting membrane potential of the post-synaptic cell. There is a constant interplay of such activity which may or may not lead to the threshold level for firing of the post-synaptic cell being reached. If excitatory influences are predominant, action potentials will arise in the post-synaptic cell. An inhibitory post-synaptic potential arises if inhibitory influences are predominant, so the possibility of an action potential arising in the post-synaptic cell is reduced.

The post-synaptic cell, in turn, influences many other neurons through the process of divergence. Here the terminal branching of its axon allows it to make multiple connections, often with several hundred other neurons.

Some idea of the complexity of neurological functioning may be obtained by considering these processes of convergence and divergence.

Signalling in the nervous system

All signalling in the nervous system is by uniformly sized impulses or action potentials, irrespective of the source of the information being transmitted. The information is coded by varying the rate and spacing of these impulses.

One receptor can tell many things by varying the rate of impulses. For example, stimulation of a joint receptor in one position may produce a low background frequency of firing, which may increase or decrease in rate as another position is approached and remain firing at this new rate until a third position is adopted.

The reflex arc

The reflex arc is the basic unit of integrated neural activity. It consists of: (1) A sensory organ; (2) An afferent sensory neuron; (3) A central nervous mechanism which may involve a number of interneurons, spread over many levels of the nervous system; (4) An efferent (motor) neuron; (5) A peripheral effector organ which produces the observed response.

When an appropriate stimulus is given, a reflex response occurs. This may be described as a characteristic – often stereotyped – involuntary response which can be elicited with some regularity on the presentation of an appropriate stimulus. Relatively simple reflexes are integrated in the spinal cord, whereas more complicated motor responses are controlled by much higher levels of the nervous system, such as the brainstem, midbrain or even the cerebral cortex.

There are a number of postural reflexes (Table 2.6) involving many levels of the central nervous system which contribute towards the positioning of the body segments relative to one another. Where balance is also necessary there is a complex interaction of these reflexes with conscious control of muscle activity to keep the person upright.

Sensory receptors and sensation

The different sensory receptors in the body are exquisitely sensitive to a particular energy form. Receptors whose primary activity is to respond to one form of stimulation, may respond to other types if the stimulus is intense enough, although the signal will be interpreted by the brain as if a stimulus of the type it is specifically designed to register had been present. For example, if the receptors of the eyes are stimulated by light or pressure, impulses are still projected to the visual cortex, so the message is ultimately interpreted as a visual sensation regardless of the mode of stimulation.

The sensory receptors most directly involved in skeletal muscle activity include:

1. Proprioceptors. These are concerned with the:

a. Orientation of the head in space – labyrinthine receptors of the ear.

b. Angle of the joint – joint receptors.

c. Degree of shortening of the skeletal muscle – muscle spindles; golgi tendon organs. Information from these muscle receptors also contributes towards awareness of joint position.

An individual's awareness or perception of his position in space and how rapidly any changes are occurring, arises from his ability to integrate information from these sources with tactile and visual information. This involves the cerebral cortex. Awareness of bodily motion is called kinaesthesis.

2. Exteroceptors. These are concerned with monitoring the events occurring in the:

a. Immediate environment to the body – skin receptors recording touch, pressure, warmth, cold, pain; taste receptors.

b. Distant environment – receptors of the eyes, ears and nose. These are sometimes called teloreceptors.

The area over which stimulation can influence the firing of one sensory neuron is called its receptive field. Only some of the massive amount of sensory information to which the individual is subjected eventually reaches the cerebral cortex. Much of this information has been filtered on the way by various mechanisms, as a sensory overload on the cortex would interfere with its efficiency.

Representation of the various areas of the body found in the sensory projection area of the postcentral gyrus – somaesthetic cortex – (Fig. 4.5) is such that the trunk only occupies a small area of this region, whereas projections related to the hands and mouth occupy a relatively much larger area. This highlights the importance of the hands and mouth as sensory organs.

The eyes also project to a relatively large area of the cortex (Fig. 4.5) reflecting vision's dominance over so many activities.

Perception is made possible through the

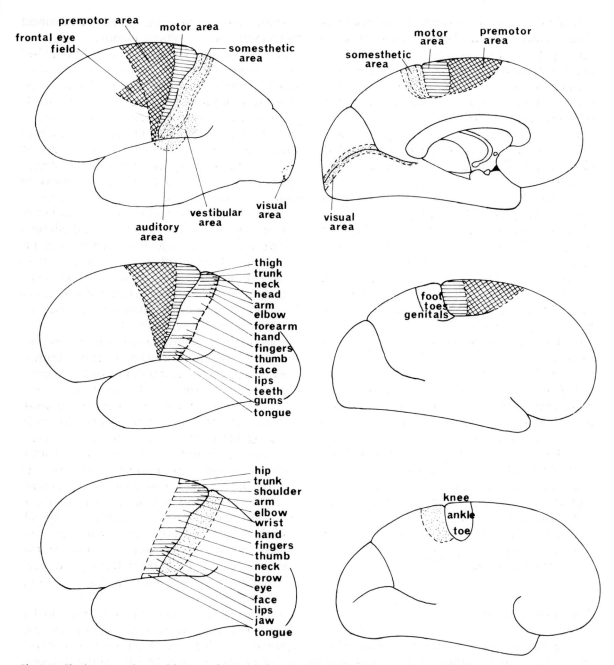

Fig. 4.5 The location of several functional areas of the cortex (top). The representation of the body parts on the somatic sensory cortex (middle) and primary motor cortex (bottom) are also shown. Note the larger areas for the hands, fingers, thumb and mouth. *The top figures are redrawn and simplified from Barr, M.L. (1979) The Human Nervous System – An Anatomical Viewpoint, 3rd edn. Hagerstown: Harper & Row Publishers Inc, p. 188.*

various association areas of the cerebral cortex. Information from various sensory sources is brought together and interpreted in the light of past experience which is stored in the memory. In this way a mental picture of the body and how it is moving in space is formed.

Sensory receptors may be:

1. Slowly adapting or tonic, if they discharge at a steady rate while the same stimulus continues to be applied. Such receptors provide a source of background information about the environment which may never reach consciousness. Examples of slowly adapting receptors include:

a. The muscle spindles, which contribute to the maintenance of posture over long periods of time by responding to alterations in muscle length.

b. The joint receptors of the capsule, which have a low threshold for firing. A proportion of these receptors is always active in every position of the joint. This type of joint receptor is more densely distributed in the proximal limb joints and the joints of the cervical region of the spine. Other joint receptors, which are found in the ligaments and have a high threshold for firing, are slowly adapting and only become active at extremes of range.

c. The pain receptors.

2. Fast adapting or phasic, if their discharges soon cease when the same stimulus continues to be applied. Should the intensity of the stimulus again be altered in any way, the fast adapting receptors will again discharge. Examples of fast adapting receptors are:

a. Joint receptors which are present in the capsules of all joints but are more numerous in the distal joints. They are inactive in immobile joints but become active for a brief period only at the onset of a change in joint motion.

b. Touch receptors.

THE SPINAL CORD

The spinal cord is a much more complex and important structure than is often appreciated. Basic movement patterns are integrated at this level although higher centres are needed to refine them.

The anterior grey matter of the spinal cord may be considered as a long motor neuron pool. Here a multitude of alpha and gamma motor neuron cell bodies are to be found as well as some interneurons.

Alpha motor neurons have large fast conducting fibres which synapse with the extrafusal muscle fibres of the muscle belly itself. One alpha motor neuron and the muscle fibres it innervates is called a skeletomotor unit or motor unit (Fig. 3.11). The small gamma motor neurons synapse with the intrafusal muscle fibres of the muscle spindle forming a fusimotor unit.

Interneurons are spread out through all the spinal grey matter. They are more numerous than the anterior horn motor cells and have multiple connections with one another. Most sensory signals coming from the periphery terminate on these interneurons rather than on to the anterior horn cells.

The interconnections between the interneurons and the anterior horn motor neurons, form the basis of the important integrative function of the spinal cord.

One particularly important interneuron is the Renshaw cell. An excited alpha motor neuron, through a Renshaw cell, inhibits motor cells nearby. In this way motor responses can be refined even at the spinal level and fatigue of the muscle fibres delayed.

The spinal cord also provides for linkages between different levels of the central nervous system. Propriospinal fibres run up and down the spinal cord from one segment to another forming a basis for those reflex responses which involve a number of spinal segments. For example, stimulation at one segmental level can influence the motor response at another segmental level, as occurs in a mass response such as withdrawal from a painful stimulus.

Sensory information entering the spinal cord gives rise to two ascending sensory systems carrying information to the brain (Fig. 4.6). These are: (1) The spino-thalamic system which conveys information about pain and temperature (lateral spinothalamic tract) and light touch and pressure (ventral spinothalamic tract) and (2) The dorsal system, which conveys touch, pressure and proprioceptive information (dorsal column).

These sensory tracts are to be found in the white matter of the spinal cord. Another

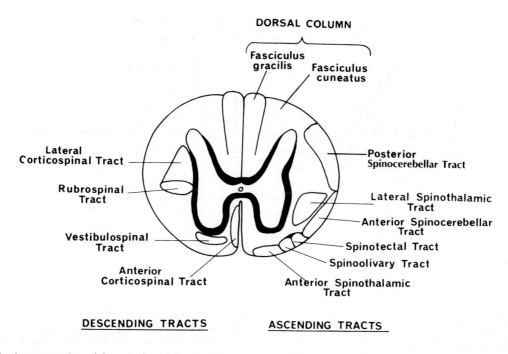

DORSAL COLUMN

Fasciculus gracilis

Fasciculus cuneatus

Lateral Corticospinal Tract

Rubrospinal Tract

Vestibulospinal Tract

Anterior Corticospinal Tract

Posterior Spinocerebellar Tract

Lateral Spinothalamic Tract

Anterior Spinocerebellar Tract

Spinotectal Tract

Spinoolivary Tract

Anterior Spinothalamic Tract

DESCENDING TRACTS   **ASCENDING TRACTS**

Fig. 4.6 A cross-section of the spinal cord showing the major ascending tracts on the right, and the major descending tracts on the left. The black area surrounding the grey matter consists of ascending and descending fibres connecting different spinal segments. The reticulo-spinal pathways are not shown because they are diffuse. *Based on material used with kind permission from Barr, M. L. (1979) The Human Nervous System – an Anatomical Viewpoint, 3rd edn. Hagerstown: Harper & Row Publishers Inc, pp. 63, 64.*

important ascending tract is the spinocerebellar tract which forms part of an elaborate feedback mechanism which controls the activity of the muscle spindles.

Information is also relayed down the spinal cord from the brain to the appropriate motor neurons via a number of descending tracts (Fig. 4.6).

The myotatic reflex system

The basic mechanism underlying posture and movement, the myotatic reflex system, is actually built into the spinal cord, although higher levels of the nervous system are still needed to refine the motor responses.

The most basic reflex involved in human movement is that which responds to a stretch stimulus. The sensory receptor involved is the muscle spindle.

Muscle spindles

Muscle spindles are small, encapsulated, fusiform, slowly adapting sensory receptors which are found lying in parallel with the skeletal – extrafusal – muscle fibres (Fig. 4.7).

Each spindle is made up of six to fourteen intrafusal muscle fibres surrounded by a connective tissue capsule. There are two types of intrafusal muscle fibre. These are:

1. Nuclear bag fibres, in which the nuclei are clustered towards the centre of the fibre, whereas the contractile portions are to be found at each end. The nuclear bag fibres extend beyond the connective tissue capsule and are attached to the endomysium of the extrafusal muscle fibres.

2. Nuclear chain fibres, in which the nuclei are spread out along the fibre. The ends of the nuclear chain fibres are attached to the capsule or to the sheaths of the nuclear bag fibres.

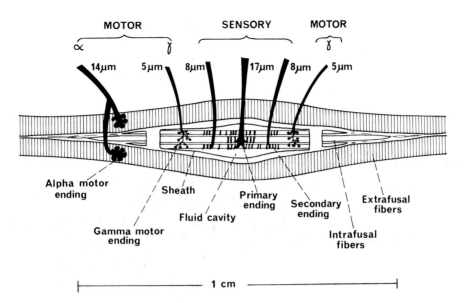

Fig. 4.7 A muscle spindle, showing its relationship to the large extrafusal skeletal muscle fibres. Note also both the motor and the sensory innervation of the muscle spindle. Those nerve fibres with large diameters are faster conducting. *Reproduced with kind permission from Guyton, A.C. (1976) Textbook of Medical Physiology, 5th edn. Philadelphia: W. B. Saunders Co, p. 680.*

The intrafusal fibres receive their own motor innervation through the small gamma motor neurons. There are two types of gamma motor neuron, tonic and phasic. Most are tonic. These neurons terminate as gamma plate endings, predominantly on the nuclear bag fibres and gamma trail endings mainly on the nuclear chain fibres. The former are mainly phasic whereas the latter are mainly tonic.

When the intrafusal muscle fibres are stimulated their ends contract, which has the effect of stretching their mid-sections. Wrapped around the mid-section are the spindle's sensory endings. These are:

1. The primary – annulospiral – endings, which are wrapped around the central regions of both the intrafusal fibre types. The afferent nerve in this case is a fast conducting fibre.

2. The secondary – flower spray – endings, which are found predominantly on the nuclear chain fibres. Their afferent nerve is a slower conductor than that of the primary endings.

Both the primary and secondary endings are sensitive to changes in muscle length.

Changes in velocity and vibration are registered by the primary endings.

Stretch may be applied to the muscle spindle by actually stretching the muscle belly in which it lies (Fig. 4.8) or by contracting the intrafusal muscle fibres themselves through the excitation of the gamma motor neurons (Fig. 4.9).

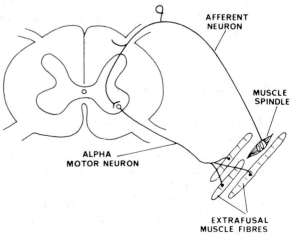

Fig. 4.8 The tendon jerk.

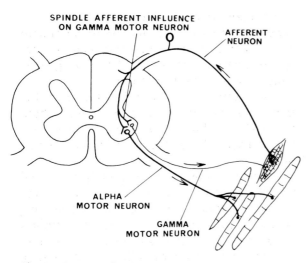

SPINDLE AFFERENT INFLUENCE
ON GAMMA MOTOR NEURON

AFFERENT
NEURON

ALPHA
MOTOR NEURON

GAMMA
MOTOR NEURON

Fig. 4.9 Gamma reflex loop.

The tendon jerk

When the muscle belly is suddenly stretched as occurs with a tendon tap, the sensory endings of the muscle spindle are also stretched. This information is relayed by the fast conducting afferent neuron to the motor neuron pool, where it synapses with an alpha motor neuron. An impulse is then relayed to the extrafusal muscle fibres of that motor unit, which in turn contract, thereby off-loading the stretch on the spindle so its activity ceases. This is the only monosynaptic reflex in the nervous system and its exact function is rather obscure (Fig. 4.8).

The gamma reflex loop

If the tendon jerk was all that occurred in response to stretch, maintaining or altering one's posture would be awkward because the spindle would be undergoing regular complete unloadings when the muscle contracts. Unlike the momentary stimulus applied in the tendon jerk, the 'stretching' effect of gravity on the muscles is always present.

The necessary modulation of the muscle spindle's activity takes place through the gamma reflex loop, in which the gamma motor neurons control and balance the sensitivity of the muscle spindle by either stepping up or stepping down the amount of contraction the intrafusal muscle fibres undergo. The gamma motor neurons are influenced by many factors acting on the motor neuron pool, particularly the afferent fibres from the muscle spindle, peripheral cutaneous stimulation through interneurons, the brainstem reticular formation and cerebellar feedback loops.

Ordinary gross background movements are initiated in the neurons of the motor cortex, which send impulses to the gamma motor neurons. The spindle contracts and impulses from its receptors go back to the cord activating the alpha neurons, which then bring about the contraction of the muscle fibres producing the desired movement. Due to the many other connections of the spindle afferents, relaxation of the antagonist muscles, changes in tone in the muscles of other limbs or even synchronised movements of the other limbs as in walking, is brought about by integration in the spinal cord. This gamma loop system is therefore most economical, saving the higher centres much otherwise complex regulation (Fig. 4.9).

Spinal integration

When afferent impulses from the muscle spindle arrive at the spinal cord, they not only influence the activity of the muscle in which the spindle is placed but also influence other muscles such as the antagonist, or even muscles on the other side of the body. This influence is mediated by interneurons and may be localised to one spinal segment or may be widespread.

Reciprocal inhibition

When an afferent neuron from an activated muscle spindle enters the spinal cord it also branches and synapses with an inhibitory interneuron. This inhibitory neuron in turn synapses with the alpha motor neuron of the antagonist muscle causing that muscle to relax thereby allowing the original prime mover to produce the movement required.

The golgi tendon organ – autogenic inhibition

Golgi tendon organs, like muscle spindles, are sensory receptors lying in muscles. They are placed along the musculo-tendinous interfaces as well as in the tendons themselves.

These sensory receptors are responsive to tension changes which may occur from contraction of the inserting muscle fibres or traction on the tendon itself. The impulses arising inhibit the activity of the muscle with which the golgi tendon organ is directly associated. This is called autogenic inhibition.

MUSCLE TONE

Muscle tone is a completely involuntary phenomenon. It comes about through signals regarding the individual's current state being relayed to the motor neurons of the anterior horn of the spinal cord.

This background signalling ensures that the various muscles of the body are always ready to spring into action when the situation demands. The ability to take up, hold and move within a posture depends on the background alteration of tone.

During life this background signalling never completely shuts down, so even in resting positions of the body, muscles will exhibit tone. Under normal conditions tone is temporarily absent in muscles when acting as antagonists to a contracting muscle. Another situation is in deep sleep.

Normal muscle tone depends on an intact gamma loop and the effects of the gamma loop on the neuronal pools in the spinal cord. In the normal human being this gamma loop system is depressed by influences from the inhibitory part of the reticular system. This inhibitory effect is lost when the spinal cord is cut in paraplegia. Now the gamma loop is released from higher control so, after the period of shock subsides, tone becomes excessive so even a small stimulus to the thigh can lead to a total response or mass reflex. In this case the gamma loop system is overactive and out of control.

Inhibition through the reticular system is varied by impulses from the vestibular system which increases tone, the cerebellar system which decreases tone and the basal ganglia which normally decreases tone.

If the cerebral cortex is isolated from the inhibitory part of the reticular system, there is usually an abnormal increase in tone. This mechanism will be discussed in more detail later.

Tone in a muscle is completely abolished when the gamma loop is destroyed. For example, this occurs if the dorsal root carrying sensory information from the muscle spindles is cut, or the anterior horn cell is destroyed as occurs in acute anterior poliomyelitis. As tone is essential for proper nutrition and blood flow, wasting is a characteristic of muscles in which tone is absent.

SUPRASPINAL CONTROL OF MOVEMENT

The basic reflexes which control muscle activity are present in the spinal cord but the movements so produced are relatively crude and lack versatility. Higher levels of the nervous system such as the reticular system, basal ganglia, cerebellum and cerebral cortex influence this activity to produce movements having greater quality and variety.

These higher influences act mainly through the gamma reflex loop, modulating the activity of the muscle spindles, thereby influencing the activity of the muscles themselves so they act in a highly co-ordinated manner. This is a beautiful and economic system. Only in very fine, precise, learned movements do these higher centres have a direct influence on the muscle fibres via the alpha motor neuron.

The reticular formation

The reticular formation, which forms the core of the brain, is made up of a complex 'net like' arrangement of a large number of small neurons. It runs from the upper end of the spinal cord, extending upwards into the thalamus, hypothalamus and their adjacent

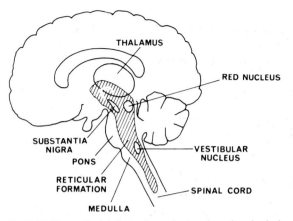

Fig. 4.10 The reticular formation, depicted as the shaded area, runs from the upper end of the spinal cord extending upwards into the thalamus, hypothalamus and their adjacent regions.

regions. These neurons are receptive to sensory input arriving from a wide variety of sources (Fig. 4.10).

The reticular formation has an important integrative function. It plays a major role in regulating sensory input to the higher centres, consciousness and learning. Within it are located areas which regulate the cardio-vascular, respiratory, endocrine and gastrointestinal systems. It has an important regulating function in movement by modulating muscle tone. Emotions influence and are influenced by the reticular formation through connections with the limbic system and hypothalamus.

Most of the reticular formation is facilitatory, although a small area in the lower part of the medulla is inhibitory. Continuous impulses are transmitted via ascending and descending pathways from the facilitatory area, although this activity can be inhibited by the basal ganglia, cerebellum and cerebral cortex.

The ascending pathways alert the individual and have an arousing function, whereas the descending pathway – the reticulospinal tract – influences the motor neuron pools, particularly the gamma motor neurons.

The facilitatory area fires spontaneously but the inhibitory area of the reticular formation cannot discharge of its own accord, so it relies on other areas of the brain such as the basal ganglia, cerebellum and cerebral cortex to drive it. Diffuse stimulation of the inhibitory area causes a decrease of muscle tone throughout the body whereas an increase of tone occurs with stimulation of the facilitatory area. Under normal circumstances these facilitatory and inhibitory impulses to the gamma motor neurons of the spinal cord are balanced so that a state of normal muscle tone exists.

When the driving action of the basal ganglia, cerebellum or cerebral cortex on the inhibitory area of the reticular formation is reduced through injury to any of these areas or their pathways, the balance between facilitatory and inhibitory influences on the motor neuron pool is tipped towards greater facilitation of gamma motor neuron activity. This leads to excessive tone – hypertonia – being present and is one of the usual causes of spasticity.

Vestibular function

The vestibular nuclei which are associated with the reticular formation, though not part of it, are influenced by information arriving from the vestibular apparatus. This information has importance in maintaining body equilibrium. The vestibular apparatus detects changes in the direction of movements of the head, particularly when the movement starts and stops. It also records the amount of forward, backward or sideways tilting of the head, as well as its movement when the whole body moves in a linear direction.

Impulses from the vestibular nuclei pass down the vestibulospinal tract and have a facilitatory effect on the tone of the antigravity muscles. There is a close interplay between the influence of the reticulospinal and vestibulospinal tracts on the motor neuron pools in the control of muscle tone.

Movements of the eyes are influenced by impulses passing upwards from the vestibular nuclei (Fig. 4.11).

Information from the vestibular apparatus eventually reaches the cerebral cortex where it is combined with information from other sensory receptors, particularly the eyes, to

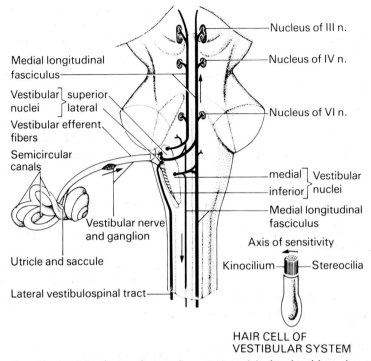

Fig. 4.11 Information from the semicircular canals regarding rotation of the head and from the utricle regarding linear motion of the head is relayed to the vestibular nucleii. Information is then relayed to the nucleii of those cranial nerves concerned with movements of the eyes – III, IV and VI. Information is also passed downwards to influence the motor neuron pools via the vestibulo-spinal tracts. *Figure from The Human Nervous System by Noback, C.R. & Demarest, R.J. copyright (c) 1967, 1975, used with the permission of McGraw-Hill Book Company.*

give the individual an awareness of his position in space.

The basal ganglia

The basal ganglia comprise the caudate nucleus, putamen, globus pallidus, subthalamic nuclei, substantia nigra, red nucleus and parts of the thalamus (Fig. 4.1). The interconnections between the various nuclei as well as the feedback circuits between the basal ganglia and the motor cortex are very complex.

In lower animals the basal ganglia are the highest functional part of the whole motor system and all voluntary movements are initiated in the region. In man, this function has been largely taken over by the motor cortex, although the basal ganglia have retained a modulating function, forming an integral part of human motor control. It seems that the basal ganglia are involved in the planning and programming of movements.

The function of the basal ganglia cannot be demonstrated experimentally, so the only evidence available in man is seen clinically in disturbances such as athetosis and parkinsonism. The oscillating tremor in parkinsonism is evidence that the damping down of the gamma loop system by the basal ganglia has been disturbed.

The cerebellum

The cerebellum – comprising the archicerebellum, paleocerebellum and neocerebellum – is concerned with co-ordinating movements. It controls the activity of the prime movers so they contract with proper timing and intensity during a movement sequence. At the same time it co-ordinates the activity of their antagonists and synergists as well as the stabilisers of the rest of the body. This beautiful interaction of the various muscles is achieved through the function of the cerebellum in setting the lengths of the intrafusal muscle fibres of the relevant muscle spindles.

Information is relayed to the:

1. Archicerebellum, from the vestibular apparatus
2. Paleocerebellum, via the spinocerebellar tracts
3. Neocerebellum, from the motor areas of the cerebral cortex.

In the normal adult under normal circumstances the archicerebellum does not play a major role in the control of movement.

The paleocerebellum forms part of a feedback circuit through which information relayed to it from the muscle proprioceptors is adjusted and fed back to the muscle spindles to control their setting.

The neocerebellum forms part of the control circuit involving the motor cortex, basal ganglia and cerebellum, which is concerned with the predictive memory function of the cerebellum. During early motor development, the cerebellum 'learns' what to anticipate if certain movements are performed. For example, a young child will tend to overshoot when he wants to touch his nose, whereas an adult automatically controls the speed and direction of his movements so they are performed delicately and can halt them if there is a danger of overshooting for any reason.

The cerebellum's function in controlling movement may be summarised as follows. When a motor command is sent from the cortex, it is passed to the neocerebellum as well as to the motor neuron pools. As the movement is executed, proprioceptive information is constantly relayed back to the paleocerebellum. The cerebellum then makes continuous comparisons between what movement was intended and the actual movement that occurred, producing adjustments when necessary. For this reason, people with injuries to the cerebellum are more likely to have difficulties when they actually move than when they remain still.

The cerebral cortex

Intentional or willed movements, in contrast to the more gross automatic movements required for the maintenance of a background posture, are initiated by the cerebral cortex. In the cortex, sensory information is collated with past experience in the various association areas. The outcome of all this activity eventually influences the firing of the motor neurons, whose cell bodies are present in the primary motor area of the pre-central gyrus, the premotor area and other areas of the parietal lobe, (Fig. 4.5). These are called the upper motor neurons, and their axons descend via the corticospinal and corticobulbar tracts to influence the lower motor neurons of the anterior horn of the spinal cord or the cranial nuclei respectively.

A map of the primary motor cortex shows that those muscles which are used for more delicate skilled actions such as those of the face, tongue and hands are relatively more widely represented than other muscle groups (Fig. 4.5).

Nerve fibres from the motor cortex of each cerebral hemisphere descend through the internal capsule, cerebral peduncle of the mid-brain and pons to the pyramids of the medulla oblongata. Here about two thirds of the fibres cross over or decussate to the other side to form the lateral corticospinal tract. The remaining fibres continue down the same side as the anterior corticospinal tract and end in the upper thoracic region. Because of the decussation, injuries to the right motor cortex will lead to deficits in motor control predominantly in the musculature of the left side of the body.

In certain forms of highly skilled activity, such as handedness or speech, one of the two cerebral hemispheres is usually dominant (Fig. 4.12). Therefore, damage to one hemisphere can lead to very specific deficits of function.

Fine movements of the hand require more

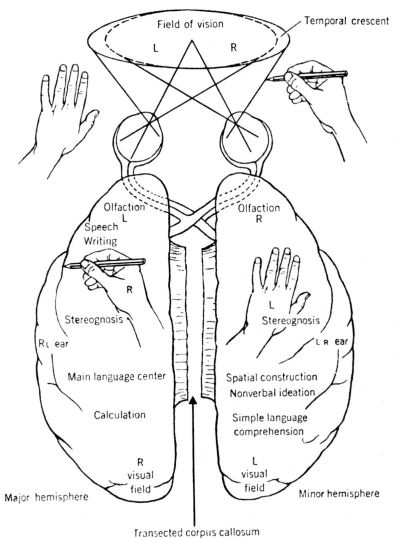

Fig. 4.12 Some of the roles of the major and minor cerebral hemispheres as established in 'twin-brain' man. General senses from one half of the visual field are projected to the contralateral hemisphere. Hearing is largely projected to the contralateral hemisphere. (*Adapted from Sperry*). *From The Human Nervous System by Noback, C.R. & Demarest, R.J. Copyright (c) 1967, 1975. Used with permission of McGraw-Hill Book Company.*

regulation from higher centres than gross automatic movements. Muscles in the forearm and hand have the advantage of being controlled directly by the cortex via both the alpha and the gamma motor neurons. The direct connection with the alpha motor neurons permits fast changes of movement, thereby allowing the many fine adjustments necessary when performing delicate manual tasks.

When a fine movement is 'willed', impulses travel from the cortex via the corticospinal tract to activate alpha and gamma motor neurons which supply the same muscle. Although the outflow of impulses along both motor neurons begins at the same time, the timing of their effects on the extrafusal muscle fibres is different. Impulses travelling via the alpha motor neurons cause the extrafusal fibres to contract before the influence of the gamma outflow comes into effect via the gamma reflex loop. This gamma outflow acts to modulate the setting of the muscle spindle and as such contributes towards controlling the movement of the fingers or hand, set in action earlier by impulses arriving via the alpha motor neuron.

Although the cortex initiates the 'idea' of the movement to be performed, it is important to remember the multitude of automatic mechanisms that are concurrently acting to control background muscle tone. This can be best illustrated by the movements involved in playing the piano. Here movements of the fingers, which are intentional, are controlled by the cortex itself but at the same time control of the local posture of the arms as well as the background posture of the rest of the body is dependent on the regulation of muscle tone, at an automatic level, involving subcortical areas.

REFERENCES AND FURTHER READING

1. Barr, M. L. (1979) *The Human Nervous System*, 3rd edn. Hagerstown: Harper and Row.
2. Basmajian, J. V. (1977) Motor Learning and Control: A Working Hypothesis. *Archives of Physical Medicine and Rehabilitation*, Vol. 58, pp. 38–41.
3. Bishop, B. (1977) Spasticity: its physiology and management. Part 1 – Neurophysiology of spasticity – classical concepts. *Physical Therapy*, Vol. 57, No. 4, pp. 371–376.
4. Bishop, B. (1977) Spasticity: its physiology and management. Part II – Neurophysiology of spasticity – current concepts. *Physical Therapy*, Vol. 57, No. 4, pp. 377–384.
5. Bishop, B. (1977) Spasticity: its physiology and management. Part III – Identifying and assessing the mechanisms underlying spasticity. *Physical Therapy*, Vol. 57, No. 4, pp. 385–395.
6. Cheney, P. D. (1985) Role of cerebral cortex in voluntary movements. *Physical Therapy*, Vol. 65, No. 5, pp. 624–635.
7. Eccles, J. C. (1977) *The Understanding of the Brain*, 2nd edn. New York: McGraw-Hill.
8. Evarts, E. V. (1979) Brain mechanisms of movement. *Scientific American*, Vol. 241, No. 3, pp. 146–156.
9. Eyzaguirre, C. & Fidone, S. J. (1975) *Physiology of the Nervous System*, 2nd edn. Chicago: Year Book Medical Publishers.
10. Ganong, L. F. (1979) *Review of Medical Physiology*, 9th edn. Los Altos: Lange Medical.
11. Geschwind, N. (1979) Specialisations of the human brain. *Scientific American*, Vol. 241, No. 3, pp. 158–168.
12. Granit, R. (1970) *The Basis of Motor Control*. London: Academic Press.
13. Granit, R. (1977) *The Purposive Brain*. Cambridge, Massachusetts: MIT Press.
14. Granit, R. & Pompeiano, O. (Eds) (1979) Reflex control of posture and movement. *Progress in Brain Research Vol. 50*. Amsterdam: Elsevier/North Holland Biomedical Press.
15. Guyton, A. C. (1981) *Textbook of Medical Physiology*, 6th edn. Philadelphia: W.B. Saunders.
16. Kots, Y. M. (1977) *The Organisation of Voluntary Movement*. New York: Plenum Press.
17. Kuffler, S. W. & Nicholls, J. G. (1976) *From Neuron to Brain*. Sunderland: Sinauer Associates.
18. Lance, J. W. & McLeod, J. G. (1981) *A Physiological Approach to Clinical Neurology*, 3rd edn. London: Butterworths.
19. Luria, A. R. (1973) *The Working Brain*. Harmondsworth: Penguin Books.
20. Matthews, P. B. S. (1977) Muscle afferents and kinaesthesia. *British Medical Bulletin*, Vol. 33, No. 2, pp. 137–142.
21. McCloskey, D. I. (1978) Kinesthetic sensibility. *Physiological Reviews*, Vol. 58, No. 4, pp. 763–820.
22. Nauta, W. J. H. & Feirtag, M. (1979) The organisation of the brain. *Scientific American*, Vol. 241, No. 3, pp. 78–105.
23. Noback, C. R. & Demarest, R. J. (1981) *The Human Nervous System*, 3rd edn. New York: McGraw-Hill.
24. Roberts, T. D. M. (1978) *Neurophysiology of Postural Mechanisms*, 2nd edn. London: Butterworths.
25. Ruch, T. & Patton, H. D. (Eds) (1979) *Physiology and Biophysics, Volume 1 – The Brain and Neural Function*, 20th edn. Philadelphia: W.B. Saunders.
26. Stein, R. B. (1974) Peripheral Control of Movement. *Physiological Reviews*, Vol. 54, No. 1, pp. 215–243.
27. Twitchell, T. E. (1965) Attitudenal reflexes. *Physical Therapy*, Vol. 45, pp. 411–418.
28. Walsh, K. W. (1978) *Neuropsychology – A Clinical Approach*. Edinburgh: Churchill Livingstone.
29. Williams, P. L. & Warwick, R. (1980) *Gray's Anatomy*, 36th edn. Edinburgh: Churchill Livingstone.
30. Wyke, B. (1972) Articular neurology – a review. *Physiotherapy*, Vol. 58, No. 3, pp. 94–99.
31. Wyke, B. (1976) Neurological mechanisms in spasticity: a brief review of some current concepts. *Physiotherapy*, Vol. 62, No. 10, pp. 316–319.

5

Basic principles of mechanics

Mechanics is the study of forces and their effects. Biomechanics is the study of the principles of mechanics as applied to living bodies. Since the human body is acted upon by a variety of forces which can lead to it moving, remaining at rest or being placed under harmful stress and strain, an understanding of the basic principles of mechanics and particularly of biomechanics is essential to the physiotherapist.

Measurement and standard units

Accurate measurement of mechanical quantities is important in the study of biomechanics. The dimensions of any mechanical quantity can be expressed in terms of the three basic units of length, mass and time.

A unit of a quantity indicates what kind of quantity it is whereas leaving a number on its own is usually insufficient. With both 1 metre or 1 kilogram the number remains the same but the unit, metre or kilogram, provides the necessary information by which to make comparisons with a relevant standard.

Any measure, to be meaningful, needs to be compared against a universally agreed standard system of units. There are two systems which are currently used: the foot-pound-second (FPS) system and the metric system. There is a trend today for more countries to adopt the metric system.

Scalar and vector quantities

There are two classes of quantity, scalar and vector. Scalar quantities are those which are completely described by a measure of their magnitude alone. Examples of scalar quantities are length, area, volume, mass and time.

There are some quantities which cannot be described by their magnitude alone. For a full description, it is necessary to know direction as well as magnitude. These are called vector quantities. An arrow placed over a letter represents a vector quantity $(\vec{F})$. Examples of vector quantities are force and displacement. These will be described in more detail later in the chapter.

MATTER, MASS, INERTIA, WEIGHT

Matter is defined as that which occupies space and may be present in solid, liquid or gaseous form. The human body is made up of matter, so when discussing the whole body or any of its segments, the unit representing the quantity of matter which is called mass can be used.

Everyday experience indicates that it is usually more difficult to change the velocity of a massive object than that of a less massive one. This reluctance of matter to change its state of motion is called inertia. Mass is a measure of this inertia. The units of mass are the:

kilogram (kg) in the metric system of units
pound (lb) in the FPS system of units.

The weight of a body is the force exerted on the body by the earth's gravitational field. This exerts a downwards force on any body mass towards the centre of the earth.

At the surface of the earth, a freely falling body in a vacuum increases its downwards speed by 9.8 metres per second in every second (metric) or 32 feet per second in every second (FPS). This is a measure of the earth's gravitational field at the surface of the earth and is seen to be constant no matter what the mass of the object. Hence the gravitational constant, g, equals:

9.8 m/s^2 (metric)
32 ft/s^2 (FPS).

The weight of a body can be expressed by the equation:

$$W = mg$$

Where W is the weight of the body
m is the the mass of the body
g is the gravitational constant.

This equation shows the relationship between mass and weight.

Centre of gravity

Whole body

It is convenient in mechanics to refer to the centre of gravity. This is the equivalent point within the body at which the whole body weight may be considered to act. It has no anatomical reality. For some positions adopted by the human body, the centre of gravity of the whole body may even be located outside its boundaries.

The centre of gravity will depend on the arrangement of the body segments. By far the greatest number of studies concerning the whole body's centre of gravity have examined the upright standing position. In this position it is generally accepted that the centre of gravity lies within the pelvis at approximately the upper sacral region, anterior to the second sacral vertebra.[10] The exact location differs between individuals.

The centre of gravity changes with every change of body position. A good example of this is during free movements. Here the body weight does not alter as the individual moves from one position to another but the centre of gravity does.

If weights are added to the body, as in the case when carrying a back-pack, the centre of gravity of the total system will need to be reconsidered. Likewise, loss of a body part through amputation alters the total body weight, so the location of the centre of gravity will be altered.

Body segments

The centre of gravity of each body segment will be found towards its heavier end (Fig. 3.1). This location is approximately 4/7ths of the distance above the segment's distal end.

Knowledge of the location of the centre of gravity of each of the various body segments is helpful to the physiotherapist in determining the leverage effect of gravity around individual joints. To help visualise gravity, a plumb line can be suspended from the centre of gravity of the body segment involved (Fig. 5.1). This plumb line represents the action line of gravity.

FORCE

A force can be simply defined as a push (compression) or a pull (tension). For a force to be produced, one object must act upon another. Motion may be caused or prevented by forces.

In the human body, forces are produced by muscle contractions. Some of the external forces acting on the body include gravity and those manual and mechanical forces used by physiotherapists when giving patients exercises. These external forces may be used either to assist or to resist a patient's own muscle contractions.

To describe a force it is necessary to know its:

1. Magnitude
2. Action line
3. Direction
4. Point of application.

Force is a vector quantity because it has both magnitude and direction. A vector is represented by an arrow. The length of the arrow shaft is proportional to the magnitude of the force; the arrow head indicates the direction of the force. Therefore vectors enable forces to be visualised.

Force systems

Any group of two or more forces is known as a force system. Two or more forces may be:

1. Coplanar – acting in the same plane
2. Concurrent – acting at the same point
3. Colinear – acting along the same action line.

For descriptive purposes when studying human movement, forces acting may be conveniently grouped together to form different types of force system. These systems are classified as follows.

1. Linear force system, when all the forces occur along the same action line (Figs. 5.5 and

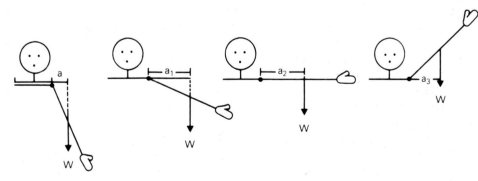

Fig. 5.1 The action line of gravity, W, does not change its direction as the arm is elevated or lowered. It does move outward or inward from the trunk but always remains vertical. *Reproduced with kind permission from LeVeau, B. (1977) Williams and Lissner: Biomechanics of Human Motion, 2nd edn. Philadelphia: W. B. Saunders. Co.*

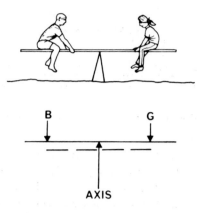

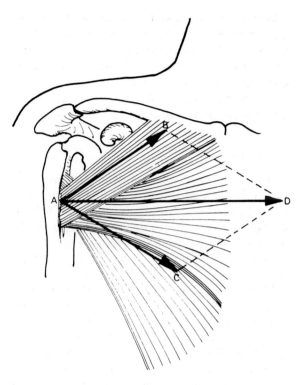

Fig. 5.2 Parallel force system.

5.6). Such forces may produce tension or compression effects.

2. Parallel force system, when all the forces are coplanar and parallel to each other but do not share the same action line. The forces in this case produce rotary effects (Fig. 5.2).

A special type of parallel force system is called a force couple. In this case the parallel forces are equal in magnitude but opposite in direction. This is illustrated in Figure 5.3 in which both forces combine to turn the steering wheel to the right.

3. Concurrent force system, when all the forces meet at the same point. There are a number of anatomical examples of this type of force system, for example, the sternal and clavicular heads of pectoralis major (Fig. 5.4).

4. General force system, when all the forces acting are in the same plane but cannot be covered by the previous categories.

Fig. 5.4 Graphical composition of the sternal and clavicular heads of the pectoralis major muscle. *Reproduced with kind permission from O'Connell, A. L. & Gardner, E. B. (1972) Understanding the Scientific Bases of Human Movement. Baltimore: The Williams and Wilkins Company.*

Composition of forces

In real life many forces may be acting on the human body simultaneously. Sometimes it is necessary to know the final effect of all these forces, or the resultant, which is the simplest force that can produce the same effect as all the forces acting together.

This process of finding the resultant is called the composition of forces. This can be expressed by using the equation:

$$R = \vec{F_1} + \vec{F_2} + \vec{F_3} \ldots + \vec{Fn}$$
$$= \Sigma \vec{F}$$

Where R means the resultant
$\vec{F}$ means a force (the arrow over the letter indicates a vector quantity)
Σ means 'the sum of'.

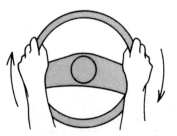

Fig. 5.3 A force couple – when turning steering wheel to the right.

When the sum of all the forces acting on the body equals zero, the force system is said to be in equilibrium. Here all the forces balance each other out and no change in place or position of the body occurs.

When the sum of all the forces does not equal zero, motion occurs.

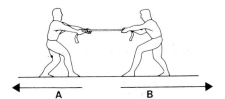

Fig. 5.6 Linear force system. Scale: ½ inch = 40 lbs wt.

Force analysis

When analysing force systems, two basic methods are used. They are the algebraic and the graphic methods. The linear force system, being the simplest to analyse, will be used to illustrate these methods, as is seen in the example of two men pulling on a rope (Fig. 5.5).

Here *A* pulls with a force of 60 lbs weight; *B* pulls with a force of 80 lbs weight. Algebraically, the resultant can be obtained by simple addition, taking into account the 'sign' – whether plus or minus – of the amounts. In this case, both the forces are directed to the right, therefore by convention these forces can be given a positive '+' sign.

To solve the present problem:

60 lbs wt + 80 lbs wt = 140 lbs wt

Therefore, the resultant force equals 140 lbs wt to the right.

Now consider the example illustrated in Figure 5.6. If *A* still pulls with a force of 60 lbs weight and *B* with a force of 80 lbs weight, the resultant is quite different. As *A* is pulling with a force of 60 lbs weight to the left, this quantity is now given a negative sign.

Therefore the resultant of this particular linear force system is:

−60 lbs wt + 80 lbs wt = 20 lbs wt

The resultant, 20 lbs wt, has a positive sign, therefore the man pulling to the right wins!

This same example can be solved graphically, using vectors. A scale is decided upon, for example ½ inch = 40 lbs wt. Vectors representing the two forces involved in the tug-o-war are drawn, the convention being to place the 'tail' of the following vector, *B*, at the tip of the arrowhead of the preceding vector, *A* (Fig. 5.7).

The resultant is found by drawing a line from the tail of the first vector to the head of the final vector. The resultant is the shaded arrow in Figure 5.7. This now gives the direction of the resultant which in this case is to the right. To find the magnitude of the resultant, this same line is also measured and reconverted using the scale ½" = 40 lbs wt. In this case, as the length of the vector is ¼", the magnitude of the resultant is 20 lbs wt.

Force analysis of concurrent force system

If two or more forces act at the same point, forming an angle with each other, some modifications have to be made to the basic algebraic approach described so far, because simple algebraic summation of the forces involved will not produce the resultant. A number of methods can be used to solve this problem.

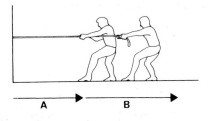

Fig. 5.5 Linear force system. Scale: ½ inch = 40 lbs wt

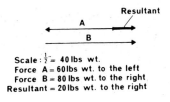

Scale: ½" = 40 lbs wt.
Force A = 60 lbs wt. to the left
Force B = 80 lbs wt. to the right
Resultant = 20 lbs wt. to the right

Fig. 5.7 Graphic solution.

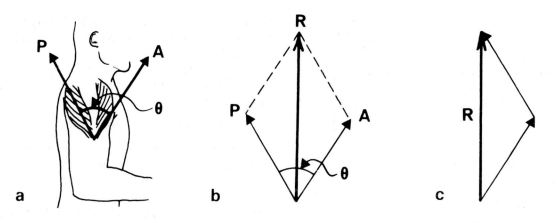

Fig. 5.8 Force analysis of the action of the anterior and posterior fibres of the deltoid muscle. (a) P and A are vectors representing the pull of the posterior and anterior fibres of the deltoid muscle, θ (theta) is the angle formed between them. R is the resultant. Scale 1‴ = 20 lb weight. (b) Parallelogram method (R = 1¾″ = 35 lbs weight). (c) Triangle method (R = 1¾″ = 35 lb weight).

1. *The parallelogram method* is used when only two forces are applied to the same point simultaneously. In Figure 5.8 the action of the anterior and posterior fibres of deltoid illustrates this situation.

After a scale is decided upon, vector A, representing the force produced by the anterior deltoid, and vector P, representing the force produced by the posterior deltoid, are drawn to scale from the same point. In this case the point represents the deltoid insertion. Both arrows are directed away from this point (Fig. 5.8b).

The other two sides of the parallelogram are now constructed. A line is then drawn from the point representing the deltoid insertion to the opposite corner of the parallelogram. This line indicates the magnitude and direction of the resultant force.

2. *The triangle method* is also used when two forces are involved (Fig. 5.8c). Here vector A is drawn to scale and in its original direction. Vector P is then drawn from the tip of vector A, also to scale and following its original direction. The resultant vector, R, is found by joining the tail of the first vector to the head of the last.

As seen in Figure 5.8 both these methods give the same solution.

Where more than two vectors are involved in a concurrent force system (Fig. 5.9a) the triangle method can be extended. Here vectors are placed end to end in the manner already described. The resultant is found by joining the tail of the first vector to the head of the last (Fig. 5.9b). This is termed the polygon method of force analysis.

3. *The trigonometric method* can be used if the value of the angle between the vectors of forces A and P is known. This method gives an algebraic solution.

Suppose the angle between the anterior and posterior fibres of deltoid is θ (theta), as shown in Figure 5.8a.

The resultant is found using the following equation:

$$R = \sqrt{P^2 + A^2 - 2PA \cos \theta}$$

Where R is the resultant
      P is the length of vector P
      A is the length of vector A

$\cos \theta$ is the relationship $\dfrac{\text{side adjacent}}{\text{hypotenuse}}$

(its value may be found by consulting the relevant mathematical table)
    $\sqrt{}$ is the square root.

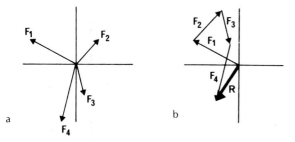

Fig. 5.9 Polygon method of force analysis.

Concurrent forces acting at 90°

A special situation occurs if the angle between two concurrent forces is 90°. The Pythagoras theorem is used to find the resultant.

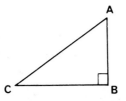

Fig. 5.10 A right-angled triangle *ABC*.

In the right-angled triangle *ABC* (Fig. 5.10) $(AC)^2 = (AB)^2 + (BC)^2$. AC is the hypotenuse and the square of the hypotenuse is equal to the sum of the squares on the other two sides.

Now suppose two forces *P* and *Q* act at right angles to each other (Fig. 5.11).

The resultant is calculated by one of the following methods.

1. Completing the parallelogram *abcd* and drawing in the resultant *R* (Fig. 5.11b). Now

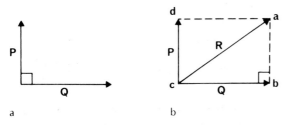

Fig. 5.11 Two forces *P* and *Q* acting at a right angle to each other.

the length *ab* is equal to length *P*, length *bc* is equal to length *Q*, and length *ac* is equal to length *R*.

2. Using Pythagoras theorem, because the triangle *abc* in Figure 5.11b is a right-angled triangle. Here:

$$(ac)^2 = (ab)^2 + (bc)^2$$

R can now be substituted for *ac*; *P* for *ab* and *Q* for *bc* to give the equation:

$$R^2 = P^2 + Q^2$$

The resultant can now be calculated by finding the square root of the value $(P^2 + Q^2)$:

$$R = \sqrt{P^2 + Q^2}$$

Resolution of forces

Sometimes it is useful to replace a single force by two or more equivalent force components. This process is called resolution of forces and enables a wider appreciation of the effects of any one force.

One useful application of this type of force analysis is in determining the effectiveness of a particular muscle force in moving a bony lever or body segment. This will vary depending on the angle of pull of the muscle, which is defined as the angle between the line of pull of the muscle (action line) and the mechanical axis of the bone or segment involved.

The mechanical axis of a bone or segment is defined as a straight line connecting the midpoints of the joints at both ends of the bone or segment, *X–X* in Figure 5.12. The angle of pull of biceps brachii is labelled θ in Figure 5.12.

Figure 5.12, illustrates different positions of the forearm as the elbow joint is moved through its range of joint motion. The angle of pull, θ, changes as the elbow is increasingly flexed. In this example, the magnitude of the force produced by the muscle remains the same.

The force produced by biceps brachii, *AB*, can be resolved by finding its rectangular components, *AC* and *AD* (Fig. 5.12). It is important to note that each of the component forces is less in magnitude than the original force, *AB*.

The component *AC*, is called the rotary component. It causes the forearm to rotate around the axis of the elbow joint.

The component *AD*, is called the non-rotary, secondary component. It may have either a stabilising (compressive) effect when the angle of pull is less than 90° (Figs. 5.12a and b) or it may have a distracting (traction) effect at angles of pull greater than 90° (Figs. 5.12d and e).

When joint movement takes place, the magnitude of the two force components *AC* and *AD* changes, as the angle of pull changes.

1. As the angle of pull approaches 90°, the rotary component *AC* increases in magnitude.

2. When the muscle force *AB*, is applied to the bony lever at a right angle, the effect of this force is entirely rotary (Fig.5.12c). This is the position of greatest mechanical efficiency for producing rotary motion.

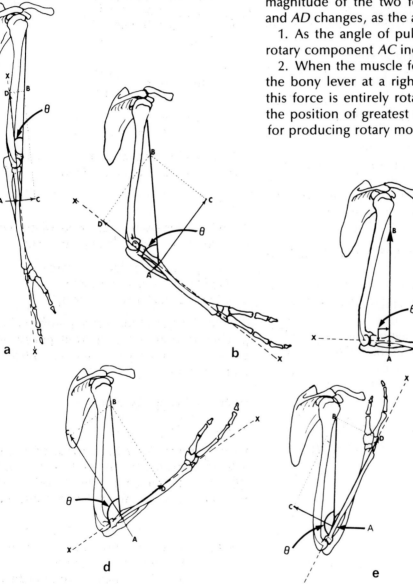

Fig. 5.12 Resolution of total muscle force of biceps brachii into rotary and secondary components. *AB*, total muscle force of biceps brachii. *X–X*, long axis of the forearm; *AC*, rotary component; *AD*, secondary component. Note the change in direction of the secondary component when the angle of pull θ, increases beyond 90° as in d and e. *Used with kind permission from O'Connell, A. L. & Gardner, E. B. (1972) Understanding the Scientific Bases of Human Movement. Baltimore: The Williams and Wilkins Company.*

3. At small angles of pull, the mechanical efficiency of the muscle is low because of its large stabilising component *AD* (Fig. 5.12a).

The effects of gravity or any other external resistance applied to a body segment, also can be determined by resolution of forces. The angle at which the force is applied is called the angle of resistance. The most effective angle of resistance is when the resisting force is applied at 90° to the body segment being rotated.

Trigonometry can be used to solve problems related to resolution of forces. For example, in Figure 5.13, the components of the muscle force *AB* can be determined if the magnitude of the muscle force and its direction given by the angle of pull of the muscle, θ, are known or can be estimated.

When the force components have been resolved as shown in Figure 5.13a, the force situation can then be presented by the geometrical representation as in Figure 5.13b. Here:

ADB represents the right-angled triangle of force.

ADBC represents a four sided figure (parallelogram) formed by completing the lines *BC* and *AC*.

Now, for the resolution of forces, *ADBC* is rectangular and all four angles are 90°.

Using the relationships:

$$\text{Sin} = \frac{\text{side opposite}}{\text{hypotenuse}}$$

$$\text{Cos} = \frac{\text{side adjacent}}{\text{hypotenuse}}$$

the required force components *AC* and *AD* can be inferred from the geometric representation (Fig. 5.13b).

$$\text{Thus sin } \theta = \frac{AC}{AB}$$

$$\text{Thus cos } \theta = \frac{AD}{AB}$$

$$\text{Hence } AC = AB \sin \theta$$
$$AD = AB \cos \theta$$

In this way, the magnitude of each force component may be determined.

Pulleys

A pulley consists of a grooved wheel with a rope running over it. Pulleys are used to:

1. Change the direction of a force
2. Modify the effect of a force
3. Obtain a mechanical advantage.

In the body, the tendon of peroneus longus is a good example of a fixed pulley which changes the direction of muscle pull but not its magnitude.

WORK, POWER, ENERGY

Work

When a force, for example that arising from a muscle contraction, is used to move a load through a distance, mechanical work is said to be done. This is expressed by the equation:

$$W = Fd$$

Where *W* is the symbol for work
F is the force acting
d is the distance through which the load is moved.

Work is done by muscles when they actively shorten to move an external load. This is termed positive work.

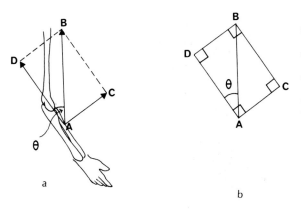

Fig. 5.13 Resolution of forces. Where *AD* is the stabilising component; *AC* is the rotating component. (*AC* and *AD* act at right angles to each other). θ is the angle of pull; *AB* is the muscle force.

However, when muscles are actively lengthening, work is being done on them by an external force, for example, gravity, to produce movement. This is called negative work in relation to the muscles.

If movement does not occur at all when a muscle contracts, as would be the case with an isometric contraction, no mechanical work is done. This is not to say that there is no energy expenditure and that the muscle does not fatigue but this is not work in the strict mechanical sense.

Power

Power is the rate of doing work. The work capacity of any muscle is related to the amount of force, or tension, it can generate, as well as the distance through which it can actively shorten. Muscle power, then, is the rate at which work can be done by a muscle or muscle group. It should not be confused with muscle strength, which refers to the amount of force the muscle can actively produce.

$$\text{Power} = \frac{\text{Work}}{\text{Time}} = \frac{Fd}{t}$$

Where F is the force acting
d is the distance through which the load is moved
t is the time taken.

$$\text{Muscle power} = \frac{\text{Work done by the muscle}}{\text{Time}}$$

Energy

Any object which has the capacity to do work possesses energy. Energy cannot be created or destroyed but it can be converted from one form to another. Chemical energy used to produce a muscle contraction is transformed into mechanical and heat energy – no energy is lost.

Mechanical energy may take the forms of potential energy or kinetic energy.

1. Potential energy refers to a body's capacity to do work as it possesses stored up energy because of its position or deformation. For example, the greater the distance an object is raised above the floor, the more potential energy it possesses by virtue of its position relative to the floor. A man standing on a box placed on the floor has more potential energy than when he is just standing on the floor.

2. Kinetic energy is the energy of a body due to its motion. Only moving bodies possess kinetic energy. The amount of energy possessed by a body depends on its velocity. Therefore if more muscles are made to contract during a movement so that the velocity of the movement is increased, the body part concerned will possess an increased capacity to do work – it has increased kinetic energy.

There are many examples in human movement where energy is transformed from potential energy to kinetic energy and vice versa. In standing on the ground, an individual possesses greater potential energy than when he lies upon it, because in the former case, his centre of gravity is higher. If a person who is standing suddenly falls, the potential energy he possessed when in the upright position, is now converted to kinetic energy as he moves towards the floor. When he reaches the floor all the potential energy has been converted to other energy forms.

BALANCE AND EQUILIBRIUM

Mechanical principles underlying the behaviour of rigid objects can be applied to the study of the human body's state of balance in any position it may adopt. For each position it is necessary to know:

1. The centre of gravity of the body.
2. The line of gravity (gravity's action line which is visualised as a vertical line projecting downwards from the centre of gravity).
3. The base of support, which refers to the supporting area beneath the body. It includes the points of contact with the supporting surface and the area between them.

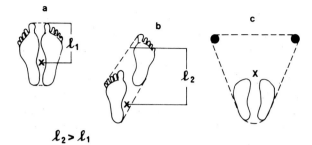

$$\ell_2 > \ell_1$$

Fig.5.14 Base of support. *X* is the point of intersection of the line of gravity of the body with the base. ---- marks the boundaries of the base.

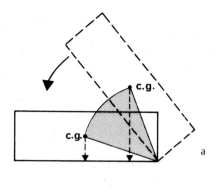

These 'points' may be body parts such as the feet shown in Figures 5.14a and b, buttocks or hands, etc., or they may be extensions of body parts such as crutches or other walking aids (Fig. 5.14c).

Equilibrium

A body is said to be in equilibrium when the resultant of all the forces acting upon it is zero. When a rigid body in static equilibrium is acted upon by a suitable force, its state of balance will be indicated by its subsequent behaviour and may be described as one of the following:

1. Stable
2. Unstable
3. Neutral.

Stable equilibrium

If after a force is applied to a body at rest, the body tends to return to its original starting position, equilibrium is said to be stable. In this case, the centre of gravity has to be raised before the line of gravity will fall outside the original base of support. The more the centre of gravity has to be raised, the more stable the body. So the most stable position for a body is when its centre of gravity is the lowest it can be, for example, in the lying position, where the body's potential energy is minimal. Figure 5.15a shows the conditions necessary for stable equilibrium.

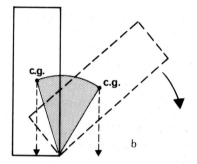

Fig. 5.15 Conditions necessary for a. stable and b. unstable equilibrium. Notice that although the block has moved through the same arc (shaded) in both cases, the consequences, as represented by the heavy arrow, are different.

Unstable equilibrium

When displaced by a force a body is said to be in unstable equilibrium if it then tends to increase its displacement. The centre of gravity drops to a lower point when compared to the original starting position, as the line of gravity falls outside the original supporting base (Fig. 5.15b).

Neutral equilibrium

A body is in neutral equilibrium if it comes to rest in a new position without a change in the level of the centre of gravity, either upwards or downwards, when it is displaced. A ball bearing rolling on a hard level surface would closely fulfil these conditions.

Stability

The stability of a rigid body depends on the:

1. Area of the base of support
2. Height of its centre of gravity above the base
3. Relationship of the line of gravity to the base of support
4. Weight of the body.

The state of balance of the human body is improved if it is made more stable. It becomes more stable when the:

1. Centre of gravity of the total weight supported over the base is lowered. The total weight will include any additional weights being carried.
2. Total weight of the body and any weights being carried is increased.
3. Line of gravity is projected to the centre of the base of support.
4. Area of the base of support is enlarged.
5. Shape of the base of support is broadened in the direction of the force being applied to the body. When a force is applied from behind, the shape of the base, as in Figure 5.14b, will allow for greater stability than the shape of the base, as in Figure 5.14a.

LEVERAGE

The human body can be considered as being a complex system of levers. By definition, a lever is a rigid bar, or mass, which rotates around a fixed point called the axis or fulcrum. Rotation is produced by force applied to the lever.

The force may be one that overcomes a resistance. This is called the effort and the part of the lever between the point where this force is applied and the fulcrum is called the effort arm. The resisting force called the resistance or load, tends to rotate the lever in the opposite direction to that produced by the effort. The part of the lever between the fulcrum and the point of application of the resisting force is called the resistance arm (Fig. 5.16).

The efficiency of a lever depends on where

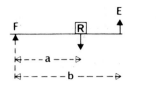

F – Fulcrum
R – Resistance
E – Effort
a – Resistance arm
b – Effort arm

Fig. 5.16

the forces are located in relation to the fulcrum. It is determined by calculating the mechanical advantage (MA), which is done by dividing the length of the effort arm by the length of the resistance arm. When the MA is greater than one, effort arm > resistance arm, the lever is said to be built for force; whereas when the MA is less than one, resistance arm > effort arm, it is built for speed. Most of the levers in the body have a MA <1.

Human equivalents

1. The 'rigid' bar – a body segment, of no particular shape.
2. The fulcrum – the joint axis about which the body segment rotates.
3. The effort force – that produced by the contracting muscles.
4. The resistance force or external load – that produced by gravity acting through the centre of gravity of the segment being moved – the weight of the segment – plus any weights attached to the segment.

The effort arm and resistance arm will be dealt with in more detail in the section discussing torque.

Classification of levers

Three orders of lever are possible depending on the way in which the effort, resistance and fulcrum are arranged spatially.

First order levers, where the fulcrum is placed between the effort and the resistance (Fig. 5.17). This type of lever may be used for force if the fulcrum is closer to the resistance (Fig. 5.17a); or it may be used to gain speed if the fulcrum is closer to the effort (Fig. 5.17b).

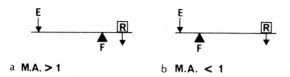

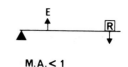

a **M.A. > 1**   b **M.A. < 1**

Fig. 5.17 First order levers.

M.A. < 1

Fig. 5.19 Third order lever.

Anatomical examples of first order levers include:

1. The action of the muscles of the neck against the weight of the head in the upright position, with the atlanto-occipital joint acting as the fulcrum.
2. The action of the triceps muscle in extending the forearm. Here the effort is applied at the olecranon process, the resistance at the centre of gravity of the forearm if no extra weight is being held and the fulcrum is at the axis of the elbow joint.

Second order levers, where the resistance always lies between the fulcrum and the effort (Fig. 5.18). It is used for force.

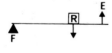

M.A. > 1

Fig. 5.18 Second order lever.

Anatomical examples of second order levers remain a very controversial subject. Some writers have suggested that rising on to the ball of the foot in a weight bearing position constitutes a second order lever. Here the big toe is said to act as the fulcrum, the effort is applied by way of the muscles inserted into the heel and the resistance is the body weight acting through the ankle. Arguments have been presented to refute this interpretation.

Third order levers, where the effort is always placed between the fulcrum and the resistance (Fig. 5.19). It is used for achieving speed at the expense of force. Most levers in the human body are of this type.

The action of the biceps brachii muscle in flexing the elbow is an anatomical example of a third order lever.

Torque or moment of force

When dealing with levers, the amount of rotation or turning about the fulcrum that a particular force can produce, is a major concern. This turning effect, or the tendency of a force to cause turning, is called torque or moment of force. Figure 5.20 represents a parallel force system in which force *B* produces movement in an anticlockwise direction, whereas force *W* produces movement in a clockwise direction.

A *moment of force* about any point is equal to the magnitude of the force multiplied by

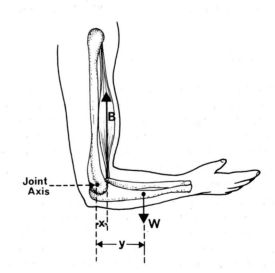

Fig. 5.20 A parallel force system acting on the forearm. Where *W*, is the weight of the forearm acting downwards; *B* is the upward force of biceps contraction; *x*, is the perpendicular distance from the action line of *B* to the axis; *y*, is the perpendicular distance from the action line of *W* to the axis.

the perpendicular distance from the action line of the force to that point.

$$M = Fd$$

Where M is the moment of force
F is the force
d is the perpendicular distance from the action line to the point.

Therefore in Figure 5.20:

The moment of force $B = Bx$
The moment of force $W = Wy$

When considering human movement, the forces acting on the body segments often act at an angle other than 90°. The moment arms of the effort and resistance forces could be described using the definition of moments as in Figure 5.21. Here the moment arm of the effort is the perpendicular distance x from the joint axis of the elbow to the line of action of the muscle force B; and the moment arm of the resistance is the perpendicular distance y from the fulcrum to the action line of gravity W.

This is one way of applying moments to body leverage.

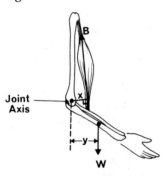

Fig. 5.21 A parallel force system acting on the forearm when the angle of pull of biceps brachii is less than 90°. *Bx* is moment of force produced by muscle contraction. *Wy* is moment of force produced by forearm weight. For equilibrium: *Bx = Wy. Bx* = moment of force B; *Wy* = moment of force W.

Another approach can be used to describe the levers of the body. In the earlier discussion on resolution of forces, mention was made that not all that force was given to producing rotation of the segment, except in cases where a force, for example that

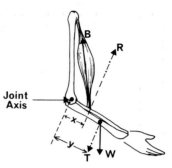

Fig. 5.22 A parallel force system acting on the forearm when the angle of pull of biceps brachii is less than 90°. Where R = Rotary component of biceps muscle contraction; T = Rotary component of weight of forearm; Rx, is the moment of force of the rotary component of biceps muscle contraction; Ty, is the moment of force of the rotary component of the weight of the forearm.

produced by a muscle contraction or gravity, is applied at 90° to the segment being moved. Another way of defining torque is that it is the product of the force component perpendicular to the lever arm (rotary component) and the distance from the line of this force component to the fulcrum (Fig. 5.22). It is important to remember that the rotary component in this case is less in magnitude than the total force being produced by the muscle contraction.

Torque curves

The magnitude of the rotary component of a muscle contraction can be found for a series of joint angles by using a number of methods. When these readings are plotted on a graph, a curve is obtained showing the change in magnitude of the rotary component with each change in joint angle. These are called torque curves.

Torque curves have been reported in the literature for a number of muscle groups. Earlier studies obtained their readings by plotting maximal isometric contractions obtained at different joint angles against the angle at which the reading was obtained.[25] With the increasing use of isokinetic dynamometers, torque curves can now be obtained for muscles contracting at different velocities

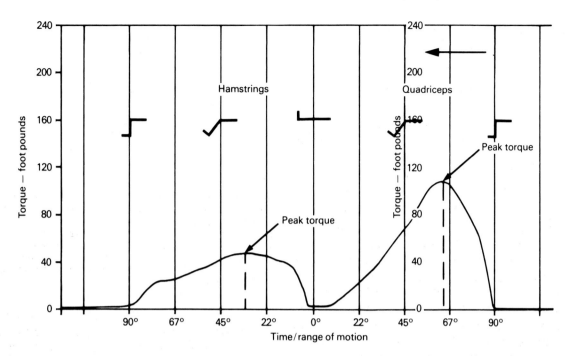

Fig. 5.23 Torque curves of quadriceps and hamstring muscle groups of normal subject performed at a constant velocity of 22.5 degrees per second. *Reprinted from Physical Therapy, vol 49, No. 7. p. 740, (1969) with the kind permission of the American Physical Therapy Association.*

(Fig. 5.23). The findings of such studies are useful to the practising physiotherapist in providing acceptable, objective and scientific data.

Equilibrium in a parallel force system

In a parallel force system, by convention all clockwise moments are labelled positive '+', and all anti-clockwise moments are labelled negative '−'.

For equilibrium, the sum of all the positive moments must equal the sum of all the negative moments. Relating this to the situation in Figure 5.20:

If $Wy = Bx$, the system is in equilibrium
$Wy > Bx$, there will be motion in the
clockwise direction
$Wy < Bx$, there will be motion in the
anti-clockwise direction.

With all classes of lever, equilibrium is achieved if the following equation is satisfied:

effort × effort arm
= resistance × resistance arm   (1)
or written another way
effort × effort moment arm
= resistance × resistance moment arm   (2)

When gravity is the only force acting on the body mass, which occurs in the classical free exercise situation, it is obvious that only three elements of this equation can readily be altered.

1. The effort – for the magnitude of the force of the muscle contraction may be changed at will.
2. The effort arm – for the moment arm of the muscle pull changes as the joint position alters.
3. The resistance arm – for the centre of gravity of the part being moved can be altered in relation to the fulcrum by changing the position of the segments in space.

However, the resistance or weight of the body segments involved cannot be significantly altered in this case.

Additional forces may be added to the classical free exercise situation to resist ($\vec{R}$) or assist ($\vec{A}$) the muscle contraction or effort force (Fig. 5.24a, b).

The effectiveness of these forces will depend on:

1. The distance of their point of application from the fulcrum.
2. The angle at which they are applied – angle of resistance. (This was discussed in the earlier section on Resolution of Forces.)

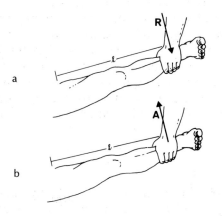

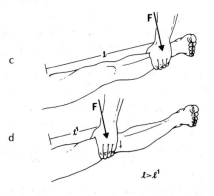

Fig. 5.24 a. Manual resistance and b. manual assistance applied to the right hip adductors. The effects of a constant force F will vary depending on the distance it is applied from the hip joint. Therefore exercise c. is much harder than d. for the hip adductors. *Figures a. and b. are after and Figures c. and d. are reproduced from Le Veau, B. (1977) Williams and Lissner: Biomechanics of Human Motion, 2nd edn. Philadelphia: W. B. Saunders Company.*

The longer the moment arm of these applied forces the greater will be their effectiveness. This principle can be used by physiotherapists to conserve their own efforts, (Fig. 5.24c).

MOTION

Motion is a process involving continuous change in place or position of a body with respect to some agreed frame of reference.

Dynamics, the study of motion, is subdivided into two areas:

1. Kinematics – which is concerned with the description of motion in precise mathematical terms
2. Kinetics – which is concerned with the forces affecting motion of a body so that it behaves in the particular way it does.

Classification of motion

Although there is considerable variety in the way human beings move, all motion can be described as being translatory, rotary or a combination of the two.

1. Translatory or linear motion occurs where the motion of any given point in or on the body is along a straight line. Further, the motion of all points in the body describe parallel straight lines. An example of translatory motion occurs when an ice skater maintains the same body position as he slides across an ice surface.

2. Rotary or angular motion occurs when all points of a rigid body describe independent circular paths about a common fixed axis. In a pure rotation, all parts of the body describe the same angular movements within the same time.

Most joint movements are rotary in nature.

3. Combined translatory and rotary motion. Many everyday movements involve a combination of translatory and rotary motion. For example, in walking, the body as a whole may be said to undergo translatory motion, as a direct result of the rotary motion occurring around the joints of the lower limbs (Fig. 5.25).

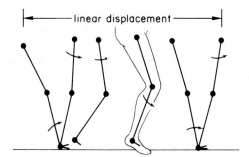

linear displacement

Fig. 5.25 Rotation of the limbs to obtain translation of the body. *Reproduced with kind permission from LeVeau, B. (1977) Williams and Lissner: Biomechanics of Human Motion, 2nd edn. Philadelphia: W. B. Saunders Company.*

Description of motion

Both linear and angular motion can be described in terms of displacement, velocity and acceleration.

Linear kinematics

Displacement is the distance a body is moved from its starting point. It is a vector quantity, which indicates both the direction and distance a body has moved. This is different from distance, for distance only conveys the amount travelled.

In Figure 5.26, an ant crawling on a table covers a path between S and F, as shown by the dotted line, in five minutes. This is the distance he travels. In the time interval of five minutes he has moved from S to F. The straight line SF is the ant's displacement during the five minutes' time interval. Conventionally, displacement is drawn as an arrow because it is a vector quantity.

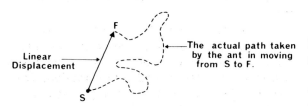

Linear Displacement

F

The actual path taken by the ant in moving from S to F.

S

Fig.5.26 Linear displacement of an ant crawling on a table top. *S* is the starting position. *F* is the finishing position.

When motion is described reference needs to be made to time. Therefore some form of time-keeping clock is necessary.

Certain quantities need to be defined quite specifically. These are velocity and acceleration.

Velocity is the amount of displacement which takes place over a specific or given time interval. It is measured quantitatively in such units as:

feet per second — ft/s
metres per second — m/s
miles per hour — mph

Suppose an athlete walks a short distance event on a straight track (Fig. 5.27).

x_1 and x_2 are his positions at the beginning, t_1, and at the end, t_2, respectively, of the time interval (t_2-t_1) he takes to complete the race.

The ratio of the displacement in an interval of time, to the length of the interval, is defined as the average velocity. The average velocity of the athlete can be written as:

$$\bar{v} = \frac{x_2 - x_1}{t_2 - t_1}$$

Where $\bar{v}$ is the average velocity (the bar placed over the v is the convention for writing an average value)
$x_2 - x_1$ is the displacement occurring in the time interval $t_2 - t_1$
$t_2 - t_1$ is the interval of time over which the race is completed.

Speed is often used interchangeably with velocity. However, speed is a scalar quantity, it indicates amount but not direction. Speed is calculated by using the equation:

$$\text{Speed} = \frac{\text{Distance covered in an interval of time}}{\text{Time interval}}$$

It is expressed in units similar to velocity: ft/s, m/s.

Acceleration is the rate of change of velocity. As a body moves from one location to another, its velocity may not remain constant. The changing velocity – in ft/s or m/s – is divided by time to give the unit of accel-

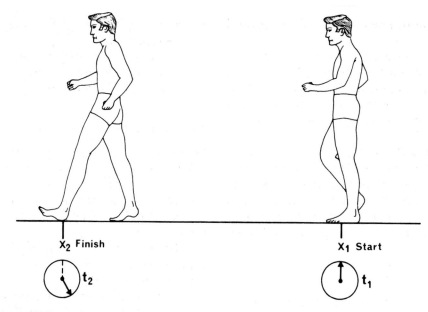

Fig. 5.27 Athlete walking a race.

eration. The unit of acceleration then may be expressed as:

feet per second per second – ft/s/s (ft/s²)
or
metres per second per second – m/s/s (m/s²)

In the previous example of the athlete in the walking race, suppose his velocity at the position x_1 at the beginning of the race, t_1, is, v_1; and his velocity at the point x_2 at the end of the race, t_2, is v_2. His average acceleration, $\bar{a}$, can be defined as the change in velocity during the time interval, divided by that interval. This may be written in the form:

$$\bar{a} = \frac{v_2 - v_1}{t_2 - t_1}$$

Where $\bar{a}$ is the average acceleration
$v_2 - v_1$ is the change in velocity
$t_2 - t_1$ is the time interval.

Rotary or angular kinematics

The kinematics of rotary motion are important for the physiotherapist, because so much human movement involves rotation of body segments around joint axes. Describing rotary motion requires the use of units related to a circle, such as degrees, radians or revolutions.

Angular displacement refers to an angular change in position during movement of a body about its axis of rotation. The angular displacement of a body is specified by an angle in relation to a reference line. In Figure 5.28 the reference line is dotted and the magnitude of change in position is found by subtracting the angle made with this reference line and the first position, θ_1, from the angle

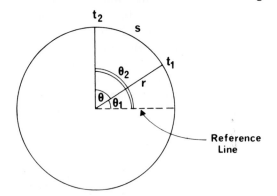

Fig. 5.28 Angular displacement. The angle measured in radians is represented as $= \frac{s}{r}$, where s is the length of the arc and r is the radius of the circle. (A radian is the relationship of an arc sub-tending a particular angle to the radius).

made with the reference line and the second position, θ_2.

It may be necessary to consider motion occurring between the positions θ_1 and θ_2. If θ_1 is the position at the beginning, t_1, and θ_2, is the position at the end, t_2, concepts of angular velocity and angular acceleration will need to be considered.

Angular velocity is the rate of change of angular displacement which takes place over a particular time interval. It is expressed as degrees per second, radians per second and revolutions per second. The average angular velocity is found by using the following equation:

$$\bar{\omega} = \frac{\theta_2 - \theta_1}{t_2 - t_1}$$

Where $\bar{\omega}$ (omega) is the average angular velocity
$\theta_2 - \theta_1$ is the angular displacement occurring during the time interval $t_2 - t_1$
$t_2 - t_1$ is the time interval during which the motion took place.

Angular acceleration is the rate of change of angular velocity. It is expressed in units of radians per second per second, and so on.

The average angular acceleration is found by using the following equation:

$$\bar{\alpha} = \frac{\omega_2 - \omega_1}{t_2 - t_1}$$

Where $\bar{\alpha}$ (alpha) is the average angular acceleration
$\omega_2 - \omega_1$ is the change in angular velocity during the time interval $t_2 - t_1$
$t_2 - t_1$ is the time interval.

Practical applications

By measuring angular displacements of the various body segments at set time intervals using high speed photography, angular velocities and angular accelerations can then be calculated at different points during the movement sequence.

In Figure 5.29, the time intervals between each dotted line is 0.02 s. Even from a quick visual inspection, it is possible to recognise that there are differences in angular velocities and accelerations in both examples, as well as within each example particularly (a) the unloaded forearm.

Such methods of recording are useful in the analysis of gait.

Force and motion

Many forces act on the human body. These may be classified as being:

1. Internal – muscle contraction
2. External – gravity, friction, air and water resistance, exercise weights, etc.

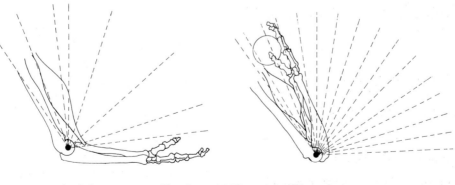

a. unloaded   Time interval 0.02   b. 10 lb. load

Fig. 5.29 Tracings of forearm during elbow flexion from stroboscopic photographs. a. Unloaded. b. With a 10 lb load. *Reproduced with kind permission from LeVeau, B. (1977) Williams and Lissner: Biomechanics of Human Motion, 2nd edn. Philadelphia: W.B. Saunders Company.*

These forces may cause or prevent motion, the final outcome being governed by those laws that relate force to motion, first discovered by Sir Isaac Newton.

Law of inertia

Newton's first law states that a body remains at rest or continues in a state of uniform motion unless acted upon by an unbalanced set of forces.

If $\Sigma \overrightarrow{F} = O$, the forces are balanced, so the body remains in equilibrum

If $\Sigma \overrightarrow{F} \neq O$, the forces are unbalanced, so change occurs.

Mention has already been made that inertia is the reluctance of a body to change what it is doing, which may be to remain at rest or continue to move in exactly the same way. A body with a larger mass when compared to another has a greater inertia. Mass is a direct measure of a body's inertia in respect to linear motion.

However, when considering rotary motion, it is necessary to take into account how the mass is distributed in relation to the axis around which the body moves. This gives the moment of inertia of the body.

Moment of inertia may be expressed by the equation:

$$I = m_1 r_1^2 + m_2 r_2^2 + m_3 r_3^2 + \ldots m_n r_n^2 \quad (1)$$
$$I = \Sigma \, mr^2 \quad (2)$$

The derivation of this equation is illustrated in Figure 5.30.

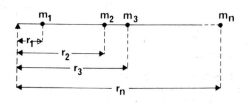

Fig.5.30 Method of determining the moment of inertia of a body. Theoretically every mass particle is accounted for in the equation $I = mr^2$. Where I = Moment of inertia; m = Mass particle; r = The perpendicular distance of the mass particle, m, from the axis.

Muscle bulk is usually concentrated towards the proximal end of many body segments so most of it is closer to the axis of joint rotation. This anatomical distribution of body mass helps reduce the moment of inertia of that segment.

By changing body positions, the mass distribution around any axis can be altered, consequently its moment of inertia is also changed. This forms the basis of selecting suitable starting positions for exercises which make initiation of movement – over-coming inertia – easier or more difficult.

Momentum

Once motion is initiated, a body which already has mass now has velocity as well. The product of these two factors is known as momentum.

$$\text{Momentum} = mv$$

Where m is the mass
v is the velocity.

Momentum can be thought of as the quantity of motion a body possesses. If two bodies are travelling with the same velocity, the one with the greater mass will have the greater momentum. Likewise, if two bodies have the same mass and one is travelling at a greater velocity than the other, the former has greater momentum.

Law of acceleration

Newton's second law deals with factors affecting acceleration of a body. It relates force, mass and acceleration (rate of change of velocity).

The acceleration of a body is proportional to the unbalanced force acting upon it, inversely proportional to the mass of the body and takes place in the direction of the acting force. A large push on a small object accelerates it rapidly. A small push on a large object will accelerate it slowly.

$$\text{Acceleration} \propto \frac{\text{Force}}{\text{Mass}}$$

or

$$a \propto \frac{F}{m} \tag{1}$$

This equation can also be written thus:

$$\text{Force} = \text{Mass} \times \text{acceleration}$$
or
$$F = ma \tag{2}$$

In the previous section the equation for acceleration was:

$$\text{Acceleration} = \frac{\text{Change in velocity}}{\text{Time interval}}$$

$$a = \frac{v_2 - v_1}{t_2 - t_1} = \frac{v_2 - v_1}{t} \tag{3}$$

Where t refers to the single quantity of time obtained when t_1 is subtracted from t_2.

This equation can be substituted for acceleration in the equation $F = ma$ to give:

$$F = m\,\frac{v_2 - v_1}{t} \tag{4}$$

$$= \frac{mv_2 - mv_1}{t} \tag{5}$$

$$\text{or } Ft = mv_2 - mv_1 \tag{6}$$

The equation: $Ft = mv_2 - mv_1$, is called the 'impulse-momentum equation'.
Note: The analysis in this section refers to linear motion.

Impulse

If a force is applied to a body over a period of time, the product of the force and time is called the 'impulsive force' or 'impulse'.

$$\text{Impulse} = Ft$$

Where F is the applied force
t is the time interval.

With reference to the impulse-momentum equation ($Ft = mv_2 - mv_1$), $mv_2 - mv_1$ is

termed the change in momentum or change in the amount of motion which occurs.

The impulse-momentum equation can be used to help describe in more detail what happens when a force is applied to a body over a given amount of time (impulse) and how this changes the amount of motion (momentum) a body will have. For example, a person usually wants to decrease the force involved in changing the momentum of the body when landing after jumping from a height, so that injury is prevented. This is done by increasing the time factor over which the change in momentum ($mv_2 - mv_1$) acts, when the individual continues the motion by 'giving at the knees'. In this way the possible damaging effects of the force produced by the body weight are reduced, for in this case there is not an abrupt change in momentum. Rather, it takes place over a longer time period than if the landing occurred with the knees held stiffly.

Law of reaction

Newton's third law states that for every action there is an equal and opposite reaction. When a force is applied to an object, the object will push back with an equal amount of force. The magnitude of the reaction force will be the same but it will act in the opposite direction (Fig. 5.31). These two forces are called an action-reaction pair.

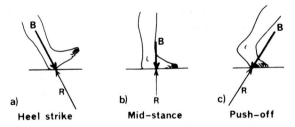

Fig. 5.31 Ground reaction force, R, during stance phase of gait at, (a) heel strike, (b) mid-stance and (c) push off. B is the force exerted by the foot.

Ground reaction

In standing and walking, the supporting

surface pushes up against the feet with the same amount of force and along the same action line as the downward thrust of the feet. This is called the ground reaction (Fig. 5.31).

During the walking cycle, ground reaction alters. It is greater at heel strike than in mid-stance because of body momentum (Fig. 5.31a). It is also greater at push-off than at mid-stance due to the contraction of the plantar flexors. When these muscles contract, they produce a backward force on the ground, which in its turn pushes the body forward (Fig. 5.31c).

For this reason, the type of surface over which the individual is walking needs to provide an adequate counterforce. This is normally supplied by friction between the sole of the foot and the ground.

Friction

Friction is the special name given to the resisting force that arises when one body moves or tends to move across the surface of another. Ability to walk and to grip various objects with the hands is dependent on frictional forces.

Frictional force (a) is independent of the area of contact between the bodies and (b) increases steadily until it reaches a maximum value when slipping is just about to occur. This value is called limiting friction.

The behaviour of frictional force can be illustrated by what happens when an attempt is made to slide a box along the floor from its original position of rest. When the horizontal force is applied, a resistance is experienced which increases until the box starts to move. Then it is found that once the box actually starts moving the force necessary to keep it moving is much less than that required to set it in motion. The resistance to motion experienced when the box is actually moving is called sliding friction.

The maximal frictional force (limiting friction) depends on (a) how firmly the surfaces are pressed together and (b) the nature of the materials in contact and their effects on each other due to their degree of roughness. This is called the co-efficient of friction and is represented by the symbol μ (mu). The co-efficient of friction μ for a rubber crutch tip on a clean tile is 0.30–0.40; whereas the co-efficient of friction of a rubber crutch tip on rough wood is 0.70–0.75. The greater the value of μ, the more the surfaces cling together.

In practice, friction between two bodies may be modified by:

1. Altering the nature of the surfaces in contact by using materials with different co-efficients of friction. Rubber soles on shoes may be more effective than hard leather soles although the co-efficient of friction of even rubber soles will depend on the walking surface.
2. Changing the forces that hold the surfaces together. A back pack may be strapped to an individual so that the total weight pressing down on the supporting surface is increased.

Pressure

When two bodies are in contact they exert a force on each other. The distribution of force over the area of contact relates to the concept of pressure.

Pressure is defined as the total force applied per area of force application and may be expressed by the equation:

$$P = \frac{F}{A}$$

Where P is the pressure
F is the applied force
A is the area over which the force is applied.

The unit of pressure is pounds per square inch (FPS).

By enlarging the area of contact, the same force, for example body weight, can be spread over a much larger area hence reducing the pressure. In standing, the area of contact is less than in the lying position (Fig. 5.32), hence the pressure exerted by the body weight in standing is greater than in lying. Note that the area of contact is not the same as the base.

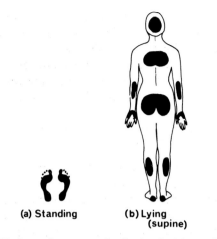

(a) Standing   **(b) Lying (supine)**

Fig. 5.32 Area of pressure distribution in (a) standing and (b) supine lying. (Area of pressure is shaded in black.)

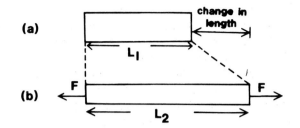

Fig. 5.33 Linear tensile stress and strain.

It is often necessary to increase the area of contact for patients, who are bedridden, to prevent skin breakdown due to pressure. This can be done by using yielding materials which fit the body contours and distribute body weight over an even wider area.

STRESS AND STRAIN

When a force is applied to a body it sets up stresses that result in deformation of the body. This deformation may be a change of shape, size or both and is measured by the strain in the body.

Stress is expressed as: force per unit area. The unit of stress is Newtons per square metre – N/m² (mks) or sometimes other units can be used e.g., kilogram weight per square inch – ksi.

There are no units of measurement for strain as it is a geometric concept.

For each stress there is a corresponding strain. Two kinds of stress each with their corresponding strain will be described here.

Linear tensile stress and strain

Suppose a bar of length L_1 (Fig. 5.33a) is subjected to equal and opposite forces applied perpendicular to the surfaces at its opposite ends as shown in Figure 5.33b, where the span has now a uniform internal stress. The value of stress is calculated using the formula:

$$\text{Stress} = F/A$$

Where F is the applied force

A is the cross sectional area of the bar.

This stress has the effect of changing the length of the bar to a new length, L_2. The fractional increase of the length of the bar – $\left(\frac{L_2 - L_1}{L_1}\right)$ – is called the linear tensile strain.

If the direction of both forces is reversed (Fig. 5.34), the bar will now decrease in length and the two quantities now relevant are termed the linear compressive stress and strain respectively.

Shear stress and strain

When a force tends to produce sliding between two planes this is called shear.

Shear stress and strain arise when a torque (Fx) is applied to a solid body (Fig. 5.35). Here

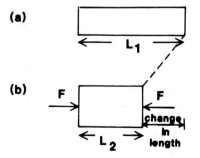

Fig. 5.34 Linear compressive stress and strain.

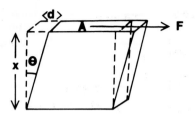

Fig. 5.35 Shear stress and strain.

F = Force applied tangentially to the block
A = Surface over which force is applied
x = Height of the block
d = The distance moved by the top face of the block
  when F applied
θ = Angle of shear strain

force is applied tangentially to the surface A rather than perpendicular as was the case for linear tensile stress.

Figure 5.35 shows a rectangular block fixed to a rigid base. (This prevents rotation of the block which would otherwise occur.) The force F acting on the block produces a deformation where the top face of the block moves a slight distance (d) to the right, relative to the bottom face.

In this situation, the angle θ, shown in Figure 5.35, measures the resultant geometrical deformation of the block under the applied tangential stress. It is also known as the angle of shear strain. This can be seen as follows. The shear strain is calculated from the ratio of the distance moved by the top of the block (d) to its dimension (height) – x.

i.e., Shear strain, $S = \dfrac{\text{displacement}}{\text{height}} = \dfrac{d}{x}$

$$= \theta \text{ provided } d << x$$

An everyday example of shear stress is in the use of scissors. Their mechanism consists of equal and opposite forces being applied to the material being cut by means of two blades which are so placed as to create a shear stress in the material (Fig. 5.36).

Stress/strain diagram

The amount of deformation produced in a

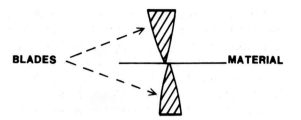

Fig. 5.36 The use of scissors as an example of shear stress.

body depends on the mechanical properties of the material of which it is made. Suppose a metal wire or spring which is rigidly supported at one end is progressively loaded by adding weights at its lower end (Fig. 5.37).

A plot can be made to show the amount of stretching of the wire (strain) which occurs as each weight is added. This is called a stress/strain diagram (Fig. 5.38).

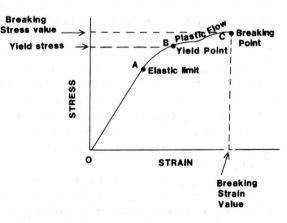

Fig. 5.37 Loaded spring.

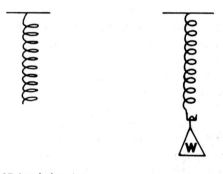

Fig. 5.38 A stress/strain diagram.

If the stress is not too large it can be shown that the amount by which the wire is stretched is proportional to the weights applied, i.e., stress and strain bear a linear relation to each other as shown by the straight line *OA* in Figure 5.38. This is called Hooke's Law.

This factor of proportionality is expressed for linear and shear stress as follows:

1. Young's modulus $Y = \dfrac{\text{Linear stress}}{\text{Linear strain}}$

$$= \dfrac{F/A}{(L_2 - L_1)/L_1}$$

2. Shear modulus $n = \dfrac{\text{Shear stress}}{\text{Shear strain}} = \dfrac{F/A}{\theta}$

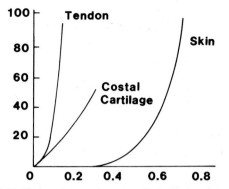

Fig. 5.39 The response of some soft tissues to uniaxial loading, *after Barbenel, J. C., Evans, J. N. & Jordan, M. M. (1978) 'Tissue Mechanics'. Engineering in Medicine, Vol. 7, No. 1, pp. 5–9.*

and is called a modulus of elasticity. A is here the area of cross-section of the wire before it was stretched.

The modulus of elasticity will vary for different materials depending on whether large or small displacements are produced by the same amount of stress.

The elastic limit of the wire is shown as the point *A* in Figure 5.38. If all the weights are removed before this point is reached the wire will return to its original length. However, when this limit is exceeded, the wire will not return to its original length as it has become permanently strained. For a stress corresponding to point *B* (the yield point) and beyond, the wire begins to exhibit what is termed plastic flow until it breaks – *C*.

In biological materials, such as skin and tendon, the arrangement of the collagen fibres determines, in part, the behaviour of these tissues when a load is applied to them. In skin, collagen is present as a dense network of fibres running in different directions, whereas in tendons the arrangement is more orderly with collagen having regular undulations that tend to run in parallel with each other. As might be expected, the elastic properties of skin and tendon tissues are widely different (Fig. 5.39).

When a moderate stress is applied across a specimen of skin or tendon tissue for example, it stretches with little resistance – like a woven fabric – until its collagen fibres have become straight and aligned. This, in more technical terms, is referred to as the 'initial lax phase of elastic behaviour'. When stress is applied to stretch the skin, there is a longer initial lax phase during which the collagen fibres become straight and aligned in the direction of the load than is the case with tendon. However, once this point is reached both tissues tend to stiffen in response to increasing stress and behave in the more expected linear fashion (Fig. 5.39).

The tensile and compressive strengths of these tissues can then be obtained by determining those stresses which are just sufficient to break them. However, this will vary depending on the direction of the applied load, as tissues tend to be strongest in the direction of normal stress situations through morphological adaptation.

Deformation

Deformation refers to the change of shape or dimensions produced by applied forces. For moderate stress, many materials exhibit 'elastic' deformation in that they return to their original shape and size after removal of stress. However, for larger stress, permanent deformation results.

Stiffness

Stiffness is a measure of the resistance offered by a structure as it deforms. It depends on the

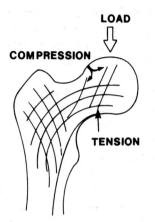

Fig. 5.40 Lines of principal stress in the head and neck of the femur.

type of materials as well as the size and shape of the structure involved. For example, materials with a high modulus of elasticity, such as bone, are stiffer than those with a lower modulus of elasticity, such as collagen.

The structure of the bones of the skeleton is optimised for normal load-bearing functions. For example, the bone structure of the femur is relatively hollow and is formed to meet the applied stress so that the bone filaments lie along the internal stress lines (Fig. 5.40). Such a design offers considerably more stiffness than a homogenous structure of the same weight. However, an abnormally applied stress may produce a lower breaking point and the bone fractures.

Viscoelasticity

Another factor which affects the stiffness of biological materials is the rate at which the stress forces are applied. This property of a material to show sensitivity to rate of stress loading is called viscoelasticity. With viscoelastic materials a quickly applied force meets with a higher resistance. For example, this phenomenon allows the spine to withstand much greater impact forces without excessive deformation of the vertebral bodies than would be the case if the same force was applied more gradually. This means that conceivably landing after a jump from a height

can have a less deforming effect on the vertebral bodies than prolonged poor lifting and carrying activities.

Creep

When a constant force is applied to a material, there is an immediate deformation which depends on the force applied and the stiffness of the material. Viscoelastic materials such as tendon and ligament will continue to deform while the load is being applied until they eventually reach a steady state (Fig. 5.41). This phenomenon is called creep and is used by physiotherapists when they apply serial plasters to increase range of motion which has been limited by tightened soft tissues. The procedure is one where after stretching the tightened soft tissue during a treatment session, a plaster is applied to maintain its new length, and kept on until the next treatment when it is removed and further stretch applied. A new plaster is made to maintain this increased length. This process is repeated until the required tissue length is achieved and is able to be maintained by normal functioning of the body part.

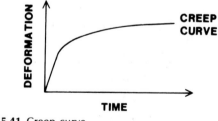

Fig. 5.41 Creep curve.

FLUID MECHANICS

Buoyancy

A body floating motionless in water is in a state of static equilibrium. Here the downward force of the body's weight is equal to the upward force that the water exerts on the body. This upward force or upthrust is called buoyancy.

Buoyancy produces an apparent loss of

weight of the body or body part when it is immersed in water. This phenomenon can be used by the physiotherapist to make active movement easier for a patient as the load (weight of the body part) that a patient's muscle force has to overcome is now reduced.

According to Archimedes principle, when a body is wholly or partially immersed in a fluid, the magnitude of the upthrust – buoyancy – is equal to the weight of fluid displaced.

When a body is placed in water, it will sink until the weight of the fluid it displaces (Fig. 5.42b) is equal to the weight of the body (Fig. 5.42a).

Specific gravity

A body will float in water only if the ratio:

$$\frac{\text{weight of the body}}{\text{weight of an equal volume of water}}$$

is less than one.

This ratio is called the specific gravity of the body. The specific gravity of water = 1.

Different tissues in the human body have different specific gravities – fat has a lower specific gravity than muscle and bone. As

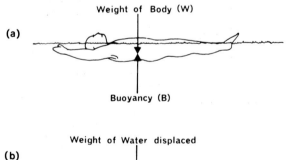

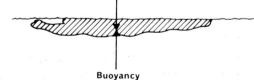

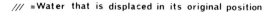

/// = Water that is displaced in its original position

Fig. 5.42 a. Forces acting in a balanced horizontal float showing body weight, *W*, and buoyancy, *B*. b. Buoyancy is equal to the weight of water displaced.

individuals differ in their body composition, their ability to float will vary; those individuals with a greater proportion of fatty tissue are generally the better floaters.

The distribution of the tissues is also important. Body parts like the lower limbs, which contain predominantly muscle and bone will tend to sink, as the specific gravity of muscle is about the same as water; whereas the specific gravity of bone is greater.

The amount of air in the lungs will also determine the specific gravity of the human body. During inspiration, the volume of the body is increased as the chest inflates, although there is a correspondingly negligible increase in body weight as air does not weigh much. Therefore the ratio:

$$\frac{\text{weight of the body}}{\text{weight of an equal volume of water}}$$

is reduced.

Centre of gravity, centre of buoyancy

When a body is immersed in water, its weight acts through its centre of gravity (Fig. 5.43).

The centre of gravity of the weight of fluid that the body displaces is called the centre of buoyancy of the body. It is defined as the centre of gravity of the displaced fluid before its displacement. Figure 5.42b illustrates the water displaced by a human floater in its original position. The centre of gravity of the weight of this water is called the centre of buoyancy.

If a body is of uniform density, the centre of gravity and the centre of buoyancy coincide. However, since the human body is not of uniform density because of tissue distribution, the centre of gravity and centre of buoyancy do not coincide. The centre of buoyancy is to be found closer to the head than the centre of gravity which is towards the heavier end of the body in the pelvic region. This situation then sets up a force couple when an individual attempts to float horizontally in the water (Fig. 5.43a). Rotation of the body occurs until the centre of gravity and the centre of buoyancy are in the same vertical

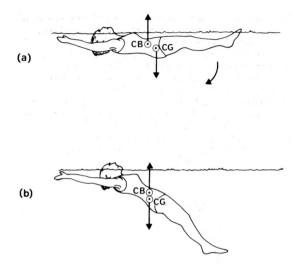

(a)

(b)

Fig. 5.43 Floating positions are governed by the relative positions of the lines of action of body weight and buoyancy. Equilibrium is achieved when they are on the same vertical line. CG = Body's centre of gravity; CB = centre of buoyancy.

line. When this happens, the body is in equilibrium and no further sinking occurs (Fig. 5.43b). Muscle forces are therefore necessary if the individual is to keep his limbs at the surface as in Figure 5.43a.

Pressure in a fluid

A body submerged in a liquid will be subjected to a hydrostatic fluid pressure determined by the depth at which it is immersed. In consequence, any surface which forms a liquid–solid interface experiences an inwardly directed force. The net result is that the body experiences compressive forces from all sides, which increase proportionally with the depth of immersion. However, there are exceptions where the body is completely permeable to the fluid (e.g. sea-sponges), where inside and outside pressures are equalised.

The principles of hydrostatic fluid pressure may be applied, for example, when in therapy the compressive forces are utilised to help to reduce oedema which tends to accumulate distally in the lower extremities. The patients are here given walking exercises in a hydrotherapy pool. The pressure is greatest distally all around the foot and gradually lessens as one moves proximally up the limb, giving a desirable graduated compression effect.

REFERENCES AND FURTHER READING

1. Barbenel, J. C., Evans, J. H. & Jordan, M. M. (1978) Tissue mechanics. *Engineering in Medicine*, Vol. 7, No. 1, pp. 5–9.
2. Barham, J. H. (1978) *Mechanical Kinesiology*. St Louis: C. V. Mosby.
3. Cooper, J. M. & Glassow, R. B. (1976) *Kinesiology*, 4th edn. St Louis: C. V. Mosby.
4. Cornwall, M. W. (1984) Biomechanics of non-contractile tissue-a review. *Physical Therapy*, Vol. 64, No. 12, pp. 1869–1882.
5. Dyson, C. (1977) *The Mechanics of Athletics*, 7th edn. London: Hodder and Stoughton.
6. Gowitzke, B. A. & Milner, M. (1980) *Understanding the Scientific Bases of Human Movement*, 2nd edn. Baltimore: Williams & Wilkins.
7. Grieve, D. W., Miller, D., Mitchelson, D., Paul, J. & Smith, A. J. (1975) *Techniques for the Analysis of Human Movement*. London: Lepus Books.
8. Hay, J. G. (1978) *The Biomechanics of Sports Techniques*, 2nd edn. Englewood Cliffs, N. J: Prentice-Hall.
9. Hellebrandt, F. A., Fries, C., Larsen, E. M. & Kelso, L. E. A. (1943) The influence of the Army pack on postural stability and stance mechanics. *American Journal of Physiology*, Vol. 140, pp. 645–655.
10. Hellebrandt, F. A., Tepper, R. H., Braun, G. L. & Elliott, M. C. (1938) The location of the cardinal anatomical orientation planes passing through the centre of weight in young adult women. *American Journal of Physiology*, Vol. 121, pp. 465–470.
11. Knuttgen, H. G. (1978) Force, work, power, and exercise. *Medicine and Science in Sports*, Vol. 10, No 3, pp. 227–228.
12. Laird, C. E. & Rozier, C. K. (1979) Toward understanding the terminology of exercise mechanics. *Physical Therapy*, Vol. 59, No. 3, pp. 287–292.
13. Lehmkuhl, L. D. & Smith, L. K. (1983) *Brunnstrom's Clinical Kinesiology*, 4th edn. Philadelphia: F. A. Davis.
14. Le Veau, B. (1977) *Williams & Lissner: Biomechanics of Human Motion*, 2nd edn. Philadelphia: W. B. Saunders.
15. Macdonald, F. A. (1973) *Mechanics for Movement*. London: G. Bell and Sons.
16. Macdonald, S. G. G. & Burns, D. M. (1975) *Physics for the Life and Health Sciences*. Reading, Massachusetts: Addison-Wesley.
17. Moffroid, M. T. & Kusiak, E. T. (1975) The power struggle. Definition and evaluation of power of muscular performance. *Physical Therapy*, Vol. 55, No. 10, pp. 1098–1104.

18. Moffroid, M., Whipple, R., Hofkosh, J., Lowman, E. & Thistle, H. (1969) A study of isokinetic exercise. *Physical Therapy*, Vol. 49, No. 7, pp. 735–747.

19. Murray, M. P., Baldwin, J. M., Gardner, G. M., Sepic, S. B. & Downs, W. J. (1977) Maximum isometric knee flexor and extensor muscle contractions, normal patterns of torque versus time. *Physical Therapy*, Vol. 57, No. 6, pp. 637–643.

20. Murray, M. P., Gardner, G. M., Mollinger, L. A. & Sepic, S. B. (1980) Strength of isometric and isokinetic contractions. *Physical Therapy*, Vol. 60, No. 4, pp. 412–419.

21. Rasch, P. J. & Burke, R. K. (1978) *Kinesiology and Applied Anatomy*, 6th edn. Philadelphia: Lea & Febiger.

22. Rodgers, M. M. & Cavanagh, P. R. (1984) Glossary of Biomechanical terms, concepts and units. *Physical Therapy*, Vol. 64, No. 12, pp. 1886–1902.

23. Tichauer, E. R. (1978) *The Biomechanical Basis of Ergonomics*. New York: John Wiley and Sons.

24. Wells, K. F. & Luttgens, K. (1976) *Kinesiology*, 6th edn. Philadelphia: W. B. Saunders.

25. Williams, M. & Stutzman, L. (1959) Strength variation through range of joint motion. *The Physical Therapy Review*, Vol. 39, No. 3, pp. 145–152.

26. Winter, D. A. (1979) *Biomechanics of Human Movement*. New York: John Wiley & Sons.

6
Posture

Posture may be considered as the relative arrangement of parts of the body – it changes with the positions and movements of the body throughout the day and throughout life. It is essentially a matter of body alignment.

'Good posture', as defined by the Posture Committee of the American Orthopaedic Association (1946), 'is that state of muscular and skeletal balance which protects the supporting structures of the body against injury and progressive deformity irrespective of the attitude in which these structures are working or resting. Under these conditions the muscles will function most efficiently and the optimum positions are afforded for the thoracic and abdominal organs'.[19]

Posture is influenced by general health, body build, sex, adequate strength and endurance, visual and kinaesthetic awareness as well as personal habits, the demands of the work place, and social and cultural traditions.

A description of posture includes:

1. The so-called static or rest posture – that is posture at rest or without anticipated action, such as when lying, sitting or standing and the many variations of these positions.
2. Dynamic posture, which can be considered as posture in action or in anticipation of action.[17]

All efficient movement consists of a posture adequate for a particular task. As the body is multi-segmental almost every movement a healthy person makes will set off a reaction throughout many parts of the body, so that the parts are acting in harmony and a balanced posture achieved.

As one watches a person move it is the movement itself which catches the eye. The joint stability which allows the movement to occur and forms the background of the movement, tends to pass unnoticed. As the movement proceeds the muscle work round the joints forming the postural background will change – at one moment a muscle may act as a stabiliser, then as movement proceeds as a synergist and perhaps later as a prime mover.

All the time the background alignment will be held, though it may be continuously adjusted as stabilisation of one joint after the other proceeds down the limb, regulating and allowing movement of the most distal segments which are more concerned with skill. This is a trained control, though as experience grows it may become almost automatic.

NORMAL POSTURE

Posture and the life cycle

One of the distinguishing characteristics of man is that he stands in the upright position far more effectively than other animals. In so doing, he has released his hands to perform more complex tasks.

The upright standing posture is inherently unstable because the body's centre of gravity is situated high above a relatively small base. Thus the body as it moves is constantly challenging and neutralising the force, gravity.

When the human infant first assumes the upright position, his ability to maintain it for very long is limited because his postural reactions although now present, still need to be perfected. This occurs with practice during play and other activities of the early childhood years. Parallel to these developments, the child becomes increasingly able to perform more complex skills, both with his hands as well as with his total body.

Body proportions alter during the life cycle

(Fig. 2.1) and in addition there are changes in the curve of the spine. In the neonate, the whole spine is flexed, forming a long 'C' curve convex posteriorly from the sacrum to the occiput. When the child begins to gain head control a counter-curve evolves in the cervical spine. Later as the child begins to sit and stand a second curve evolves in the lumbar region.

Once the standing position is achieved and during adult life the following four curves are present:

1. Cervical curvature – convex anteriorly
2. Thoracic curvature – convex posteriorly
3. Lumbar curvature – convex anteriorly
4. Sacral curvature – convex posteriorly.

An increase in the anterior curve is called a lordosis; in the posterior curve – a kyphosis. Any lateral curvature is called a scoliosis.

In old age, the shape of the spine tends to revert back to the long 'C' shaped curve. However, in many elderly people the cervical curve may increase as they try to keep their eyes directed parallel to the floor, so that they can look ahead. When compared with the neonate, spinal flexibility is now greatly reduced.

These structural changes of the spine and their accompanying effects on neighbouring soft tissues, account in part, for the characteristic appearance of the posture typical of different age groups (Fig. 6.1).

Posture and human communication

Each individual, irrespective of build, will have a distinct body contour. A balanced posture

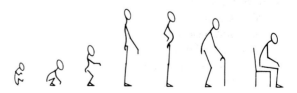

Fig. 6.1 The seven ages of man. Postural changes. *Reproduced with kind permission from MacLeod, J. (1973) Clinical Examination, 3rd edn. Edinburgh: Churchill Livingstone.*

can be aesthetically pleasing, being both graceful and efficient in repose and movement.

The posture adopted by an individual indicates much about his self-esteem as well as the state of his musculoskeletal system and the neurophysiological mechanisms controlling it. Through 'body language', involving changes in facial expression and body position, people convey various signals about their feelings and moods to onlookers – a factor exploited by actors and others involved in the visual arts. Very often, the postural shifts involved in body language do not reach the consciousness of the person emitting the signals or for that matter the onlooker, although he will subconsciously respond to them.

Basic positions

Three basic positions will be discussed in this section, namely standing, sitting and lying.

These basic positions may be modified by:

1. Adjusting the position of the head and limbs in relation to the trunk
2. Adjusting the trunk in relation to the head or limbs when these are fixed
3. Making finely adjusted vertebral movements.

When discussing these basic positions the assumption is usually made that the position to be analysed must be symmetrical. However, most people have a dominant eye, hand and foot. In daily life it is common to adopt asymmetric attitudes, shifting the body weight from time to time from one side to the other. For example, if people are observed standing at a bus stop it will be noticed that few of them maintain a symmetrical stance for long.

This shifting of weight helps prevent fatigue and contributes towards maintaining adequate circulation particularly in the postural muscles of the legs when standing. By alternating the main support from one leg to the other, the muscles become periodically unloaded and relax.

Similar observations can be made for any position. Remaining in any one position for too long may lead to ischaemia of the tissues particularly those under pressure, for example, the buttocks in sitting. People who cannot naturally make these postural shifts, for example, those with paraplegia, have to be trained by the physiotherapist to change their posture regularly.

Standing – body alignment

In standing, the body segments may be considered as being like movable blocks stacked and linked one on top of the other. Ideally the line from the centre of gravity of each of these segments should be centred over its supporting base – the segment below – for balance to be maintained with minimal muscular effort.

The composite of all these 'lines' is the body's line of gravity which passes through a point on a level with and immediately in front of the second sacral vertebra. This point is the centre of gravity for the whole body and is found at a distance above the ground of 55–57 per cent of the total body length – approximately at the level of the second sacral vertebra.[16]

Body balance depends to a large extent on the weight distribution on each foot and between the two feet as well as the balance of the pelvis over the feet, the trunk over the pelvis and the head over the trunk. At the same time the weight should be evenly distributed between the two sides of the body (Fig. 6.2).

On examination the body should be viewed from four aspects, front and back, and right and left sides.

The ideal 'normal' erect posture is one in which the vertical line drawn through the body's centre of gravity – the line of gravity – when viewed from each side runs:

1. Approximately 5 centimetres in front of the ankle joint
2. Just in front of the centre of the knee joint
3. Through the hip joint or just behind it
4. Just in front of the shoulder joint
5. Through the mastoid process.

When viewed from either the front or the back the vertical line passing through the body's centre of gravity should theoretically bisect the body into two equal halves with body weight evenly distributed between the two feet.

Pressure distribution over the soles of the feet will vary, depending on whether shoes are worn or not. Although there are large individual variations, some recent research into foot ground pressure patterns of a limited number of 'normal' subjects has shown that when bare-footed, approximately 45–65 per cent of the body weight is carried on the heels, whereas 30–47 per cent is carried on the forefoot and only 1–8 per cent over the mid-foot.[4] These proportions may be markedly altered following injury or disease, by prolonged mechanical stress or the wearing of high-heeled shoes.

The body weight is supported on the legs with the patellae facing directly forwards. The pelvis should be balanced on the femora in an arbitrary neutral position neither too far forward nor too far back. In the lateral view, in the vertical plane, the pubic symphysis and the anterior superior iliac spines are aligned; in the horizontal plane, the anterior superior

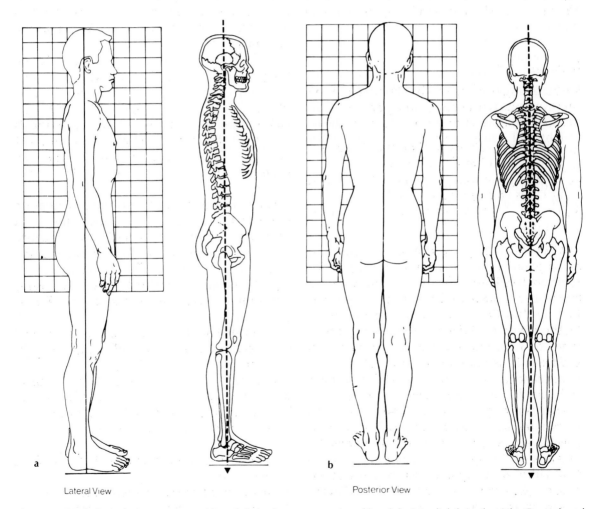

a
Lateral View

b
Posterior View

Fig. 6.2 A well aligned erect posture, although in b, the upper trunk and head deviate slightly to the right. *Reproduced with kind permission from Kendall, H.O., Kendall, F.P. & Wadsworth, G.E. (1971) Muscles – Testing and Function, 2nd edn. Baltimore: The Williams and Wilkins Company.*

iliac spines and the posterior inferior iliac spines are aligned (Fig. 6.2).

The position of the pelvis is important, for the sacrum which is part of the spine also forms part of the pelvis. Because the connection between the sacrum and the iliac bones is so firm, a change in position of the pelvis leads automatically to a realignment of the spine, particularly in the lumbar region. Obviously when there is limitation of motion in the lumbar spine as a result of pain or degeneration, this will have a marked effect on the possible postural adjustments available.

In the trunk, the abdomen should be flat and relaxed, neither sagging nor retracted. The chest should be erect without being tense or fully expanded.

The weight of the shoulder girdle and the arms should be centred over the spinal column with the arms relaxed. The head should be erect and well balanced on the neck so that the eyes can function most effectively. If the head is held too far forward or back, its heavy weight will cause tension, strain and often pain in the neck muscles, headache and eye strain. The weight of all these structures should be supported by the spine and carried down through the pelvis to the supporting legs.

The balanced posture of the body reduces to a minimum the work done by the muscles in maintaining the body in an erect position.

Through the use of electromyography,[5] it has been demonstrated that in general:

1. The intrinsic muscles of the feet are quiescent – support is provided by the ligaments.
2. Soleus is continuously active in all cases because gravity tends to pull the body forward over the feet (Fig. 6.3); whereas gastrocnemius and the deep posterior tibial muscles are less frequently active.
3. Tibialis anterior is quiescent, although this alters when high heels are worn.
4. Quadriceps and the hamstrings are generally quiescent, although they may show slight activity from time to time.
5. Iliopsoas remains constantly active.
6. Gluteus maximus is quiescent.

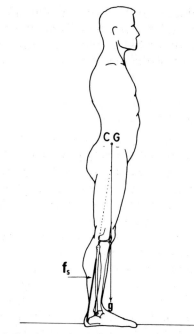

Fig. 6.3 Gravity tends to pull the leg forward over the foot. This is counteracted by the activity of the soleus (f_s) to maintain the upright posture. *Reproduced with kind permission from O'Connell, A. L. & Gardner, E. B. (1972) Understanding the Scientific Bases of Human Movement. Baltimore: The Williams and Wilkins Company.*

7. Gluteus medius and tensor fascia lata are active to counteract lateral postural sway.
8. Erector spinae is active, counteracting gravity's tendency to pull the trunk forward.
9. The abdominal muscles remain quiescent although the lower fibres of the internal obliques are active in order to protect the inguinal canal.

In the standing position, with the arms hanging loosely by the side, gravity pulls on the structures surrounding the joints of the shoulder girdle and upper limbs, tending to distract them. Muscular activity does not play a major role in controlling gravity's effects here, although it has been shown that minimal activity does occur in:

1. The upper fibres of trapezius
2. Serratus anterior
3. Supraspinatus
4. The posterior fibres of deltoid.

Supraspinatus and tension in the superior part of the joint capsule prevent downward dislocation of the head of the humerus on the glenoid cavity while the body is in the upright position.

Postural sway[13,14,15]

Standing is not a static position – a person does not stand completely still even if trying to do so. The upright position is maintained by the alternating action of antagonistic muscle groups which prevents overbalancing. This results in a continuous slight sway of the body, keeping the total body centre of gravity over the area covered by the feet – the 'base'.

A line projected vertically downwards from the centre of gravity to the supporting surface falls slightly posterior and to the left of the geometrical centre of the base when adopting a natural stance. This position is consistent for all ages. The magnitude of the sway about the centre of the base, as shown by the path traced out by the vertical projection from the centre of gravity (Fig. 6.4), tends to be larger in the very old and the very young.

The constant shifting of the body's centre of gravity during standing, leads to the muscle spindles being pulled upon irregularly, which causes alternating activity and inactivity of the various motor units. This helps prevent fatigue as well as assisting venous return.

Vision appears to be primarily involved in controlling fine balance in the standing position. It has been shown, for example, that an individual's balance can be manipulated by

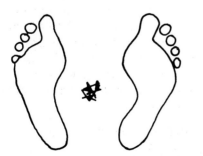

Fig. 6.4 Oscillating path traced out by the constant shifting of the body's centre of gravity during standing.

altering his visual surroundings without him being aware that this is going on.[21]

The ankle and foot proprioceptors also make an important contribution to the control of balance.

Sitting

Sitting is one of the most frequently adopted positions used during waking hours if one considers the amount of time spent by many people sitting at work, studying, sitting in vehicles or watching television or spectator sport.

There is a wide variety of sitting positions dependent on the person and the surface on which he sits.[2,7,8,11,17] It is essential in all positions that the basic vertical alignment of trunk and head is maintained unless the person is resting with the back and head supported in an easy chair.

Compared with standing, the sitting position is the more stable position as the total body's supporting surface is greater and generally allows relaxation of the muscles of the lower limbs (Fig. 6.5).

Sitting on the floor

This position is one constantly used by the young child and very often by the adolescent. The body posture to a large extent will be dependent on the position adopted by the legs, for example, cross-legged sitting, sitting knees bent, sitting with the lower legs bent under the body and side sitting with the legs either to the right or left of the body. If taken to alternate sides, the total 'C' curve is reversed and therefore the side sitting positions can be used with safety.

Sitting on a chair or stool

In sitting on a chair or stool, the base extends from the anterior part of the soles of the feet to the posterior edge of the buttocks. The weight of the trunk is transferred to the supporting surface of the chair, mainly by the ischial tuberosities and their surrounding soft tissues. The weight of the legs and part of the thigh is transferred to its supporting surface – the floor – via the feet.

The height of the chair should be equal to the length of the leg from the back of knee to the base of the heel with the knee bent to 90° and the feet flat on the floor. The seat, with the person sitting well back on it, should reach to within a few inches of the knee joint. If too long there will be pressure behind the knee joint; if too short, there will be pressure on the posterior surface of the thigh against the anterior border of the seat, the base will be lessened and more pressure placed on the feet.

The type of support given to the back, by

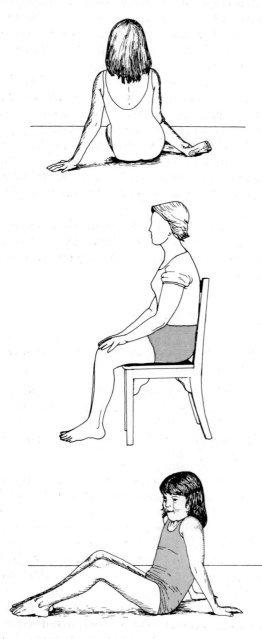

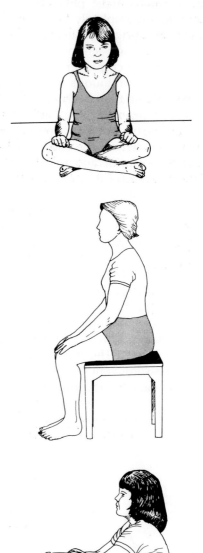

Fig. 6.5 Different sitting postures.

a chair or by a cushion, is important in altering the amount of muscle activity and intradiscal pressure occurring in any position.[1,2] With increasing inclination of the back-rest, muscle activity necessary for supporting the trunk decreases, as does the amount of intradiscal pressure. When possible the arms should be rested either on the arm rest, on a table or in the lap. If a patient is sitting up in bed it is necessary to ensure that the lower back is adequately supported by pillows.

Lying

Lying, with its many variations of position, including supine, prone and side lying is a much used posture during the daily cycle of activity, rest and sleep. It should be a position of ease and comfort and allow complete relaxation. It is the normal day to

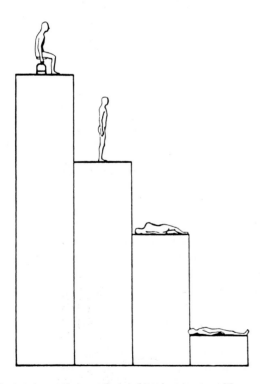

Fig. 6.6 Approximate relationships between position and total pressure on normal third and fourth lumbar discs. *Reproduced with permission from Nachemson, A. M. & Morris, J. M. (1964) In vivo measurements of intradiscal pressure. The Journal of Bone and Joint Surgery, Vol 46A, No. 5, p. 1089.*

day posture adopted by infants during the early months of post-natal life.

It is the easiest position in which to maintain the body equilibrium because the centre of gravity of the total body is low. It requires very little muscle activity to maintain, the force, gravity, being counteracted by mechanisms that are mainly passive. Therefore, it is the least energy consuming of the three basic positions discussed in this chapter. Intradiscal pressure in the lumbar region is also less when compared with other positions (Fig. 6.6).[22]

It is a position of rest provided that the supporting surface is firm and comfortable so that sagging of the body is prevented and maximum relaxation gained. In side lying a small pillow is advisable to keep the head in line with the body and depending on the person's posture, it may be necessary to maintain the head in a good position in supine lying.

Whatever the position assumed at the commencement of rest, the extremities will change position frequently and the body turn, at intervals, during sleep.

POSTURAL RE-EDUCATION

'Poor' posture, whatever the individual's build, involves:

1. A faulty relationship of the various parts of the body which produces increased strain on the supporting structures
2. Inadequate balance over the base of support.[9]

Postural deviations will occur with an increase or decrease of the normal body curves. There may be an upset of the body mechanics leading to uneven pressure within the joint surfaces, ligaments will be under strain and the muscles holding the body upright may need to work harder. Pain may occur.

It is seldom that only one part of the body is involved, normally the total posture is at fault. Most patients with 'poor' posture will have

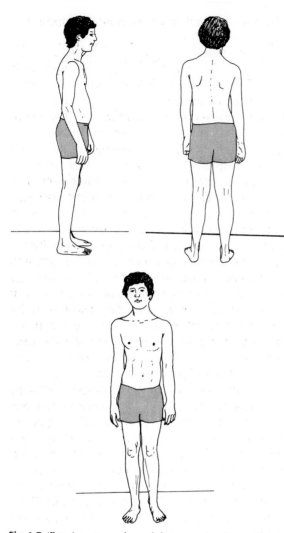

Fig. 6.7 'Poor' posture of an adolescent schoolboy. There is poor balance with abnormalities of both antero-posterior and lateral alignment of the body on the feet. Weight is unevenly distributed and there is poor alignment of the pelvis, spine, shoulder girdle and head.

little or minimal structural change, the fault is one of body alignment.

The causes of poor posture are many and varied. Each person will have individual problems. Some of the factors which cause mal-alignment are a lack of knowledge concerning posture, poor habits or environment, injury or illness and in some patients lack of strength, flexibility, stability or minor neurological damage.

In the case of the young child it is difficult to know if the posture will correct itself. As development occurs there will be changes in the proportional relationship of trunk and limbs, of body flexibility and muscular control and in the curves of the spine. The flexibility of the infant will gradually lessen as the child grows and stability becomes necessary. Gradually a balance will be struck between stability and mobility.

Provided growth and development are watched carefully and the advice given to parents on the need to establish a good level of nutrition and good habits of play and rest is followed, there is probably little need for a corrective programme.[27]

As the child grows older, bilateral sports such as swimming, ball games and dance, with their variety of movements, all provide useful and necessary activities as movement becomes increasingly restricted by school or work and the fatigue of travel.

Adolescence, if it brings a period of rapid growth together with inactivity and poor habits, can bring with it problems of control particularly in the tall slender girl, who may be less active than the male.

It can be said that patients of all ages have postural problems and many can be helped towards correcting or preventing a worsening of the problems.

Self motivation

The correction of poor postural habits will depend largely on self-motivation. This will be greatly influenced by the approach and personal posture of the physiotherapist; the attention given to detail in examining, analysing and explaining the problem; as well as the setting up of an interesting and relevant treatment plan.

The patient must gain an appreciation that a balanced posture is an asset. It is attractive and it improves self-confidence. It makes for movement efficiency, easier working habits and lessens fatigue so that leisure time can be more fruitfully spent.

The physiotherapist must understand the

limits placed on the gaining of postural efficiency by the patient's build.

The gaining of knowledge

The knowledge of posture may be given in the form of an explanation of the structure and function of the body and what constitutes an effective balanced posture. Photographs of 'good' and 'poor' posture in a person of similar build and age are often useful. Photographic or video-tape records of the patient's own posture provide a continuing stimulus.

The detection of errors

The problems involved in the correction of the patient's own posture and their relevance to both living and working situations need to be sensitively approached.

It is necessary that the patient gains a knowledge and an increased awareness of his own postural state and that he learns to detect and correct faults by adjusting and controlling the relevant postures.

The relief of abnormal tension and pain

Many patients with minor postural faults report for treatment because of pain. Abnormal tension may be present. The muscles usually affected are those of the posterior neck, shoulder girdle and/or dorso-lumbar region. The abnormal tension built up causes muscle imbalance so both the background on which movement takes place and the movement itself may be affected. Extra and unnecessary muscles come into play to overcome this imbalance causing inefficiency, fatigue and pain.

The patient must learn to feel the difference between abnormal tension and relaxation in a muscle or muscle group in order to learn to relax them. If there is a state of general tension then general relaxation needs to be taught to and mastered by the patient.

Other physiotherapy measures to relieve pain may go hand in hand with the relaxation techniques.

The establishment of neuro-muscular control

Although postural control is an automatic or reflex function, correction will be necessary at two levels. These are the gaining of:

1. Conscious control
2. Automatic control.

Conscious control

It is thought that conscious correction made often enough will help to form a good habitual posture. It is a matter of the patient gaining an awareness of the position of his body in space and of learning a new motor skill through constant and regular practice.

The correction of such 'static' postures as lying, sitting and standing forms a basis for the start of treatment. They are key positions from which many intermediate postures, particularly those most commonly used are derived, and from which many movements of the trunk, arms and legs take place.

The emphasis will be on a correct base with weight evenly divided between both sides and a systematic correction of all segments involved in the posture. In standing, the emphasis will be on the correct balance of the pelvis over the feet, the trunk on the pelvis and the head on the trunk, so that the patient gains the feeling of a correct alignment.

A long mirror used in early treatment provides a useful reinforcement as the unaccustomed positions often feel uncomfortable and abnormal. The patient will see the improvement and gain the feeling of the correction. Gradually kinaesthetic and visual awareness will be built up as the correction is repeatedly made and the gaining of correct alignment becomes more automatic.

Automatic control

A controlled movement will start from a more or less static position. The attention of the person will be concentrated, in the main, on the carrying out of the movement – a movement with a purpose. A mostly automatic, dynamic control allows the body to move from a more or less static position to one of readiness for movement and provides both general and local stability. Adjustments will be necessary to maintain balance and to overcome natural forces such as gravity as well as other forces involved in the movement itself.

The movement may be one involving the whole body on its base or may involve a changing base. Even if the movement is a small one the total body will react to it.

The regaining of mobility and strength

Some patients will have a slight loss of flexibility through muscle and soft tissue tightness which makes the gaining of correct alignment difficult. There may be some co-existing muscle weakness in the antagonists of the tightened muscles.

A few exercises given in carefully chosen starting positions in which the patient can concentrate on the localised contraction of the antigravity muscles, will be useful. They will aid local control and at the same time flexibility, by relaxing the tight antagonists. The exercises should be upgraded as control improves.

Good working and resting habits

Working postures and conditions both at home and at work should be carefully evaluated and where possible necessary improvements made. Particular emphasis should be placed on checking the suitability of equipment in daily use such as bed, chair, desk height, lighting and so on.

Occupational and recreational activities may be included in the programme with the emphasis on efficient posture and smooth rhythmical movement with well-controlled respiration.

The need for a constant change of position, even if momentary, will help to cut down fatigue with its consequent inefficiency.

The achieving of a balanced posture will come from constant awareness and correction throughout the day with a co-operative and highly motivated patient.

REFERENCES AND FURTHER READING

1. Andersson, B. J. G., Örtengren, R., Nachemson, A. & Elfstrom, G. (1974) Lumbar disc pressure and myoelectric back muscle activity during sitting. *Scandinavian Journal of Rehabilitation Medicine*, Vol. 6, pp. 104–114.
2. Andersson, B. J. G., Örtengren, R., Nachemson, A. L., Elfstrom, G. & Broman, H. (1975) The sitting posture: an electromyographic and discometric study. *Orthopaedic Clinics of North America*, Vol. 6, No. 1, pp. 105–120.
3. Argyle, M. (1975) *Bodily Communication*. London: Methuen & Co.
4. Arcan, M., Brull, M. & Simkin, A. (1975) Mechanical parameters describing the standing posture, based on the foot-ground pressure pattern. In *Biomechanics V-B*, Komi, P. V. (Ed.) pp. 415–425. Baltimore: University Park Press.
5. Basmajian, J. V. & Deluca, C. J. (1985) *Muscles Alive*, 5th edn. Baltimore: Williams & Wilkins.
6. Barlow, W. (1954) Posture and the resting state. *Annals of Physical Medicine*, Vol. 2, No. 4, pp. 113–122.
7. Broer, M. R. & Zernicke, R. F. (1979) *Efficiency of Human Movement*, 2nd edn. Philadelphia: W.B. Saunders & Co.
8. Carlsöö, S. (1972) *How Man Moves*. London: Heinemann.
9. Daniels, L. & Worthingham, C. (1977) *Therapeutic Exercise for Body Alignment and Function*. Philadelphia: W.B. Saunders.
10. Dornan, J., Fernie, G. R. & Holliday, P. J. (1978) Visual input: Its importance in the control of postural sway. *Archives of Physical Medicine and Rehabilitation*, Vol. 59, pp. 586–591.
11. Grandjean, E. & Hunting, W. (1977) Ergonomics of posture – Review of various problems of standing and sitting posture. *Applied Ergonomics*, Vol. 8, No. 3, pp. 135–140.
12. Hasselkus, B. R. & Shambes, G. M. (1975) Aging and postural sway in women. *Journal of Gerontology*, Vol. 30, No. 6, pp. 661–667.
13. Hellebrandt, F. A. (1938) Standing as a geotropic reflex. *American Journal of Physiology*, Vol. 121, pp. 471–474.
14. Hellebrandt, F. A. & Franseen, E. B. (1943) Physiological study of the vertical stance of man. *Physiological Reviews*, Vol. 23, pp. 220–255.
15. Hellebrandt, F. A. & Fries, E. C. (1942) The constancy of oscillographic stance patterns. *The Physiotherapy Review*, Vol. 22, No. 1, pp. 17–23.
16. Hellebrandt, F. A., Tepper, R. H., Braun, G. L. & Elliott, M. C. (1938) The location of the cardinal anatomical orientation planes passing through the centre of weight in young adult women. *American Journal of Physiology*, Vol. 121, pp. 465–470.
17. Howarth, B. (1946) Dynamic posture. *Journal of the*

American Medical Association, Vol. 131, No. 17, pp. 1398.

18. Joseph, J. (1960) *Man's Posture*. Springfield: Charles C. Thomas.

19. Kendall, H. O., Kendall, F. P. & Boynton, D. A. (1952) *Posture and Pain*. Baltimore: Williams & Wilkins.

20. Kendall, F. P. & McCreary, E. K. (1983) *Muscles, Testing and Function*, 3rd edn. Baltimore: Williams & Wilkins.

21. Lee, D. N. & Lishman, J. R. (1975) Visual proprioceptive control of stance. *Journal of Human Movement Studies*, Vol. 1, pp. 87–95.

22. Nachemson, A. & Morris, J. M. (1964) In vivo measurements of intradiscal pressure. *Journal of*

Bone & Joint Surgery, Vol. 46A, No. 5, pp. 1077–1092.

23. Purdon – Martin, J. (1977) A short essay on posture and movement. *Journal of Neurology, Neurosurgery, and Psychiatry*, Vol. 40, pp. 25–29.

24. Rasch, P. J. & Burke, R. K. (1978) *Kinesiology and Applied Anatomy*, 6th edn. Philadelphia: Lea and Febiger.

25. Shambes, G. M. (1976) Static postural control in children. *American Journal of Physical Medicine*, Vol. 55, No. 5, pp. 221–252.

26. Wells, K. F. & Luttgens, K. (1976) *Kinesiology*, 6th edn. Philadelphia: W.B. Saunders.

27. Wiles, P. & Sweetnam, R. (1965) *Essentials of Orthopaedics*, 4th edn. London: J. A. Churchill.

7

Relaxation

Relaxation is a state of rest of mind and body; relaxing, the achieving of that state.

Life has a basic rhythm with periods of greater or lesser arousal–both mental and physical–and with effort and rest interspersed at more or less regular intervals each day. On a gross level this is illustrated by the wake-sleep cycle.

The basic rhythm is also evident in the various functions of the body, for example, in the rhythmical contraction and relaxation of the heart; during the inspiratory and expiratory phases of the breathing cycle as well as in movement with one muscle group contracting while the antagonist relaxes to allow the movement to take place. This alternating rhythm can be speeded up or slowed down in response to both internal and external stimuli, depending on the needs and demands of the particular situation. Such fluctuations are normal.

Coping with stress

Everyone has times of both personal and environmental stress. Challenges and difficulties as well as stimulating events, both pleasant and unpleasant, must be faced and lead to a rise in the level of arousal in the brain – a stress response. Normally, with fatigue, the level of arousal falls and sleep occurs.

A certain level of arousal is necessary to help the individual meet the challenges of life

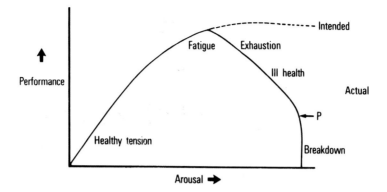

Fig. 7.1 The human function curve. P = the point at which even minimal arousal may precipitate a breakdown. *Reproduced with kind permission from Nixon, P.G.F. (1976) The Human Function Curve. The Practitioner, Vol. 217, p. 766.*

and living efficiently. Trouble occurs only when the response to stress becomes excessive and out of control.

The capacity to cope with stressful events varies from person to person. Some have the ability to recognise excessive stress and deal with these situations or prevent them occurring. Alternatively, if excessive stress is not recognised and a solution found, fatigue and disturbance of sleep will result.

With fatigue and loss of sleep, work inefficiency occurs leading to further muscle tension, causing even greater fatigue. The individual will attempt to make up for the loss of efficiency incurred by again increasing the level of arousal, which if allowed to continue can lead to depression and ill health. Thus a self-perpetuating cycle is established (Fig. 7.1).

Pattern of stress

Stress in daily life is reflected in the over-activity of the general body musculature. This excessive tension in various muscles forms a well recognised pattern.[12] The face is tense. The forehead is creased, with the eyes held tightly closed or held widely open. The lips are tightly closed with the teeth often clenched firmly together. The tongue is held rigidly on the roof of the mouth.

In depression, the posture of the head is one in which either the head is carried forward with the chin tucked in or the head moves forward on the neck, with the chin jutting out in an aggressive fashion. The shoulders are raised and the neck appears shortened.

The upper limbs are held rigidly and close to the chest, with the elbows flexed. The body generally is held stiffly, with breathing principally in the upper chest region.

If seated, the person sits either slumped back in the chair or on the edge of the chair with the legs crossed. The foot and leg will often be moved in a pumping up and down action.

Many students suffer from increased tension which can interfere with their performance. The stress of study, fear of failure, desire to succeed and pace of work, as well as poor environmental conditions and working habits, may all contribute to this condition.

If the student learns to recognise these tensions and understands their cause and their effects on her, she will be able to gain from the use of active relaxation methods. Her own personal experience will enable her to help others to live and work more efficiently.

Muscle relaxation

Muscle relaxation involves a diminution of neuro-muscular excitability, leading to a decrease in that tension produced by the contractile components of the muscle. In complete relaxation there is little or no apparent activity involving these components, although muscle tone is present.

The use of relaxation therapy

The goal of relaxation therapy for a person will be to encourage control over the level of muscle contraction so that it is not excessive for the needs of the work to be done or the situation to be faced.

In physiotherapy, the gaining of general relaxation may be either a treatment in itself or a treatment component in an overall plan. For example, for a patient with a known condition whose whole recovery is being hampered by excessive psychological and physical tension, relaxation will be a preparatory part of the physical retraining programme.

Other uses of relaxation therapy are more specific. It may be aimed at gaining differential or selective relaxation, as the individual learns to control background activity, by eliminating unnecessary tensions and movements, so that an activity can be performed with a minimal effort, for example, typing. It is an aid to the cultivation of good working habits.

The gaining of localised relaxation is often used in conjunction with other pain relieving methods, leading to a lessening of pain and increased movement potential.

To obtain general relaxation the individual should learn to appreciate his excessive tension, to discriminate between a tense and relaxed state and produce relaxation at will. This involves an understanding of the causes leading to excessive tension, the ability to tolerate stress and remain calm, to work with an economy of effort and therefore less fatigue, as well as the knowledge that the solution lies within his own control.

The emphasis in the gaining of relaxation will be on the growth of an awareness of a muscular or positional change and an appreciation of a new sensation of internal control. It demands regular practice and intense concentration. It is an acquired skill.

In the early stages the patient's concentration will be aided if he works in a quiet atmosphere with his eyes closed. The starting position is usually lying or sitting, in a fully supported position. The aim is not to produce a sleeping state but rather one of 'alert tranquility'.[6] As soon as possible the work is upgraded and other positions are added particularly those most frequently used in daily life, such as typical working positions.

The words used in the training of relaxation are important. They should be few, short, positive and meaningful, and spoken in a calm, quiet manner, so that they give a mental concept of what is required of the person and so help to shorten the time of learning. They could be considered 'trigger' words for they are giving a positive command.

Timing is also important. The release of tension, particularly in the early stages, takes time. Therefore there must be a sufficient pause for allowing relaxation to take place; for the person to gain an appreciation of a new feeling or a new position and to realise some success has been achieved. This will contribute to further motivation.

The choice of a technique

There are many approaches to the training of relaxation. Five well known techniques used by physiotherapists are outlined. The choice of a technique often depends on the patient's condition, his personality and/or the specific skills of the individual therapist.

1. a. The 'contract-hold-relax' or 'tension release' technique of Jacobson.[8] This technique consists of a systematic sequence of isometric contractions followed by relaxation. It seeks to achieve increased control over skeletal muscles until the subject is able to induce very low levels of tension in major muscle groups. The programme concentrates in the first two weeks on achieving all possible relaxation of one arm. It gradually proceeds over a period of many weeks to involve the total body. The words used are 'tense-hold-release'.

b. The 'contract-hold-relax' technique of Fair and Basmajian.[6] This technique also consists of the use of the 'contract-hold-relax' technique but proceeds much more quickly. For example, the first treatment may involve the arm, face, neck and chest so that a considerable though varying degree of relaxation, including some relaxation of breathing, may occur. An area in which relaxation is achieved easily may be used as a starting point from which a spread of relaxation can be gained. Biofeedback may be used early in treatment.

2. The self-directed relaxation of Fink.[7] This technique involves the recognition of excessive tension and emphasises relaxation – 'a letting go'. Slowly over many weeks a certain control is gained over all parts of the body. It is an effective but slow and demanding technique. The words used are 'let go, more – more and more'.

3. The reciprocal relaxation technique of Mitchell.[12] This technique uses the antagonists of the tense muscles to bring about a movement in the opposite direction to that of the tension, thereby taking up a new position and lessening neuromuscular activity in the tense muscles. Here the words used are 'gently push (or pull) and feel – stop – feel – and feel –'.

4. Yoga and meditation. This is used by some physiotherapists who are suitably qualified in these techniques.

5. Biofeedback, using electromyography.[3] This method has been shown to be effective. Here, the patient is given auditory and/or visual signals indicating the existing level of tension in the target muscles. Feedback allows the individual to further adjust his response to achieve even greater relaxation.

The early teaching sessions should be long enough to ensure that the patient knows what to do and feel. The practice sessions are then progressively shortened but increased in frequency particularly utilising working positions in an effort to learn control in tense working situations; for example, in driving a car.

Books on methods of relaxation are most useful in helping a person to analyse and overcome psychological difficulties and in setting out a method of gaining relaxation. It is possible for the person to undertake the training programme by himself or herself. Others will find early guidance by the therapist helpful and may use a book or tapes for reinforcement.

At the finish of a session it is helpful to sit quietly for a few minutes and enjoy the sensation of relaxation.

REFERENCES AND FURTHER READING

1. Anderson, T. McClurg (1951) *Human Kinetics.* London: W. Heinemann.
2. Basmajian. J. V. (Ed.) (1984) *Therapeutic Exercise,* 4th edn. Baltimore: Williams & Wilkins.
3. Basmajian, J. V. & De Luca, C. J. (1985) *Muscles Alive,* 5th edn. Baltimore: Williams & Wilkins.
4. Benson, H. (1975) *The Relaxation Response.* New York: William Morrow & Co.
5. Davidson, T. D. (1978) Stress in the elderly. *Physiotherapy,* Vol. 64, No. 4, pp. 113–115.
6. Fair, P. L. & Basmajian, J. V. (1976) Physical Therapy in Physical Rehabilitation. In *A New Method of Physical Rehabilitation Series.* New York: (Cassette Tape Cat. No. T82) Basmajian, J. V. (Ed.) Biomonitoring Applications Inc. N. York.
7. Fink, D. H. (1957) *Release from Nervous Tension.* London: George Allen & Unwin.
8. Jacobson, E. (1962) *You Must Relax,* 4th edn. New York: McGraw-Hill Paperbacks.
9. Matthews, P. B. C. (1977) Muscle afferents & kinesthesia. *British Medical Bulletin,* Vol. 33, No. 2, pp. 137–142.
10. Metheny, E. (1952) *Body Dynamics.* New York: McGraw-Hill.
11. Mills, I. H. (1978) Coping with the stress of modern society. *Physiotherapy,* Vol. 64, No. 4, pp. 109–112.
12. Mitchell, L. (1977) *Simple Relaxation.* London: John Murray.
13. Nixon, P. G. F. (1976) The human function curve, with special reference to cardio-vascular disorders: Part 1. *The Practitioner,* Vol. 217, November 1976, pp. 765–770.

8
Skilled performance and learning

Motor behaviour is a concern of the physiotherapist. Traditionally psychologists have also been involved in the study of perceptual motor skills producing a rich literature which is a potentially useful reference source for physiotherapists.[10,12,15,18,19,21,22,25,26,27]

Performance, learning and skill

During each treatment session, the physiotherapist monitors a patient's performance in a particular task. This is done to gain some estimate of the amount of learning that has occurred if the objective of that treatment is for the patient to acquire a particular level of skill. It is important to realise that this is only an estimate each time, because the level of skill that a patient may have acquired over a number of treatment sessions may be depressed, at any one performance, by such temporary factors as fatigue and boredom.

The level of performance does not necessarily reflect the actual capacity of the patient to move skilfully although performance, under optimal conditions, should accurately reflect the level of skill learning already attained.

Learning has permanent effects. Performance is more affected by temporary factors. If skill in a particular task has been attained, it should be retained over relatively long periods of time – time during which temporary factors such as fatigue will come and go.

The patient learns desired skills during

treatment. Therefore, when the physiotherapist comes to assess the patient's performance on any particular day, an estimate of how the performance may have been affected by such factors as fatigue, time of day, emotional state and motivation needs to be made. In this way a true picture of the actual amount of skill learning that has taken place, emerges.

Skilled performance

A skilled person is one who knows exactly the right method to use in each situation that arises when performing a particular task. His muscles contract with appropriate force in proper sequence with respect to other muscles. His movements flow easily together in an organised spatial and temporal sequence so the task is done smoothly and economically.

A skilled performer is able to select the right signals to which he will respond, choose the right course of action, make precisely the right movements and check these by reliable means. He is adaptable. All this is achieved through learning.

When the term 'skill' is used, the implication is that learning has taken place. Therefore, movements which occur as a stereotyped response to a particular stimulus, for example reflexes, are not usually classified as skills. Reflexes are better thought of as component parts of more complex perceptual-motor skills.[13]

Skilled behaviour is intentional and has purpose. It is goal oriented and flexible. In order to determine whether an individual is skilled it is necessary to know what his goal is and how he intends to achieve it. A patient may perform a beautiful sequence of movements but not achieve what he intended to do. His performance in this case cannot be called skilled.

Movements are the means by which the goal is achieved, though these will never be exactly the same on apparently identical tasks performed at different times. However, this will not alter the fact of an individual's current level of skill.

Specific movement is not the distinguishing factor of a perceptual-motor skill,[2] although movements are the means by which a goal is achieved by the performer. For example, quite different sets of muscles and movements are involved in the skill of writing one's name with a pencil, one's finger or with a long stick in the sand. Despite the differences in muscle action, there is a remarkable similarity in the form of the writing produced in each case. A complex motor programme for 'writing' behaviour apparently guides each of these situations. This is an economical concept because it seems unlikely that the nervous system is able to store individual programmes for each and every movement that will be needed for all possible situations the individual will meet throughout life.[2]

How such complex motor programmes are learned and how this involves central nervous system mechanisms are intriguing questions. The answers to these questions are not yet clearly understood.

Reaction time, Movement time

The physiotherapist, in attempting to analyse a patient's skill in performing a particular task, must also take into account such psychological processes as perception, decision making and movement organisation which all take place in the central nervous system prior to the movement sequence being performed.

These processes take time, a fact which has been used by research workers in their attempts to understand their nature. Two useful measures are shown in Figure 8.1.

1. *Reaction time* – which is the time taken from the presentation of an unanticipated signal until the beginning of the observed movement response.

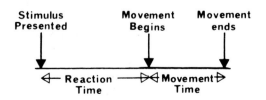

Fig. 8.1 Reaction time and movement time.

2. Movement time – which is the time taken to complete the movement programme.

A problem at any of the stages along the way may contribute to an observed lack of skill. If the offending stage can be identified, treatment methods aimed at the cause of interference with skilled movement performance may be started. The underlying causes of poor performance may then be related to a wider range of possibilities than the more obvious deficits in muscle, bone or joint function alone.

Information processing models of perceptual-motor skills

Skilled behaviour has been defined as: 'Complex intentional actions involving a whole chain of sensory, central and motor mechanisms which through the process of learning have come to be organised and co-ordinated in such a way as to achieve predetermined objectives with maximum certainty.'[25]

One useful aid in helping organise the many factors involved in skilled performance is to use a model of the human organism, as an information processing system,[4,15,17,24] whose channel capacity is limited. What this means is that not all the information to which the human being is exposed is processed as he attempts to solve problems which involve body movement. Much sensory information of both the internal and external environment impinges on the individual. Only a limited proportion of this is ever used.

Such models (Fig. 8.2) attempt to depict in a simplified form the chain of events leading from sensory input to motor action; showing how information about what is to be achieved, the task itself and the results from the performer's own actions, is integrated. How this information is used is dependent, in differing ways, on the functions of both long and short term memory. (This is not shown in Figure 8.2.)

Such models depict some of the functions presumably occurring in the nervous system. They are not meant to represent actual anatomical structures although certain parts of the model in Figure 8.2 such as sense organs and muscular system, are more anatomical in nature. There have been many models produced by different workers in this field which are variations on the same basic theme. Although differing in detail they include the following components:

1. A perceptual mechanism: which identifies and classifies sensory information in the light of past and present experience. Memory is important here.

2. A decision mechanism: which receives information via the perceptual mechanism and decides on a plan of action. This is done by searching the long term memory, where information has been stored in a more permanent form as a result of practice, in order to choose an appropriate response. This takes time – more time being necessary if there are more responses to choose from and the individual is less certain of the type of response

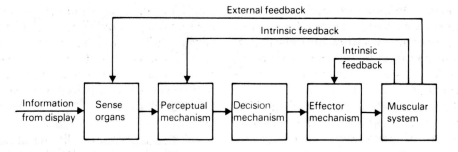

Fig. 8.2 The human information processing model. *Reproduced with kind permission from Marteniuk, R. G. (1975) Information processing, channel capacity, learning stages and the acquisition of skill. In Whiting, H. T. A. (Ed.) Readings in Human Performance. London: Lepus Books, p. 9.*

required. Such is the case with the novice performer. Through practice the time involved is lessened; just as through practice certain stimuli come to be matched with certain responses.

With the decision mechanism, information is processed sequentially.[23] If information arrives at too fast a rate so the mechanism cannot cope with it, subsequent information is held for a short period in short term memory after it has passed through the perceptual mechanism. It then moves on in an orderly sequence, when the decision mechanism is free to deal with it.

3. An effector mechanism: which uses the plan of action chosen by the decision mechanism to organise appropriate responses. This is done in the light of the goal being sought and specific environmental conditions. It sends the necessary motor commands to the appropriate muscles in correct sequential and temporal order.

4. A feedback mechanism: which feeds back information to the system about (a) the movements themselves while the performance is underway, called 'knowledge of performance' and (b) the effect the movement had on the environment called 'knowledge of results'.

Feedback allows the performer to compare what he planned to do with what he did. This forms the basis of his decisions concerning his next move.

The environment and skill

'Man moulds his movements to his environment'.[7] Different environments place variable demands on individuals. The environment contains much information, some of which is relevant to the performance of skilled movement for a task, whereas much of this information is not.

An individual needs to learn to selectively attend to those cues which are relevant, because of the human being's limited capacity to cope with too much information at any one time. What he decides to attend to will, in part, depend on many personal factors including expectations, preferences and past experience.

All his attention will be focussed on the feedback arriving from his own responses in the early stages of learning. Anything else happening in the environment will probably be ignored because his information processing capacity is already stretched to the limit. If at this stage he does allow his attention to wander to features in the environment which are not allied to the task, his performance is likely to be unsuccessful.

Through practice the individual learns to reduce the uncertainty of what cues he should be attending to for a successful performance. This lessens the attention demands of the particular skill, freeing him to attend to other environmental features while still performing skilfully.

This has relevance when considering the development of perceptual-motor skills in the very young. 'Catching a ball' is a complex skill for the young child, though relatively simple for the older child and adult. The young child's environment is less predictable to him because he has had such little experience comparatively about the results of his own performances within that environment. He is easily distracted. Experience is necessary to guide him as to the relevance of the many possible environmental cues with which he is confronted at any one time.[2,9]

Cues arising in the environment are said to be either 'fixed' or 'changing'.[16] When cues which are important for the performance of a skill are relatively fixed in one position, such skills are called 'closed skills'. For example, when an individual sitting at his desk reaches forwards to pick up a cup placed on the desk's surface, this would be classified as a closed skill. To some extent such an environmental situation limits the spatial organisation of the motor pattern – much the same groups of muscles being used each time he makes the attempt. Within this closed skill, the timing and the organisation of the motor pattern can still be varied widely. With practice, fixation of the motor patterns involved tends to occur.

An 'open skill' is one in which important

cues for performance constantly change, for example, when objects move through space such as a ball approaching a player in a game of tennis. Obviously an open skill is much more complex than a closed skill. With practice, a closed skill develops a fixed motor pattern. An open skill with practice, leads to the development of a larger repertoire. Practice ensures that the performer, in this case, will be able to cope with the many possibilities the environment may present to him. He will become more versatile in performing the skill in different circumstances.

It would be useful for the physiotherapist to attempt to classify skills as 'open' or 'closed' when planning treatment programmes. Both types should be represented in a fully rounded programme, because this more accurately reflects the real-life environment.

The organisational structure of skilled movement

In considering the organisation of skilled movement, it is useful to think in terms of a broad general plan or programme of action which guides the movements involved in achieving the goal. This plan would include the idea of what the purpose of the movement is, what stages are involved and how they are arranged.

For example, if an individual wants to throw a ball at a target, the thought of throwing the ball becomes the idea. The broad plan, 'throw a ball at the target' can be broken down into an ordered sequence (Fig. 8.3):

1. Grip the ball
2. Stance
3. Back swing of the upper limb
4. Forward swing of the upper limb
5. Release the ball
6. Follow through.

Each of these 'larger' stages in the sequence can then be broken down in turn into even more specific components.

Acquisition of perceptual motor skills

Skilled motor performance is developed through the process of learning. This process varies as the learner makes progress, for learning itself leads to changes in the structure of the skill being learned, as its various operations become increasingly refined through practice.

It is thought by some that all motor learning is over at a very early age, although this notion has not been proved conclusively. During the first four years individuals are said to acquire a repertoire of basic movements. These then become the building blocks for the more complex motor skills which are learned later by children and adults. It is thought that the learning of 'new' skills later on involves a recombination of these basic operations under a new broad plan or programme of action.

An optimal level of arousal, which is neither

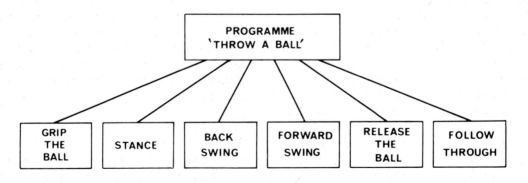

Fig. 8.3 The hierarchical and sequential organisation of motor skills. *Based on material used with kind permission from Marteniuk, R.G. (1975) Information processing, channel capacity, learning stages and acquisition of skill. In Whiting, H.T.A. (Ed.) Readings In Human Performance. London: Lepus Books.*

excessive nor inadequate, is considered necessary to prepare the individual to receive the information on which learning will depend. However, adequate arousal does not mean that he will automatically receive and process the correct information.

Learning a new perceptual-motor skill is considered to cover a number of phases. The three phases of learning suggested by Fitts and Posner[5] will be discussed here.

1. Early or cognitive phase. Here the learner attempts to identify and understand what is to be done as he develops a plan of action. Therefore early in the learning process he has to pay great attention to cues and events in his environment as well as to his own responses. For this reason, feedback is particularly important in helping him structure his future behaviour. In this manner he learns what information is most pertinent for the task in hand.

Because the emphasis in this early phase is on the learner deciding what to do much of his activity is said to be mental or 'cognitive'. For this reason, mental practice of the skill, rehearsing the moves to be performed in his mind before actually doing them is useful here, as are instructions and demonstrations by the physiotherapist. There is usually a large amount of improvement in performance in this early phase.

2. Intermediate or associative phase. Here there is a shift from what to do, to how to do it. Through practice, the movements required become established and errors are gradually eliminated. Those components of the skill which earlier were independent, become increasingly combined within an overall plan of action.

This phase, as in the early phase, lasts for varying periods of time depending on the complexity of the skill and the past experience of the learner.

3. Final or autonomous phase. This is an extremely advanced phase which some learners may never achieve. In this phase, the activity has become so well learned that the performer can now devote his attention to other events occurring in the environment without his performance being disturbed. His behaviour has become automatic.

Certain innate abilities of the learner may be more or less useful during the various phases of skill learning. It has been shown, for example, that sensitivity to exteroceptive (visuo-spatial) cues is critical early in the learning sequence, whereas sensitivity to proprioceptive cues is more important later on when some practice has already occurred.[6] Therefore, it could be argued that those individuals high in visuo-spatial abilities have an advantage in the earlier phase of learning but at the later phases this ability may not have such a strong effect on the eventual learning outcome.

Feedback

Learning cannot occur without information being supplied to the learner about the errors he makes when he performs the movements required. If errors are detected, this allows for corrections to be made at his next attempt.

Information that a performer receives about the performance of a skill, whether while he is performing it (knowledge of performance) or after the skill is completed (knowledge of results), is termed feedback.

Success as indicated by knowledge of results, does not necessarily mean that the performance has been skilful, for a goal still may be achieved through the use of a poor movement pattern.

Feedback is received through one or more of the sensory systems at any one time. Major sources are visual, auditory, vestibular, tactile or proprioceptive. This feedback which is available to the patient may be augmented through the physiotherapist's own monitoring skills and her response. Biofeedback provides another method of doing this.[1]

Feedback should be accurate in terms of direction and magnitude of the error that has been made. It should be a form of guidance given before additional attempts at the same movements are made. Feedback about the outcome of the movement should be given to the patient each time he attempts it, so that optimum learning can occur, for frequent feedback facilitates learning.

Through this type of physiotherapist-assisted practice the patient should develop his capacity to accurately detect his own errors, so at a later stage in the learning process this assistance can be withdrawn. It is important that this withdrawal does not occur before the patient has developed this capacity.

Principle of specificity

The skilled performance of any task reflects an unique combination of basic movement related factors, for example, perception, balance, flexibility, strength and so on. Some writers have suggested that those factors which are developed on one task do not necessarily transfer well to another task.[18]

Therefore, practice conditions should be as closely related as possible to the normal living demands of the activity, whether this is an activity of daily living, a work skill or sport. For example, when retraining gait after an injury, it is useful to practise walking in a variety of situations rather than relying solely on walking up and down a single track in the physiotherapy department. Ideally, participation in the activity itself is the primary way to develop the unique set or combination of movement abilities required. Therefore gait training should include the use of different supporting surfaces, slopes and stairs, as well as activities such as stepping up into a bus or crossing a road in any full rehabilitation programme.

Sometimes a physiotherapist is not able to apply this principle when treating patients, because their medical condition may make this an unsafe course of action at the time. Wherever possible, the physiotherapist, when designing treatment practice sessions, should try to simulate the desired conditions in which specific movement combinations will be required at a later date.

Practice

Learning of a perceptual-motor skill comes about through the repeated practice of the desired activity which leads to improvement of the specific abilities required.[13,14] Much practice is necessary to perfect these abilities – improvement being more obvious in the early stages of the learning period than later.[3]

Findings related to the simple manipulative skill of cigar making illustrate these points well. Evidence has been presented that indicates that only after two years and about three million repetitions of making individual cigars, can a worker's performance be called 'skilled'.[3]

Learning may never be completed for a specific task when one considers the improvement in performance of champion athletes, ballet dancers and concert pianists over careers spanning many years. This provides a hopeful basis on which to plan long-term programmes providing many practice opportunities for the more disabled members of the community.

A physiotherapy treatment session may be considered in many instances to be providing the opportunities for guided practice of the skills to be learned. As it is through practice that learning occurs, the more attempts of the desired movement that can be accomplished in each treatment session, with appropriate feedback, the greater the amount of learning that will take place.

There are two major ways of arranging practice periods and their accompanying rest pauses. These are termed:

1. Massed practice – when the length of the rest taken between the practice periods is less than the practice periods themselves.
2. Distributed practice – when the rest periods are relatively longer than the practice periods.

Learning usually depends on the number of times the activity is performed rather than these practice arrangements.[20,28] There are some situations where the use of massed practice does interfere with learning. These are important for the physiotherapist to consider because of the low level of skill that many of their patients possess when seen initially. These situations are when:

1. Massed practice leads to the performance dropping to such a low level that the risk of

further injury becomes unacceptable. This could be the case when patients are attempting to use crutches after a long period of bed rest.

2. The patient becomes excessively fatigued.

Control of movement and memory

Memory is important for skilled performance at a later date. Through learning, a motor pattern involving the timing and sequencing of its components becomes represented in the memory. This representation is called a motor programme. There is evidence that such central motor programmes can control the movements required for well practised skills, with little reference to peripheral feedback such as kinaesthetic information from muscles and joints.

Early in the learning process dependence on such feedback is much greater. This would explain why early attempts at performing a new skill are jerky, because each component operation involved has to be checked using feedback information before proceeding to the next operation in the movement sequence. More accomplished performers' movements are efficient and can be done with speed.

Writers in the field of motor control have tended to support either a central or a peripheral control theory of movement.[11] Evidence has been produced to verify both positions. More recent thought has suggested that perhaps a view which integrates both concepts would be much more productive for those seeking the truth about motor control.[8]

This idea may be illustrated by taking the skill of driving a car. Here, the pattern of limb movements would be considered as being controlled by a motor programme – a central control view; whereas the fine adjustments needed because of a changing environment would be considered as being controlled through feedback supplied to the system – a peripheral control view. The important point is that both ideas are necessary for explaining the skilled performance of driving a car.

Once well learned, perceptual-motor skills are highly resistant to forgetting. This factor becomes significant when physiotherapists are involved in retraining adults, particularly those with more severe forms of injury. There is probably still much stored about movement in long-term memory. This can be successfully exploited when attempting to acquire the necessary new motor programmes or improving those components of skill still remaining.

REFERENCES AND FURTHER READING

1. Basmajian, J. V. (Ed.) (1979) *Biofeedback – Principles and practice for clinicians.* Baltimore: Williams and Wilkins.
2. Connolly, K. J. (1977) The nature of motor skill development. *Journal of Human Movement Studies*, Vol. 3, pp. 123–143.
3. Crossman, E. R. F. W. (1959) A theory of the acquisition of speed-skill. *Ergonomics*, Vol. 2, pp. 154–165.
4. Crossman, E. R. F. W. (1964) Information processes in human skill. *British Medical Bulletin*, Vol. 20, No. 1, pp. 32–37.
5. Fitts, P. M. & Posner, M. I. (1967) *Human Performance.* Belmont, California: Brooks-Cole.
6. Fleishman, E. A. & Rich, S. (1963) Role of kinesthetic and spatial-visual abilities in perceptual-motor learning. *Journal of Experimental Psychology*, Vol. 66, No. 1, pp. 6–11.
7. Gentile, A. M. (1972) A working model of skill acquisition with application to teaching. *Quest*, Vol. 17, pp. 3–23.
8. Glencross, D. J. (1977) Control of skilled movements. *Psychological Bulletin*, Vol. 84, No. 1, pp. 14–29.
9. Kay, H. (1969) The development of motor skills from birth to adolescence. In *Principles of Skill Acquisition*, Bilodeau, E. A. (Ed.). New York: Academic Press.
10. Kelso, J. A. S. (Ed.) (1982) *Human Motor Behavior: an introduction.* Hillsdale, New Jersey: Lawrence Erlbaum Associates.
11. Kelso, J. A. S. & Stelmach, G. E. (1976) Central and peripheral mechanisms in motor control. In *Motor Control: Issues and Trends*, Stelmach, G. E. (Ed.), Chapter 1, pp. 1–40. New York: Academic Press.
12. Kelso, J. A. S. & Clark, J. E. (1982) *The Development of Movement Control and Co-ordination.* Chichester: John Wiley and Sons.
13. Kottke, F. J. (1980) From Reflex to skill: the training of coordination. *Archives of Physical Medicine and Rehabilitation*, Vol. 61, pp. 551–561.
14. Kottke, F. J., Halpern, D., Eastern, J. K. M., Ozel, A. T. & Burrill, C. A. (1978) The training of coordination. *Archives of Physical Medicine and Rehabilitation*, Vol. 59, pp. 567–572.
15. Marteniuk, R. G. (1976) *Information Processing in Motor Skills.* New York: Holt, Rinehart, and Winston.

16. Marteniuk, R. G. (1979) Motor skill performance and learning: considerations for rehabilitation. *Physiotherapy Canada*, Vol. 31, No. 4, pp. 187–202.

17. Posner, M. I. & Keele, S. W. (1973) Skill learning. In *Second Handbook of Research on Teaching*, Travers, R. M. N. (Ed.) Ch. 25, pp. 805–831. Chicago: Rand McNally and Co.

18. Schmidt, R. A. (1975) *Motor Skills*. New York: Harper & Row.

19. Schmidt, R. A. (1982) *Motor Control and Learning*. Champaign: Human Kinetics Publishers.

20. Stelmach, G. E. (1969) Efficiency of motor learning as a function of intertrial rest. *The Research Quarterly*, Vol. 40, pp. 198–202.

21. Stelmach, G. E. (Ed.) (1976) *Motor Control: Issues and Trends*. New York: Academic Press.

22. Stelmach, G. E. & Requin, J. (Eds.) (1980) *Tutorials in Motor Behavior*. Amsterdam: North Holland Publishing Company.

23. Welford, A. T. (1974) On the sequencing of action. *Brain Research*, Vol. 71, pp. 381–392.

24. Whiting, H. T. A. (1972) Theoretical frameworks for an understanding of the acquisition of perceptual-motor skills. *Quest*, Vol. 17, pp. 24–34.

25. Whiting, H. T. A. (1975) *Concepts in Skill Learning*. London: Lepus Books.

26. Whiting, H. T. A. (Ed.) (1975) *Readings in Human Performance*. London: Lepus Books.

27. Whiting, H. T. A. (Ed.) (1984) *Human Motor Actions. Bernstein Reassessed*. Amsterdam: Elsevier Science Publishers B.V.

28. Whitely, J. D. (1970) Effects of practice distribution on learning a fine motor task. *The Research Quarterly*, Vol. 41, No. 4, pp. 576–583.

9

The patient and disability

Health is a condition of well-being where all the interlocking systems relating the individual to his environment work together in harmony. It is taken for granted by many people. Sometimes this state may be disturbed by illness or trauma to one or more of the body systems which may lead to temporary or permanent disability. The disability may be one of movement and abnormal movement results.

Most patients are extremely distressed by any disability. Probably they have never appreciated how important their health is and have taken for granted their ability to function as they wished or needed.

The physiotherapist, through her specialised theoretical and practical knowledge and her expertise in the correction of abnormal movements, can help many of these patients. She can also attempt to prevent some further movement disorders by anticipating and ensuring that they do not occur. Usually she works with other professionals in attempting to achieve these goals.

It is necessary when working with these professionals that a common language is spoken and understood. Some of the terms used are defined in this chapter.

PATHOLOGY, AETIOLOGY, DIAGNOSIS, PROGNOSIS

Pathology is the abnormal physiology of a

particular tissue; aetiology is the cause. In some patients the pathology may show itself in terms of loss or abnormality of movement. This loss or abnormality of movement is most likely due to impairment of the structure of bones, muscles, joints, nerves, blood vessels, connective tissue and skin as well as the processes which control movement and provide energy for it. These pathologies may arise from a variety of causes – they may be acquired through injury or disease or they may be congenital. The abnormalities of movement which may be present are many and varied and may include some of those shown in Figure 9.1.

The physiotherapist most commonly treats patients of all ages with pathology involving the musculoskeletal, neurological, respiratory and cardiovascular systems.

Diagnostic labels enable the physiotherapist to gain some idea as to what type of movement disturbance can be anticipated in both the short and long term, as well as the possible limitations the condition may impose on the patient's response to exercise. It is important that an adequate diagnosis be made if treatment is to be planned rationally. For example, the diagnostic label of rheumatoid arthritis indicates that movement is most likely to be disturbed by pain and stiffness. It also indicates that care must be taken by the physiotherapist in planning and carrying out exercise treatment so that the extent and degree of such exercise is sufficient to be effective without causing further inflammation and pain.

The diagnostic labels and her own clinical assessment enable the physiotherapist to predict, to a certain extent, what should be achieved by the patient in both the short and long term. This is called the prognosis and it helps, together with the examination of the patient, to form a basis for planning by the physiotherapist and to give the patient a realistic sense of hope without deceiving him or his relatives.

However, the wise physiotherapist never forgets that even when the prognosis looks bleak many patients have remarkable reserves of courage and determination which may be used to confound early predictions. It is best to keep an open mind and encourage a realistic optimism.

DISABILITY, HANDICAP

Disability is the manifestation of the pathology involved, in terms of loss or reduction of functional ability. The type of disability occurring depends on the site and extent of the pathology as well as the part or parts of the body influenced by tissue damage. For example, the disability may include loss of

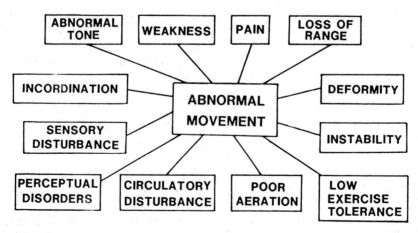

Fig. 9.1 Abnormalities of movement.

range and/or joint stability, decreased muscle strength, power, endurance, muscle balance and co-ordination, producing abnormal patterns of movement. There may be abnormalities of sensation and perception, memory and concentration, decreased or increased muscle tone and abnormal reflex activity. Decreased cardio-respiratory function may occur. Some disabilities may have widespread effects, for example a localised lesion in the brain such as a cerebrovascular accident (stroke) may have widespread effects involving paresis or paralysis of the whole of one side of the body.

The loss of function, with efficient care, may be temporary and reversible for many patients, who subsequently gain a full recovery. For others it may involve long-term treatment resulting in full independence for daily living, though with some limitations on their previous way of life. A lesser number may be left with a permanent or irreversible disability. In some pathological conditions disabilities increase as the condition progressively deteriorates. For example, the patient with a progressive and distressing long-term illness, such as emphysema, usually faces a downhill struggle with his general condition becoming progressively worse. He needs all the support that his family, friends and the medical profession can give him. The aging process itself creates loss of functional ability.

Most patients can manage all activities of daily living, though sometimes with a changed pattern. The child with a congenital deformity for whom early treatment is often not possible, may learn to make an amazing use of a severely deformed limb.

The age of onset is often an important factor to consider. Physical, intellectual, social and emotional growth may be retarded in the very young child because of some developmental disorder. In the very old, disease and injury may add to the functional limitations already present due to old age itself.

Handicap is defined as the disadvantage or restriction of activity caused by a physical, sensory or psychological impairment. A person who is disabled is not necessarily handicapped – much depends on the circumstances in which he finds himself.

The same disability may present a major handicap to one person, whereas to another the handicap may be minor if at all. For example, a concert pianist may be severely disadvantaged by a stiffened hand in his bid to return to the concert platform, whereas it would not stop a business executive from immediately resuming his occupation.

A person with a disability may be handicapped in some situations but not in others. Movement loss may produce dependency which will only show itself occasionally. For example, the business executive may still have to rely on others to perform certain tasks that he previously was able to do. Thus a knowledge of the patient's home and work situations is essential if relevant planning of the therapeutic exercise programme is to be done.

It is important to realise that many people, whether disabled or not, feel less than adequate when compared with others in certain situations – they are 'handicapped'.

People who are permanently disabled may become very disadvantaged physically, economically, socially, mentally and emotionally. Major barriers which can impose a handicap on even the most motivated person include financial, architectural, transport and educational ones as well as society's attitudes to the disabled. These very real barriers may limit a disabled person's social contacts, career opportunities and recreational activities. In this sense they place a handicap upon him compared with the able-bodied people in the community. His freedom of choice is limited.

THE PSYCHOLOGICAL AND EMOTIONAL REACTION OF THE PATIENT

The same physical impairment may cause varying degrees of emotional and psychological handicap. For example, one patient may make the best use of what function he has left, while another will be hesitant to use the disabled part and may never even use it to its best advantage. If trauma has occurred, neither the extent nor the functional result of the injury necessarily equates with the patient's psychological reaction to it. Often the circumstances under which the injury occurred and the cause of the injury have a bearing on the patient's reactions. For example, if he has been at fault he may have feelings of guilt and grief; if the poor conditions at his workplace were the primary cause, his feelings may be those of resentment, antagonism and aggression.

The question of compensation following an accident at work or on the road and the long delays often experienced in waiting for a settlement sometimes hinder the patient's will to work towards a recovery.

The patient's age may also influence his reaction. The older patient knows his freedom of choice of a job is lessened. He is also less able to change his occupation because of the additional functional limitations due to age itself as well as many employers' negative attitudes to the older worker. The young are often considered more adaptable and find other openings more readily.

The cosmetic appearance, the abnormality and obvious difficulty of function may also be a cause of grief, worry or shame. For example, a patient with a hand affected by injury or disease, may tend to hide it and be afraid to mix socially.

The emotional and psychological reaction which occurs in most people following an injury or during a long-term illness is often severe. They have a concept of loss and wonder why it should have happened to them. This is followed by a period of anxiety as the implications of the loss are realised. Disbelief, anger and fear are often observed. These effects may vary according to the personality of the patient, the disability suffered and/or his responsibilities.

Many patients may have severe bouts of depression and are apathetic and resentful so that their attitude for a certain time may be self-defeating. The reaction of a patient with a chronic condition, such as rheumatoid arthritis, is influenced by the fact that he may become weary and discouraged because of long-continued pain, often increasing general debility, the limited use of his limbs and their changing appearance, as well as seeing many around him in hospital clinics with worsening conditions. Likewise, following a stroke, the patient's inability to control his limbs fully, particularly his hand, may become a source of great frustration to him in adjusting to living. This realisation, coupled with the relatively poor prospects for full recovery of function, can prove overwhelming to him.

Usually over a period of time most patients learn to adjust to their disability and become determined to cope with their problem if full, careful, sympathetic explanations are made and positive advice and treatment are given. Emotional support from family and friends and often from other patients may help greatly. With treatment and time the patient generally realises his potential. This may be full recovery or, if he is severely disabled, a surprising adaptive capacity of the part of the body affected may be possible. A few patients do not accommodate, may lack motivation, become bitter and maximise their physical and emotional problems.

REFERENCES AND FURTHER READING

1. Anderson, E. (1973) *The Disabled Schoolchild.* London: Methuen.
2. Anderson, E. & Clarke, L. (1982) *Disability in Adolescence.* London: Methuen.
3. Blaxter, M. (1976) *The Meaning of Disability.* London: Heinemann.
4. Boswell, D. M. & Wingrove, J. M. (Eds.) (1974) *The Handicapped Person in the Community: A reader and source book.* London: Tavistock Publications for Open University Press.
5. Boswell, D. M., Jaehnig, W. B. & Mittler, P. (1975) *A Handicapped Identity.* In *The Handicapped Person in the Community, Units 1–3.* Milton Keynes: Open University Press.

6. Carver, V. & Liddiard, P. (Eds.) (1978) *An Ageing Population*. Sevenoaks: Hodder & Stoughton in association with the Open University Press.
7. Cone, J. C. P. & Hueston, J. T. (1981) Psychological aspects of hand injury. In *The Hand, Vol. 1*, Tubiana, R. (Ed.), Ch. 63, pp. 704–719. Philadelphia: W. B. Saunders.
8. Deaver, G. G. & Brown, M. E. (1945) The challenge of crutches – prescribing crutch gaits for orthopaedic disabilities. *Archives of Physical Medicine*, December.
9. Dunham, J. R. & Dunham, C. S. (1978) Psycho-social aspects of disability. In *Disability and Rehabilitation Handbook*, Goldenson, R. M. (Ed.), Ch. 2, pp. 12–20. New York: McGraw-Hill.
10. Hislop, H. J. (1976) The penalties of physical disability. *Physical Therapy*, Vol. 56, No. 3, pp. 272–278.
11. Jay, P., Livingstone, K. & Tudor, G. (1975) Aids for the physically handicapped and chronically sick. In *The Handicapped Person in the Community, Unit 7*. Milton Keynes: Open University Press.
12. Nichols, P. J. R. (1971) *Rehabilitation of the severely disabled, 2 – Management*. London: Butterworths.
13. Partridge, C. J. (1980) The Effectiveness of Physiotherapy. A classification for evaluation. *Physiotherapy*, Vol. 66, No. 5, pp. 153–155.
14. Rusk, H. A. & Taylor, E. J. (1953) *Living with a Disability*. New York: Blaikston Co.
15. Tooth, S. (1977) *Handicapped at Home*. London: Design Council.

10

The rehabilitation team

Rehabilitation involves the treatment and training of the patient so that he may obtain his maximal potential for normal living, physically, psychologically, socially and vocationally, in the shortest possible time. The emphasis is on improvement of the patient's capacity to function effectively and ensure an early patient take-over. The concepts and techniques are applicable to every phase of care of the acutely to the chronically disabled.

A team approach to treatment is often essential because of the severity of many of the conditions caused by injury or disease and the gross physical and psychological problems which can follow.

The team may be small or large. Its size depends on the type and extent of the injury or disease experienced by the patient as well as the immediate and long-term facilities available. For some patients with disorders of movement the team may consist of a doctor, therapist, family members and the patient himself. If the disability is more severe and long-term rehabilitation is necessary, many others are included in the team (Fig. 10.1).

The aim of treatment given by the team is to help the patient achieve his full potential. If improvement of the patient's disability is not possible it will involve maintaining and developing his remaining abilities. If the patient has a progressively deteriorating disease the aim will be to minimise its effects and make his life as active and comfortable as possible.

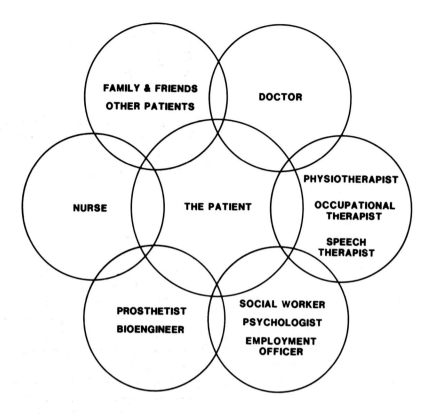

Fig. 10.1 The rehabilitation team.

Success is measured by how well the patient functions in daily life. This result is made easier if a closely integrated team with specialised knowledge, communication and technical skills works to help him.

The doctor guides the team regarding the extent of the injury or the severity of the disease, the surgical or medical treatment given and the prognosis. He discusses the aims of treatment with the patient and all those concerned with the treatment so that the team works as a whole with each member appreciating the work of the others.

The questions to be asked by team members are:

1. What does the patient want and expect from the treatment?
2. Is this considered possible?
3. Are the aims of both the patient and all team members the same so that they work

together with a positive attitude and a harmony of effort?

Regular team discussions allow team members to review progress and discuss common problems.

As treatment proceeds there usually will be a change in the relative importance of the part played by individual team members. The time for these changes needs to be recognised and accepted by all team members if the patient's rehabilitation is to proceed smoothly.

The patient in the team

The patient is helped greatly by a team approach when he can see members communicating and working together with a common purpose to aid his recovery rather than perhaps being treated by several individuals, however competent, who have no contact with other team members. The roles of the various team members need to be made clear to him.

Initially, the patient will be given information by the doctor about the extent of his injury or illness as well as the possible future steps in his treatment. As soon as possible an explanation is given to him by the other team members of the part they hope to play in his rehabilitation.

Therapists who may be involved in the treatment of the patient, sometimes over a long period, spend much treatment time with him and are often able to give appreciable help, gradually building up a good working relationship with him and helping him cope with some of his problems.

The patient's questions should be answered fully and truthfully and his part in the treatment plan stressed – he is a team member. He must be encouraged to become actively involved in the planning of his rehabilitation programme so that it is relevant to him.

The demands on the patient

The demands placed on the patient during his rehabilitation may vary greatly. Most patients want as full a recovery as possible and will work hard towards this end. Many recover fully and quickly. For others, particularly the heavily handicapped and the aged, the psychological, emotional and physical demands are heavy but most will work to gain the maximum possible recovery. A few may settle for less.

Motivation, which is important in most human behaviour, means the stimulation of an active interest through the provision of an incentive. For the patient this means an arousal; the incentive – his own recovery.

If the patient is to co-operate fully in the team he must be sure that the treatment is worthwhile. His abilities and physical capacity to improve are of little use to him unless he is motivated to work and has confidence in the people treating him. All members of the team will be involved to help the patient achieve the best possible result in his rehabilitation.

An all-out effort by the patient is needed if the fullest recovery is to be gained in the shortest possible time. He must have a knowledge and understanding of his own condition, the steps being taken to help him and his part in his own recovery. This should stimulate his interest and provide a challenge for him to respond. Encouragement will come from others but he must understand that voluntary effort on his part, provided the potential is there, will decide to a great extent the level of the recovery. Success will only come through consistent practice. Each success in achieving a goal will set a strong stimulus for him to continue to work.

Whatever the level of the disability, most patients are fearful, uncertain and anxious about their future. They fear the extent of their final handicap, pain, loss of job, perhaps the loss of independence, difficulties of meeting family and financial obligations and so on. These fears and anxieties must be understood by all in the team.

Many patients, particularly the more heavily handicapped, will need help in overcoming depression. This may require long-term counselling and sometimes psychiatric support.

Group support from others who have faced similar problems can provide help and stimulation for patients and their families and may be arranged by the rehabilitation team or through self-help organisations in the community.

Learning those skills which will help the patient cope with his present situation demands motivation, intense concentration and memorising if they are to be learnt quickly and thoroughly. Improvement of the patient's movement skills depends to a great extent on his knowledge of his own body and how and where it is placed in space so that he can know and can visualise what is happening. If the patient's previous pattern of movement can be re-established, his memory of past experiences and the advice from his therapist and family will help him decide whether his movement is correct or not. Constant practice is usually necessary if the corrected movement is to be retained.

The patient's task is much more difficult if a new pattern of movement has to be established because of limitations imposed by the extent of the injury or disease. He needs help to accept the necessity for change and to attempt to learn the new patterns required. The use of demonstrations, films and appropriate advice and physical help by the therapist as well as encouragement and support, particularly from other patients, can lead to success.

Adaptive measures may be necessary to aid in the patient's performance such as the use of special aids and appliances when the normal use of ordinary equipment is difficult. Their use can help the patient to attempt movements that he may have avoided because of his previous lack of success.

The patient's growth of understanding and his part in the planning give purpose and provide a stimulus to him to meet the demands placed on him to play an active part in his recovery by entering into his treatment programme with enthusiasm. Any improvement should be explained to him as this can help him develop a desire to succeed. He must come to appreciate that he will have to work consistently and hard if the abnormal is to become more normal and his function improved.

If the disability is so severe that a return to his own home is difficult, knowledge of self-care and the ability to do some productive work, even while he is in a home, a hospital or institution, are also worthwhile objectives. They affect the well-being of the person. They are also economically useful, in that personnel and operating costs of the institution or if the patient can return home, the cost of helpers in his home, are thereby reduced.

REFERENCES AND FURTHER READING

1. Beasley, R. W. (1981) *Hand Injuries*. Philadelphia: W. B. Saunders.
2. Bax, M. & Livingstone, K. (1975) The medical approach to handicap. In *The Handicapped Person in the Community, Unit 4*. Milton Keynes: Open University Press.
3. Evans, C. D. (1981) *Rehabilitation after Severe Head Injury*. Edinburgh: Churchill Livingstone.
4. Frazer, F. W. (1982) *Rehabilitation within the Community*. London: Faber & Faber.
5. Hunter, J. M., Schneider, L. H., Mackin, E. J. &
   Callahan, A. D. (1984) *Rehabilitation of the Hand*, 2nd edn St Louis: C. V. Mosby.
6. Illis, L. S., Sedgwick, E. M. & Glanville, H. J. (1982) *Rehabilitation of the Neurological Patient*. Oxford: Blackwell Scientific.
7. Kushlick, A., Blunden, R., Horner, D. & Smith, J. (1975) Goal setting. In *The Handicapped Person in the Community, Unit 9*. Milton Keynes: Open University Press.
8. Nickel, V. L. (Ed.) (1982) *Orthopaedic Rehabilitation*. New York: Churchill Livingstone.

11

The role of the physiotherapist

The physiotherapist may work as a clinician, educator, researcher, consultant and/or administrator. In this and the following chapters her role as a clinician is discussed. Intellectual, practical and interpersonal skills are necessary.

The physiotherapist, in fulfilling her clinical role, has a responsibility to the patient and the team to think through the nature of the patient's problems and form a reasoned judgement as to what is wanted, possible and acceptable to all concerned. Her theoretical and technical knowledge and practical abilities enable her to appreciate the possibilities available to the patient and envisage what may be done together with him and for him and then to set up and carry out a progressive treatment plan with skill and consideration and the co-operation of the patient.

A physiotherapist is needed who is a thinker, a problem-solver and at the same time a person who can put her knowledge to an essentially practical use. Good communication is essential as the therapist will work in close co-operation with the patient and other team members as well as the patient's family if this seems helpful and is approved by him.

The physiotherapist should have the ability to listen, gain an understanding of the patient's problems and respond to his queries by giving a clear explanation of her role and how she hopes to help him achieve the maximum possible function. Her interest, personal warmth and compassion should come through clearly to the patient as she talks with him. Her general appearance, facial expression and posture, as well as her energy and enthusiasm, will make an early impression for good or ill on the patient.

The patient is entitled to an explanation of the part to be played by him and by the physiotherapist in the total programme of the team as well as the short and long-term goals of his physiotherapy programme. For example, the significance of pain and oedema and the importance of early healing following trauma or surgery or of limited respiratory function in chronic airways disease, is explained to him. He should be given clear instructions on what to do and what not to do in aiding his recovery and should be made aware that much of the extent and speed of his recovery depends on his playing an active part in the treatment programme. Any improvement should be shown and explained to him as soon as it occurs. The therapist needs to help the patient build up his morale, give him the confidence so that he can help himself and motivate him to work towards his recovery. Her words should be clear and suitable to his level of understanding and her voice carry conviction.

Communication with the team

The physiotherapist must have a knowledge, understanding and appreciation of the work and responsibilities of the team as well as of how team members interact with each other, if she is to be an effective team member. She should contribute constructively by assisting in formulating the progressive programme of total management in consultation with the patient and the rest of the team, as well as by reporting regularly to the other team members on the patient's progress, static state or regression.

Immediate reporting to the team is essential if the therapist observes that the patient's condition has reached a plateau or if regression is occurring. This will allow for an immediate reappraisal of the treatment goals and the future contribution of the physiotherapist to the patient's programme.

Clinical problem-solving

In the examination, planning and carrying out of the treatment the therapist should develop the ability to collect relevant details from the patient and the team, to observe accurately and continuously, to recognise the normal as well as any abnormality of function and to select and carry out suitable tests. Details of the examination procedures are set out in Chapter 13. Following the examination she must be able to analyse and interpret the information she has collected, keeping in mind the likely prognosis as well as the present and future plans of the team. For some patients the original and possibly an ongoing cause of trauma, whether produced by an injury or following a disease such as rheumatoid arthritis, may be accentuated by the misuse of the body due to lack of knowledge, poor working habits or poor equipment, which may occur in the home, work place or sports field. This must also be investigated.

These processes form the basis of satisfactory planning which then can be undertaken in conjunction with the patient and other team members. During this planning the therapist must gain a knowledge of the total management programme and the likely result expected from the overall treatment given to the patient.

In planning an effective and imaginative exercise treatment for the patient, the physiotherapist is involved in a problem-solving situation. Problem-solving includes the identification of problems, the setting of short and long-term goals for the physiotherapy treatment and the steps necessary to achieve them. The patient must be involved in this planning so that the treatment is related to his needs and his interest gained. These goals need to be closely co-ordinated with those of other team members. This is particularly important if more than one therapist is involved in treatment so that the maximum co-operation is gained with minimal overlap – the one building on the work of the other.

Each step in the treatment programme must be carefully designed. Here the therapist is concerned with the 'thinking' process behind the selection of relevant and interesting tasks to be performed by the patient, any modifications including the 'breaking up' of these tasks and the suitability of the techniques to be used to bring about the desired result.

As she works the therapist collects and interprets information from and about the patient, selects and carries out appropriate treatment procedures and makes an appraisal of their effectiveness.

Teaching skills

Much of the success of treatment depends to a great extent on the physiotherapist's teaching ability. The specific purpose of any activity included in the treatment programme should always be explained to the patient and a clear demonstration given of the activity. These are useful teaching methods and help the patient learn more quickly. Activities need to be found in which the patient is interested and are appropriate to the stage of treatment. The use of a known skill is often helpful.

In these ways it is hoped to gain the patient's confidence, to give him the belief that he plays a major part in his own recovery and to motivate him to work. Any improvement occurring should be indicated to him as it provides positive feedback which should encourage him to work harder. The quality of his performance must be monitored continuously, with the speed of his recovery depending to a great extent on his playing an active part in the treatment programme and progressively taking over and increasing the scope of his activities. Progress should be continuously reviewed and treatment stepped up as soon as possible.

Practical competence

The practical competence of the therapist is necessary for a treatment to be fully effective.

It is 'thought in action' and a most important aspect of treatment. It implies that the therapist's knowledge of suitable handling techniques, the setting, teaching and supervision of suitable tasks and activities and the use of apparatus, is coupled with the ability to use them with skill, sensitivity, consideration and safety at the appropriate stage of treatment. It also implies that the therapist monitors the effects of these techniques and activities and modifies, changes or ceases them when necessary.

The use of the physiotherapist's hands

The provision of physical help to the patient is an important part of the physiotherapist's work. Her gentle, sensitive but firm hands, free from tension, can provide both physical and emotional help. They are a means of communication and a source of information to and from the patient. They can give comfort and reassurance and help promote a feeling of safety and security.

Her hands can play a definite role in the initial and continuing examination of the patient and aid in the diagnosis of movement problems. Working together with her eyes and ears, her hands – by their feeling touch – can help the therapist to collect information and to define more clearly areas of pain, the reaction of the tissues, the nature and area of swelling and abnormal muscle tone. They can help promote a knowledge of an abnormal pattern of movement and of the exact point at which difficulty occurs.

In treatment, her hands may work to ease pain, promote relaxation of the total body or its part, influence swelling, loosen soft tissues, mobilise joints, assist or resist movement or provide necessary joint stability. Her eyes and a good position of her head, neck and trunk will help give direction to the movement of her hands and allow them to work free of undue tension.

Physical help may be needed to make an action possible for the patient in an acceptable form. The therapist's hands may provide a stimulus to a movement by the patient if they are sensitively and correctly placed. Movement through range in a desired pattern can be illustrated by a relaxed passive movement. Then the physiotherapist helps to provide the initial stimulus to act by guiding, supplementing and reinforcing the movement at the point and time of need, so that the sequence and timing of the movement is correct and the patient knows the pattern and points of weakness. 'It is here the pull is to be.' A perception of correct movement is being given to the patient. As the treatment session proceeds this cycle of physiotherapist – patient interaction is repeated over and over again. Help is gradually withdrawn as progress occurs. This interaction is a skill and an art and provides a foundation for success. The process is illustrated in Figure 11.1.

A cold, limp, insensitive, indecisive hand or probing fingers can be destructive to movement. It can cause inhibition – a withdrawal by the patient.

Stretch and resistance to aid the development of strength are used as soon as possible. The aim is to promote a patient take-over and the therapist will vary the amount of assistance and resistance given accordingly.

The use of other stimuli in treatment

Effective treatment requires that the therapist uses visual, auditory, proprioceptive, tactile and vestibular stimuli to help the patient learn. They can be considered as therapeutic tools.

Vision helps the patient gain a knowledge of both his normal and abnormal movements. He may first watch a normal movement either of his own limb or a movement demonstrated to him. He then tries to reproduce this movement with his disabled limb. His memory of the feel of the normal movement will reinforce his visual picture. Associated movements of his eyes, head, neck and trunk will help to increase his knowledge of the normal as well as increasing stability. The use of a mirror as a temporary aid to help him follow a total movement, note its efficiency and make any improvement necessary, may prove helpful.

Sound is an effective stimulus. Words can be used by the therapist to stimulate or soothe a patient, to direct and shape his movements, to explain aspects of treatment and provide correction when necessary. The patient must listen and concentrate on the words addressed to him whether in explanation or direction. The words should be few, simple, carefully chosen and suitable to the patient's level of understanding. They should be clearly spoken so they are easily heard by the patient and, when possible, depict the action needed –

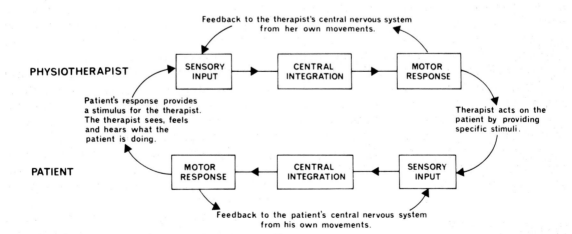

Fig. 11.1 The interaction between the physiotherapist and the patient. *Based on material and redrawn from Stockmeyer, S.A. (1972) A sensori-motor approach to treatment. In Pearson, P.H. & Williams, C.E. Editors Physical Therapy Services in the Developmental Disabilities. Courtesy of Charles C. Thomas Publisher. Springfield: Illinois.*

for example, lift, drop and relax, push and pull, stretch and squeeze. The tone should stimulate interest and be related to the desired effect. For instance, be brisk when a quick action is needed and slow and quiet for a relaxed movement. It should set the tempo for the movement.

Words can also be used by the patient to state his intentions before he performs a movement sequence and while it is under way, thereby enabling him to direct his own actions from within. This can help him as he attempts to learn a new skill or improve his performance.

Music can be used to help the patient improve the timing of his movements. Rhythmical movements done to music provide interest, relaxation or stimulation for many people and often arouse the memory of previously learned actions. Music may also add variety to a treatment.

Proprioceptive and tactile stimuli may be given by the careful use of the physiotherapist's hands as has already been discussed. The actual performance by the patient himself provides a rich source of proprioceptive stimulation as muscle and joint receptors respond to changes in length and load.

Vestibular stimulation arises from changes of head position. Head position is important in enabling the eyes and ears to be directed effectively to collect information. It is also important in influencing the alignment and tone of the rest of the body. The therapist should be aware that any activity, whether active or passive, involving motion of the head through space is providing vestibular stimulation to the patient.

All forms of stimulation can be used either separately or more often in combination with each other, to help the patient gain a knowledge of what is required of him. Similarly, correction of the patient's performance can be done in this way.

Growth of knowledge

As the physiotherapist works, a further specialised knowledge of normal and abnormal movement needs to be actively sought and steadily accumulated. It is important that any personal lack of knowledge or skill is recognised and steps taken to seek help and guidance. As her expertise grows she has the responsibility to share her knowledge with other physiotherapists and students. Her clinical experience will give relevance to her teaching.

Ongoing research into all aspects of physiotherapy is essential to ensure that current treatments being offered to patients are as effective as possible. Clinical trials, as well as the use of single case studies, are to be encouraged.

The therapist, through her understanding of the potential dangers of faulty posture and movement and their avoidance, has the capacity to advise many patients on how to avoid physical stress and accidents in the home, work place and on the sports field. This specialised knowledge of preventive medicine may lead to her working as a consultant to industry and educational and sporting bodies.

She also has an important social responsibility to foster positive community attitudes towards people who are disabled and be involved in increasing public awareness of their needs. This can be done at the individual level as well as through the skilled use of the mass media.

Some of the specialised basic body of knowledge necessary for effective physiotherapy includes knowledge of the:

1. Structure, function and control of the normal body
2. Movements of the body and how these are influenced by anatomical, physiological, mechanical, psychological and socio-cultural considerations
3. Many activities in which the body is used, varying from general daily living tasks to specific work and recreational skills, so that she can advise and treat her patients.

In addition to this knowledge of the normal, the physiotherapist must have a knowledge of and the ability to recognise:

4. An abnormal physical condition caused by trauma, disease or a congenital defect which can affect the body, the possible prognosis and the consequent emotional and psychological reaction of the patient
5. The medical and surgical procedures employed by the doctor and the work and contribution of other team members
6. Suitable tests which form part of the examination of the patient
7. The theoretical bases and the possible effects of the many techniques which can be used in treatment as well as the gaining of technical skill
8. The effects of disabilities involving other parts of the body which may profoundly, though indirectly, increase the disability currently being treated, for example, lack of vision or hearing, postural instability, low exercise tolerance, inco-ordination and poor local and general postural habits

as well as

9. A knowledge of the provision and of the fitting of certain suitable splints and the use of other equipment to help the handicapped person move more easily

and

10. The ability to recall clinical situations already experienced and to learn from these experiences.

Thus the gaining of technical skills which are an essential part of competent physiotherapy treatments can be built on a firm knowledge base.

Knowledge of one's own body

Knowledge can also be gained through an active, intellectual approach to the use of the therapist's own body. The therapist can apply this knowledge and the appreciation so gained, to aid her in the examination and treatment of her patients. It is suggested that she increases her awareness of the unique movements of her body and their sensory properties in different living and working situations by considering what her bodily movements mean to her as she explores their potential, analyses their functions and appreciates the growth of her own personal movement skills.

It is essential that she becomes aware of the:

1. Changing shape of her body when moving and at rest
2. Effect of vision and the influence of the head, neck and trunk position in facilitating the skilled use of her body in the many situations arising in daily life
3. Kinaesthetic sensations felt when a group of muscles act and the difference she feels when they are stretching, contracting or relaxing as well as the sensations produced by various joint positions
4. Differing aspects of delicate, light and heavy touch on her own body and on that of others and the dexterity, adaptability, versatility and strength needed in handling various objects
5. Use of her body in a wide variety of tasks so that the particular demands for skill, flexibility, stability and strength as well as the task's effects on the body's structure are understood
6. Changing sounds produced by light, heavy, even and uneven tread

as well as

7. Presence of environmental hazards in the treatment area, home and work place such as poor lighting, unsuitable floors, undue heat or cold and noise.

REFERENCES AND FURTHER READING

1. Anderson, T. McClurg (1951) *Human Kinetics.* London: Heinemann.
2. Currier, D. P. (1984) *Elements of Research in Physical Therapy*, 2nd edn. Baltimore: Williams & Wilkins.
3. Forster, A. L. (1975) Physiotherapy – a response to challenge. *Australian Journal of Physiotherapy*, Vol. XXI, No 4, pp 125–134.
4. Forster, A. L. & Galley, P. M. (1978) Assessment of professional competence: the clinical teacher's

responsibility. *The Australian Journal of Physiotherapy*, Vol. XXIV, No. 2, pp 53–59.

5. Hislop, H. J. (1975) The not-so-impossible dream. *Physical Therapy*, Vol. 55, No. 10, pp. 1069–1080.

6. Mennell, J. (1934) *Physical Treatment by Movement, Manipulation & Massage*, 3rd edn. London: J. A. Churchill.

7. Metheny, E. (1952) *Body Dynamics*. New York: McGraw-Hill.

8. N.U.S.T.E.P. (1967) An exploratory and analytical survey of therapeutic exercise. *American Journal of Physical Medicine*, Vol. 46, No. 1.

9. Ottenbacher, K. J. (1986) *Evaluating Clinical Change*. Baltimore: Williams & Wilkins.

10. Stockmeyer, S. A. (1972) A sensori-motor approach to treatment. In *Physical Therapy Services in the Developmental Disabilities*, Pearson, P. H. & Williams, C. (Eds.), Ch. 4, pp. 186–222. Springfield: Charles C. Thomas.

11. Watts, N. T. (1983) The privilege of choice. *Physical Therapy*, Vol. 63, No. 11, pp. 1802–1808.

12. Wolf, S. L. (1985) *Clinical Decision Making in Physical Therapy*. Philadelphia: F. A. Davis.

12

Efficient movement

The physiotherapist is concerned with helping patients to move more efficiently as they seek to achieve a desired goal.

The efficient performance of any voluntary activity depends initially on the concept the person has of the movement as well as his need and desire to do it. It is one that fulfills a specific purpose with economy of movement at the required speed and with the least expenditure of energy. Adequate strength, power, endurance, flexibility, stability and co-ordination are needed. The body adapts its posture and overall balance to suit the movement whether the movement is simple or complex, symmetrical or asymmetrical. Knowledge of the body's position in space, the judgment of distance, height, depth and path of the movement and the ability to adapt to quick changes are necessary for accuracy. The speed of the movement is set by the task and the person's movement abilities.

The ability to move and the quality of movement is governed by the efficiency of the control of the central nervous system. Adequate sensory information from the eyes and ears as well as tactile, vestibular and proprioceptive sources provide the necessary information to bring about movement. Emotions such as happiness give lightness to the movement; anxiety and fear cause unnecessary tension.

Movement patterns

When performing a purposeful movement a muscle never acts alone. Any active movement, whether simple or complex, involves groups of muscles which, acting with varying roles and intensity, co-operate with one another to produce a smooth rhythmical co-ordinated movement pattern. The pattern can usually be broken up into stages or phases of the total movement. The muscles, within or between these stages, form a rhythmical pattern suitable to the demands of the task.

As Wood Jones[20] writes in his book, *The Principles of Anatomy as Seen in the Hand*, 'to do an act of precision with the fingers, we call into play the prime movers of the action: the antagonists exert their regulating control to the utmost: the synergics prevent undesired actions of the prime movers. But as the business becomes more exacting fixation of the hand becomes necessary, fixation of the elbow may also be demanded and when all our attention is concentrated upon the performance of some very delicate act, which may require only one tiny muscle for its active performance, we may in fact have to employ a host of muscles for the immobilisation of parts, the movement of which would hinder the desired act.'

If the prime mover in a pattern is weak then an attempt will be made with any available muscle to produce the action or one that is as nearly as possible a substitute for it – a 'trick' movement occurs. Likewise if the range of movement of a joint taking part in the pattern is limited, other joints involved in the movement may increase their range to supplement the range of the affected joint.

The patterns of movement needed in daily life vary from person to person, depending on such things as age, sex, build, needs, occupation, interests and the culture in which the person lives. There are usually several ways to perform the same action and no two people move in exactly the same way.

A number of the features underlying efficient movement and their control can be identified (Figure 12.1).

It is important to recognise that functionally these features are interdependent as well as independent. They may be influenced by the patient's general health, nutrition and environment, as well as his genetic endowment.

When first learning any activity unnecessary muscles come into action and unwanted muscle tension occurs which may hinder the accuracy of the movement. This excess activity must be eliminated. If the person can visualise the form and learn the feeling of the correct movement, learning time can be reduced and an efficient movement pattern developed with practice. Versatility and rhythmic quality is gradually acquired with experience. The skill with which similar movements are carried out varies according to a person's movement abilities, dexterity, eye–hand co-ordination, motivation, training and general physical fitness.

ACTIVITIES

The needs for daily living

Most people wish for the ability to be independent, to move freely in many directions and to have the skill, strength and endurance to carry out the various activities of daily living and to enjoy recreation. Certain functions are common and necessary to all individuals. All want the ability to communicate, to be independent in toilet care, dressing and eating, to move from lying to sitting to standing, to get from place to place by walking or using some form of transport. They also want the ability to handle the many gadgets that go to make for comfort and convenience in modern living, for example, the telephone, switches, keys and so on. Socio-cultural differences can be clearly seen in the patterns of many of these activities.

When participation in daily work is considered the variations are enormous. A person may be involved in heavy or light manual labour, a sedentary occupation or in tasks involving a high level of manipulative skill. Some people, such as the housewife, will have both light and heavy duties. Just as there are differences in work load, so there will

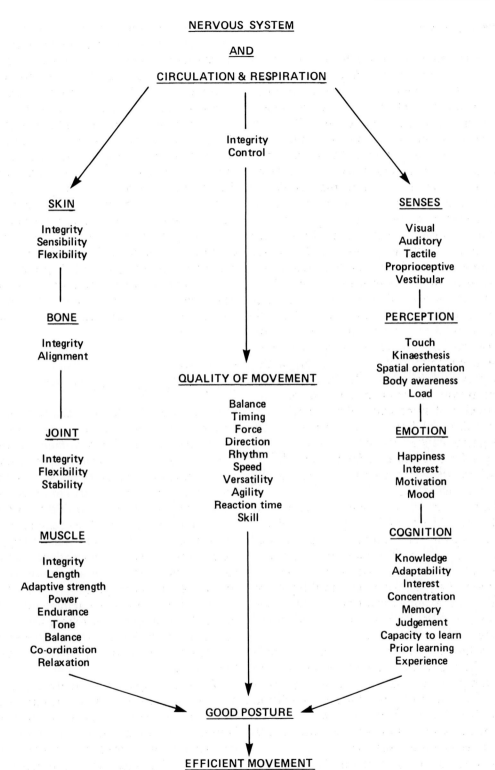

Fig. 12.1 Elements which may contribute to produce an efficient movement.

be individual differences in fitness, skill and the capacity to work.

All people need occupation of some kind or they tend to deteriorate mentally and physically. For many people in daily life the constant, varied and necessary movements involved in various activities of living, work and recreation, keep the body in a condition to cope with everyday needs. Joints are regularly moved, muscles contract, relax or stretch according to the demands of the movement and work is done. The circulatory and respiratory systems are stimulated to maintain fitness. Some people with sedentary occupations who take little physical exercise are often unfit.

Activities may be primarily:

1. Supportive, involving posture, general and local stability, ease of adjustment and the setting up of a position of readiness for movement – for example, standing or sitting and reaching for, grasping and holding an object.
2. Dynamic, involving movement of the body and its parts and the character, quality, direction and level of movement, for example, walking or swimming. Dynamic activities may also involve the giving and receiving of a force as, for example, in throwing and catching a ball.
3. Manipulative, involving grasp and release and the many diverse skilled movements of the hands, for example, doing up buttons on a shirt.
4. Protective, involving muscles acting as guardians of the body by reacting to an abnormal force which could cause injury or discomfort. Such reactions are often automatic.
5. Fitness promoting, where regular participation in sport or similar physical activities is undertaken for enjoyment and to maintain or improve health.

After injury or disease, movements become less efficient. The amount of activity which is eventually possible will depend on the extent of disability, the length of time following the onset of the disability before treatment is started and the treatment given, as well as the patient's motivation to be active.

GENERAL CLASSIFICATION OF MOVEMENT

Movements used in treatment can be classified depending on whether the physiotherapist or the patient primarily provides the driving force necessary to produce the required movement.

These movements may be active or passive.

1. Active movements may be sub-divided into:
   (i) Free active movement – used by the patient to overcome the effects of gravity, for example, rising from lying to sitting.
   (ii) Resisted active movement – used by the patient to overcome the effects of a manually or mechanically applied force, for example, lifting a load, closing a door, using a knife and fork, or digging using a spade.
   (iii) Assisted active movement – helped by an assisting force applied by the physiotherapist or in some cases the patient or by the use of apparatus such as sling suspension. For example, the physiotherapist may support the weight of the limb by her hands or suspend it in a sling or the patient may provide self-assistance to aid the movement of his weak limb.
   (iv) Assisted-resisted active movement – helped by an assisting force applied by the physiotherapist or the patient through that part of the range which is weak and resisted through the remainder. For example, in the case of a patient with a weak quadriceps who is unable to perform the last few degrees of knee extension, the physiotherapist may resist knee extension through most of the range but assist it as full knee extension is approached.

The type of muscle contraction which occurs in active movements may be:

   a. Dynamic – (isotonic; isokinetic)
      – concentric (shortening)
      – eccentric (lengthening)
   b. Static – (isometric).

2. Passive movements are those produced by an external force during muscle inactivity. All joint movements can be performed passively by manual means.

   They may be either:

   (i) A slow, steady, rhythmical, relaxed movement carried out by the physiotherapist or the patient which may be stopped by the patient

  or

   (ii) A single thrusting movement carried out by the physiotherapist which is sudden and of short duration and cannot be stopped by the patient.

3. Accessory movements are those movements which cannot be performed actively in the absence of resistance. Although not controlled voluntarily, they are important if the joint is to function normally.

There are two types:

   (i) Accessory movements which become apparent when resistance is applied. For example, the metacarpophalangeal joints rotate when a tennis ball – a resistance – is grasped.

   (ii) Accessory movements which can only be performed passively, for example, when one attempts to pull the proximal phalanx of the index finger distally, by distracting it from the second metacarpal or when performing 'joint mobilisations' as described by Mennell[16], Cyriax[8], Maitland[14,15], Grieve[11].

REFERENCES AND FURTHER READING

1. Anderson, T. McClurg (1951) *Human Kinetics*. London: Heinemann.
2. Barlow, W. (1973) *The Alexander Principle*. London: Victor Gollancz.
3. Basmajian, J. V. (Ed.) (1984) *Therapeutic Exercise*, 4th edn. Baltimore: Williams and Wilkins.
4. Broer, M. E. & Zernicke, R. F. (1979) *Efficiency of Human Movement*, 4th edn. Philadelphia: W.B. Saunders.
5. Buchwald, E. (1952) *Physical Rehabilitation for Daily Living*. New York: McGraw-Hill.
6. Buchwald Lawton, E. (1963) *Activities for Daily Living*. New York: McGraw-Hill.
7. Carlsöö, S. (1972) *How Man Moves*. London: Heinemann.
8. Cyriax, J. (1977) *Textbook of Orthopaedic Medicine – Vol. 2. Treatment by Manipulation, Massage and Injection*, 9th edn. London: Cassell.
9. Gardiner, M. D. (1963) *The Principles of Exercise Therapy*, 3rd edn. London: Bell & Hyman.
10. Grandjean, E. (1975) *Ergonomics in the Home*. London: Taylor and Francis.
11. Grieve, G. P. (1981) *Common Vertebral Joint Problems*. Edinburgh: Churchill Livingstone.
12. Hollis, M. (1981) *Practical Exercise Therapy*, 2nd edn. Oxford: Blackwell Scientific.
13. Kendall, F. P. & McCreary, E. K. (1983) *Muscles, Testing and Function*, 3rd edn. Baltimore: Williams & Wilkins.
14. Maitland, G. D. (1977) *Peripheral Manipulation*, 2nd edn. London: Butterworths.
15. Maitland, G. D. (1977) *Vertebral Manipulation*, 4th edn. London: Butterworths.
16. Mennell, J. (1934) *Physical Treatment by Movement, Manipulation and Massage*, 3rd edn. London: J. A. Churchill.
17. Muybridge, E. (1955) *The Human Figure in Motion*. New York: Dover Publications.
18. Oborne, D. J. (1982) *Ergonomics at Work*. Chichester: John Wiley & Sons.
19. Williams, P. L. & Warwick, R. (1980) *Gray's Anatomy*, 36th edn. Edinburgh: Churchill Livingstone.
20. Wood Jones, F. (1941) *The Principles of Anatomy as seen in the Hand*. London: Baillière, Tindall & Co.

13

A general outline of the examination of a patient

A thorough preliminary examination of the patient must be made by the physiotherapist to collect facts on which to base treatment. The examination processes cover five main areas, namely, the ability to question thoughtfully, to observe carefully, to palpate sensitively, to test in a purposeful and systematic manner as well as the competence to carry out the whole examination with care and consideration for the patient. These are skills that must be acquired if the maximum amount of information is to be obtained about the patient and his condition. The fundamentals of the examination remain the same though the type of questions asked and the testing procedures selected will vary depending on the patient, his condition, the particular local or general area involved and his needs.

In the examination the physiotherapist is faced with a problem-solving situation in which her knowledge of the normal and abnormal in structure, function and behaviour as well as of individual differences is put to practical use. One of the best ways of learning to examine a patient is to watch a skilled physiotherapist or doctor examine a patient either in the examination room or on videotape.

Examining will be a slow process at first but once a system is developed by the therapist, speed will increase without affecting accuracy.

Medical history and diagnosis

Most patients are referred to a physiotherapist by a doctor. The medical history, the diagnosis and prognosis together with results of tests and X-rays should be studied by the physiotherapist and all features relevant to the physiotherapy treatment noted before the patient is seen.

Preparation for the examination

Ideally the examination room or screened cubicle should be warm, light and quiet, so that the patient's privacy and comfort are ensured and the therapist's work aided. It should be large enough so that all necessary movements can be carried out and observed. The room should contain a firm treatment table of adequate size which can be approached from both sides. All relevant equipment should be in the room so that the examination can proceed smoothly without interruption.

THE PHYSIOTHERAPY EXAMINATION

The approach to the patient

The initial approach of the physiotherapist to the patient is most important. She will greet the patient by name, introduce herself and explain her role. Her approach should be warm and friendly and her manner inspire confidence to set the patient at ease. Her consideration for the patient's comfort at the start of the session will be appreciated by him. Such factors help to form an understanding on which co-operation can be built. Therapy begins here.

Following the initial introduction, if the patient is not already suitably clothed for the examination, he should undress sufficiently in the dressing room so that all relevant parts of his body can be clearly seen. The patient is watched carefully from the moment he enters the room. His general appearance, his facial expression, whether he looks ill or well, any abnormal posture or movement as well as his gait are noted.

Questioning the patient – the subjective examination

The physiotherapist should develop the ability to question, listen with understanding, respond and remember. The way her questions are posed is important. The object of the questions is not to lead the patient but rather to let him tell his story in his own way. For example, 'Why did you go to the doctor?'; 'What is worrying you most at this time?'.

The therapist should listen to the patient's account of his disability and how it affects his life-style. A knowledge of his living, work and recreational needs should be gained and present problems spelt out. The story of a typical day in the patient's life may be most useful.

The examination processes of questioning, observing, palpating and testing often go hand in hand. Each provides pointers for further examination. This is well illustrated when an attempt is made to gain a full picture of the pain suffered by the patient.

Pain is often the symptom which prompts the patient to seek professional help. Therefore it is important that the story of the pain is known by the therapist. 'Where is the pain – does it spread? What type of pain is it? Is it mild, acute or severe? Does it vary in severity? Is it constant or intermittent – where and when does it occur – what aggravates it and what relieves it? Is it getting better or worse – or has it remained the same? Have you ever had it before?' and so on.

Observing the patient's hands as he describes the pain is often a useful guide. For example, he may use his whole hand to indicate a generalised pain, point with his index finger for localised pain or jab it for a stabbing pain.

The area of pain and the contour of the part will be observed for signs of inflammation. Then the therapist proceeds to palpate the painful area, feeling for changes in temperature and tissue texture. With the muscles in the area relaxed, the therapist works from the perimeter towards the painful area which should be located with the palm and border of the hand and then sensitively palpated. Her hands should be warm, firm but gentle and the pressure light and not cause pain. If the skin is movable it should move with the fingers. Painful prodding with the fingers should be avoided.

Other questions will arise as the examination proceeds and the therapist will be able to capitalise on what she has already learnt from the medical records.

Observing and comparing – the objective examination

The ability to observe is a key factor in both the examination and treatment of the patient. To observe accurately requires practice and experience. Later it becomes easier. A basic rule in examining patients is to look before you touch.

A systematic routine helps to make observation more orderly and report writing easier. Brief notes can be taken as the examination proceeds and expanded later when the full examination is recorded. It is necessary that the therapist develops a good visual and verbal memory.

It is easy when a medical diagnosis is known to 'look for' what could be considered probable. It is important that the therapist learns to first 'look at' the patient, see, understand and be able to describe what is there, rather than to 'look for' what could be considered probable from the medical diagnosis.

During the examination, the patient's body and limbs must be correctly aligned so they can be seen and compared both at rest and in movement. A comparison can be made between both sides of the body if one side is normal but if both sides are affected, for example, following injury to both lower limbs, a comparison will be made with a known normal.

The body contours, colour, skin condition, presence or absence of muscle wasting, oedema and scars are all noted.

The patient will then be asked to show what he can do and attempt what he finds difficult or impossible to do.

Disturbances of function

The physiotherapist observes the patient's movements and notices any disturbances in their patterning and execution as well as those movements he avoids doing. To help her do this it is useful to look for such clues as:

1. The effect of pain and/or oedema on the movement
2. An abnormal posture
3. The loss of the normal sequencing and timing of the movement – lack of co-ordination
4. A disturbance in the grading and intensity of the movement
5. Inappropriate speeds of the body segments being moved
6. The presence of abnormal reflex activity
7. Any disturbance of balance
8. Undue fatigue.

The presence of such clues will assist the physiotherapist to further direct the examination. The physiotherapist's hands will be used sensitively to feel the affected part to confirm and expand on those observations she has already made and so help determine the movement problem.

Disturbances of a motor pattern may be due to many factors which often functionally overlap. These factors include: (i) pain; (ii) oedema; (iii) muscle weakness; (iv) loss or excess of joint range; (v) decreased or increased muscle extensibility; (vi) lack of mobility of soft tissues; (vii) loss of sensation; (viii) poor endurance; (ix) poor balance; (x) poor cardio-respiratory function; (xi) abnormal perception; (xii) abnormal reflex activity; (xiii) disturbances of muscle tone; (xiv) poor concentration or understanding; (xv) poor motor memory; (xvi) poor motor planning; (xvii) fear, anxiety and other psychological factors.

Where no injury or disease is apparent, the patient's general and local habitual posture should be investigated for clues as to the cause of his movement dysfunction and appropriate tests carried out.

Testing procedure

During the assessment the therapist will perform a series of quick tests to give her a general appreciation of the patient's functional abilities and provide her with pointers towards more specific tests which need to be done.

Many testing procedures are available to the physiotherapist to enable her to extend her knowledge of the patient. Some of these tests rely on the therapist's observation and manual skills whereas others require sophisticated instrumentation. Wherever possible, tests that provide an accurate measurement should be used and recorded.

A description of some of the most common tests used by physiotherapists is given in Appendix 1.

Whatever test the physiotherapist chooses to use, five factors must be considered. These are that:

1. The patient has an understanding of the test and its purpose
2. The tests are appropriate
3. Testing methods are accurate and done with skill, consideration and sensitivity
4. Modifications are made if necessary
5. The results are correctly interpreted.

Duration of the examination

If the examination is a complex one as in the case of some neurological disorders or if the patient is easily fatigued, sessions over two or three days may be necessary for the preliminary examination.

Examining is basically a continuous process. On a day-to-day basis as the physiotherapist treats, she examines. This continuous examination means that treatment may be stepped up or modified quickly as the physiotherapist is alerted to change. There is usually something more to be learned every day from the patient.

Recording and reporting

A record of the findings of the total examination should be made. It must be accurate, clear, brief and systematically set out. Technical language should be used. The use of diagrams and photographs may be included where appropriate. The record should be dated, signed and filed and be readily available.

Retesting should be done regularly and any necessary changes in the patient's status and treatment recorded. These records form the source for those written and verbal reports given from time to time to the patient's doctor and others who may be concerned with the patient.

The physiotherapist when reporting either verbally or in writing should be able to give a clear, accurate and brief description of what the patient has achieved, still cannot do and wants to do, as well as being able to discuss future plans for treatment.

Problem-solving

Once the examination is over and the recording is completed, the physiotherapist examines the findings, analyses and determines the problems and their cause in the light of her own knowledge, the probable medical prognosis and any requests by the doctor.

Priorities in treatment will be set in the light of the essential features of the patient's abilities and disabilities.

The questions to be answered following the examination are:

1. What are the present problems?
2. What is the most urgent problem at this time?
3. What is the best way to overcome the problems?
4. What abilities are present that can be put to immediate use?

She can then decide which physiotherapy procedures are necessary to help the patient and link them, when possible, with his daily routine, as well as integrate them with the work of the rest of the team.

Self-appraisal

At the end of the examination, the physiotherapist analyses how she has performed. Feedback from other staff may be possible and useful. A videotape of her performance, if the patient is agreeable, is a most useful method of self-appraisal and can form the basis for discussion with an experienced staff member.

REFERENCES AND FURTHER READING

1. Chance, A. E. & Humphries, D. A. (1967) Medical students' power of observation. *British Journal of Medical Education*, Vol. 1, pp. 131–134.
2. Cyriax, J. (1978) *Textbook of Orthopaedic Medicine – Vol. 1*, 7th edn. London: Baillière, Tindall and Cassell.
3. Forster, A. L. & Galley, P. M. (1978) Assessment of professional competence: the clinical teacher's responsibility. *The Australian Journal of Physiotherapy*, Vol. XXIV, No. 2, pp. 53–59.
4. Hoppenfeld, S. (1976) *Physical Examination of the Spine and Extremities*. Norwalk: Appleton Century Croft.
5. Johnson, M. L. (1955) Observer error, its bearing on teaching. *Lancet*, August 27, pp. 422–424.
6. Kendall, F. P. & McCreary, E. K. (1983) *Muscles, Testing & Function*, 3rd edn. Baltimore: Williams & Wilkins.
7. Macleod, J. (1979) *Clinical Examination*, 5th edn. Edinburgh: Churchill Livingstone.
8. Mainland, D. *Anatomy – Medical Students Series*. London: Hamish Hamilton Medical.
9. Mason, S. & Swash, M. (1980) *Hutchison's Clinical Methods*, 17th edn. London: Baillière Tindall.
10. McCrae, R. (1983) *Clinical Orthopaedic Examination*, 2nd edn. Edinburgh: Churchill Livingstone.
11. Parry, A. (1985) *Physiotherapy Assessment*, 2nd edn. London: Croom Helm.
12. Wolf, S. L. (Ed.) (1985) *Clinical Decision Making in Physical Therapy*. Philadelphia: F. A. Davis.

14

An exercise programme

The physiotherapy programme should be positive and interesting to the patient. It aims to regain the fullest possible function having regard to the nature of the injury or disease affecting the patient. The programme will be strongly directed towards ensuring a patient 'take-over' and closely co-ordinated with that of the overall rehabilitation team so that time is used economically. Treatment to be effective, should start at the optimum time, be competent, provide for continuity of care when necessary and be acceptable to the patient.

Therapeutic exercise, which forms a major part of most physiotherapy programmes, may be defined as the use of active bodily movements in the treatment of the patient. It may include individual movements of joints and muscles if they are indicated as well as graduated training for many of the activities involved in daily life. It is often used in conjunction with other physiotherapeutic modalities. In this chapter only the therapeutic exercise programme will be discussed.

Some of the processes involved in a progressive physiotherapy exercise programme as well as some of the outcomes which are desirable for the patient are summarised in Figure 14.1.

When planning a progressive exercise programme, the physiotherapist is faced with a problem-solving situation. The diagnosis and prognosis as well as the patient's level of activity before the onset of his disability need

THE THERAPIST　　　　　　　　　　　　　　　　THE PATIENT

Performs an effective examination　　　　　　Communicates needs, desires and
Analyses the data　　　　　　　　　　　　　　　fears to the therapist
Establishes long and short term goals　　　　Acquires knowledge of the
Selects appropriate treatment　　　　　　　　　condition
　procedures　　　　　　　　　　　　　　　　　Acquires knowledge of what to do
Selects challenging projects　　　　　　　　　　and what not to do
Designs effective independent　　—— EFFECTIVE→ Becomes motivated to work
　'home' programmes　　　　　　　← FEEDBACK—— Receives encouragement
Communicates effectively with the　　　　　　Gains confidence in himself and
　patient and team members　　　　　　　　　　those treating him
Cooperates with other team members　　　　Cooperates with those treating him
Corrects effectively
Reassesses and reports regularly
Replans when necessary
Ensures a patient takeover
Provides encouragement

TREATMENT OUTCOMES

Relief of pain
Control of oedema
Prevention of further damage and disability
Regaining of
　strength
　power
　endurance
　stability — balance
　flexibility
　co-ordination
　sensory awareness
Normalization of tone
Improved cardio-respiratory function
Reconditioned skin
Development of motor skills
Improved perception
Improved morale and patient satisfaction.

FUNCTIONAL USE

Fig. 14.1 Clinical problem-solving.

to be considered. A thorough examination forms the basis of an effective plan of treatment as it allows the problems to be identified. What is it the patient can do, cannot do, wants to do and why is he unable to do it?

The physiotherapist has the responsibility of analysing in detail the patient's movement problems. She assesses what components of efficient movement are present or absent, the effects of the present malfunction and the possible potential for improvement.

Planning, in which the patient plays an important part, is concerned with the setting of priorities, of short and long-term goals and the possibilities for any immediate improvement in his functional abilities. Using this framework the physiotherapist can plan a series of progressive programmes in which therapeutic exercise plays a major part.

The overall aims in planning an exercise programme are to:

1. Motivate the patient and improve his morale
2. Relieve symptoms, particularly pain and oedema if present
3. Regain all possible function
4. Provide a foundation to forward planning
5. Set up a programme for independent work
6. Note any restrictions, either local or general, placed on the planning as well as any special precautions
7. Prevent, if possible, further disability
8. Maintain or improve all unaffected function
9. Maintain or gain general physical fitness.

It is necessary to find the quickest method, acceptable to the patient, of gaining the greatest possible return of function with minimum energy cost in the shortest possible time.

The physiotherapist will consider the value of different approaches to exercise therapy for the patient and her personal skills in their use.

It will be a matter of selecting, testing and using various activities and methods of regaining effective movement, so that their worth for the patient can be established. These activities, may be carried out by the patient alone or with the help of the physiotherapist and/or equipment.

An effective exercise programme involves the treatment of the 'whole' patient, not just the local condition. In this way all possible functional ability is gained and poor movement habits eliminated. If the final result is to be satisfactory, the exercise programme must be co-ordinated with other physiotherapy measures and with the overall rehabilitation plan. Thus time is used economically and the frustration for the patient of unnecessary overlap in treatment is avoided.

The exercise programme, planned around the needs of the patient, should be inter-esting, stimulating and demanding of his concentration. Its purpose and the relevance of the individual exercises should be explained and understood by him.

The first priorities are to ensure the easing of pain and reduction of oedema if present, both of which inhibit active movement, as well as the encouragement of the use of any remaining function that can be carried out with safety.

In any plan, a variety of dynamic and purposeful activities is needed. Priorities, key positions and essential activities should be stressed again and again and in different ways if possible throughout the programme to bring out all the characteristics of movement necessary. Simple movements may be needed in the early stages to help gain efficiency, changing to more complex movements as control grows. Each activity will place unique demands on the starting position, muscles and joints.

Often the quickest way of training for any activity is the use of the activity itself. However, this is often not the most effective and quickest way of regaining overall function. Because of the uniqueness of each activity and the versatility of action necessary for the average patient, it is essential to ensure that all joints are moved in all directions through the available range and all muscles worked both dynamically and isometrically. In this way common movement components will be gained providing the foundations for many activities. The greater the emphasis placed on normal everyday activities, the greater the level of patient participation will be, as once learned they can be carried over into everyday life.

The ingenuity and imagination of the therapist and her wide repertoire of exercises will help to build a relevant and stimulating programme for the patient, which incorporates where possible, his own particular needs and holds his interest. The use of simple equipment, similar to that available in the home or related to his work or recreation, also adds interest and incentive and aids in the formulation of a home programme.

All programmes start with a few general

warming up exercises, gradually progressing to more difficult activities, with the exercises adjusted continuously to the changing levels of strength, flexibility, co-ordination and endurance of the patient.

A programme of independent activity which the patient can do throughout the day, will be established as soon as possible. It should be relevant, well taught, checked and progressed regularly.

How long and how often an activity should be done is a matter for the judgment of the physiotherapist. No activity demanding concentration and skill should be carried to the point of fatigue for other work is to follow. Once the efficiency of a movement lessens, it is usually an indication to change to another movement preferably in another part of the body and return to the previous movement later.

Brief periods of rest will increase efficiency. Rest implies freedom from action. The alternation of work and rest is a normal process. A change of position – standing and stretching – or a change of muscle and joint work, may provide relief.

An established skill may sometimes be used to produce a useful basis for the retraining of a lost function.

A few general conditioning exercises are helpful in any programme. They may be done in the form of circuit training and once learned demand minimum supervision although they must be constantly checked and upgraded.

Planning of the programme is a continuing process as exercises are progressed, modified, added to or discarded.

It is useful for the therapist to write down her exercise plan as this will quickly show her where emphasis is being placed and if anything is being omitted. This habit of planning on paper is also useful when the time comes to review the programme. A review should be done regularly and the questions to be answered include:

1. What has been achieved?
2. Is a measurement of achievement possible?
3. Have the aims altered?
4. What features must be added to or removed from the programme?

The psychological, physiological and mechanical demands of the programme need to be carefully assessed so that the patient works to the maximum that is possible for him at any one time.

THE CHOICE OF AN ACTIVITY

The factors to be considered in the selection, formation and analysis of an activity are complex. They include:

Psychological factors:
1. The patient's idea of what activities he needs and how they should be performed
2. His motivation to work.

Anatomical and physiological factors such as the:
1. Necessary painfree range required
2. Varying types and gradation of muscle action needed
3. Muscular and skeletal stability to hold the position
4. Strength, endurance and skill required
5. Sensory and motor components necessary to control the movement
6. Integrated joint and muscle action to carry out the activity accurately
7. Necessary sequence, timing, speed and rhythm to ensure a smooth economical performance.

Mechanical factors such as:
1. The magnitude of the muscle forces involved
2. Gravity and friction
3. Momentum
4. Conditions necessary for stability such as the size of base and so on
5. Type of supporting surface.

Environmental factors such as:
1. Noise
2. The working space
3. Lighting
4. Excessive heat or cold
5. Air pollution.

The choice of an activity is influenced by what the physiotherapist learns about her patient from talking with him, observing carefully, using her hands sensitively, assessing his movement potential, his needs, interests and motivation to work and making appropriate deductions. It also depends on the need for and purpose of the activity and its importance to the patient at this time. The questions to be asked and answered by the physiotherapist are:

1. Has the patient the desire to do the activity?
2. Does it have priority in treatment?
3. What may be achieved or changed by it?
4. Are the necessary components of strength, power, endurance, flexibility and so on and their controls present?
5. Can the mechanical demands of the movement be met?
6. Are the difficulties and the intensity of the activity set at a suitable level?
7. Is the level of general fitness – strength, endurance and cardio-respiratory efficiency adequate?
8. Is the environment like or related to home, work or recreation conditions?
9. Can the activity, if achieved, be put into immediate use or act as a stepping stone to other activities?
10. Are there any particular dangers associated with its performance?

In any activity there are two factors at work with a conflict between the need for mobility and stability and the consequent adjustment of the posture to allow the movement to take place and at the same time, ensure stability.

The safety of the patient must be ensured throughout the treatment as well as in setting a home programme.

THE ACTIVITY

An activity consists of three parts:

1. The starting position
2. Movement on a background posture
3. The finishing position.

The starting position

The starting position forms a support system – a position of readiness from which movement can be initiated and carried out. If the movement is to be accurate it is essential that the patient understands the need for good postural alignment, is conscious of the position of his head and body in space and is able to correct it if necessary. All the time minor postural adjustments will be necessary. If they are incorrect the relevant stimuli to the central nervous system will be faulty and the total movement incorrect.

The starting position may be used:

1. As a foundation for an activity
2. To provide fixation of one part of the body so that localised movement can be achieved
3. To train posture and balance
4. As an exercise to improve the stability and safety of the required posture.

There are four basic positions – lying, sitting, standing and kneeling. From these positions many other positions are derived according to the abilities and needs of the patient and the knowledge, skill, imagination and ingenuity of the physiotherapist.

In choosing a position an analysis must be made of the:

1. Movement necessary to take up and hold the position
2. Joints and their necesary range and points of fixation
3. Muscle groups involved
4. Type of contraction needed
5. Help, if any, needed.

The factors to be considered in selecting a starting position for an activity are that the:

1. Starting position is appropriate to the activity, relevant to the needs of the patient and acceptable to him
2. Supporting surface is stable, the base of support is of an adequate size and there is a correct distribution of weight
3. Position can be taken up, with or without help, held in good alignment and is

capable of quick adjustment according to the needs of the activity
4. Line of gravity falls within the base and the patient has the ability to raise or lower the centre of gravity according to the demands of the activity
5. Resistance to outside forces can be withstood
6. Position is suitable to give and receive impetus if necessary.

As soon as possible the starting position will be progressed to a more demanding one. Progression may be achieved by altering the size of the base, raising the centre of gravity, altering the speed, increasing movement stress and changing the state of the supporting surface from either firm to soft or still to mobile.

The position may fail because of:

1. An inappropriate choice
2. Muscle imbalance with weakness particularly in the rotary component
3. Joint and muscle pain
4. Lack of joint range
5. Lack of co-ordination
6. Lack of balance
7. Abnormal reflex activity
8. Disturbed perception.

Support given by a person or from apparatus such as a splint, wall bars or parallel bars or the use of a mat, may help to ensure the patient's safety and give him the confidence that this is so.

Movement upon a background posture

Each movement upon a background posture will be made up of key stages or phases which form an orderly sequence. Stage will follow stage in a regular order and at a specific time, with each stage having its own muscular and joint requirements. In any one stage a muscle may act by shortening, holding in a static position or by lengthening. Likewise the joints involved may change their action. The joint range necessary or the angle of fixation may be constantly changing.

It will be necessary to analyse each stage specifically and determine the joints involved, their points of fixation and their range, the muscles and the type of contraction necessary and the stability of the background posture.

In looking at the movement, the questions to be asked include:

1. What is to be moved? (The part or parts of the body and its shape in space)
2. Are the basic movements in the activity present?
3. Where is it to be moved? (The pattern or direction of the movement and the level, whether high or low on which movement takes place)
4. How is it to be moved? (The quality of the movement – its accuracy, efficiency, sequence, rhythm and speed)
5. How does it feel and look to the patient? (The visual, auditory and kinaesthetic image)
6. How can the physiotherapist help the patient? (Explanation, demonstration, provision of stimuli and support)
7. Can the sequence of movements within the activity be carried out completely or can parts only be done?
8. If a stage of the sequence fails, are preliminary exercises necessary?
9. Has what is wanted and expected been achieved? If not, why not?

The answers to the questions will be provided by the constant keen observation and assessment carried out by the physiotherapist together with a search for further knowledge when difficulties occur.

If a stage of the movement fails then preliminary exercises may be necessary and later that stage linked into the total movement.

The finishing position

The activity may:

1. End with a return to the original starting position
2. Be the beginning of a new phase in the total sequence of movement

3. Be the starting position for a new movement

or

4. It may end in a position of rest.

GENERAL PRINCIPLES OF TRAINING

Training may be defined as the preparation of a person to perform a purposeful activity skilfully by means of systematic exercise under supervision. It may include training for a job, independence in living or recreation. All factors applicable to the training of an athlete will need to be considered. A specific or progressive demand to bring about a desired result will be placed on the patient. It entails work, as hard and constant as his local and general condition allows. Training is an active process.

Motivation

Much of the success of any training programme depends on the motivation of the patient to succeed and the amount of effort he is prepared to make. He must understand that maximum function is restored only by his own voluntary effort. The establishment of a good working relationship with the therapist helps greatly towards achieving success.

His potential to work when challenged and under stress is as yet unknown as patients differ in their degree of motivation. The therapist must encourage the patient as he strives towards his goals and give generous praise when he succeeds. Should the patient fail, it is important that the therapist gives him positive support and encourages him to try again.

Knowledge of the activity

It is essential that the patient has a knowledge of the activity and understands its purpose. He needs to gain a clear picture of the activity as a whole, of the part or parts of the body to be moved, the path of the movement, an awareness of his body in space and how the movement is to be carried out.

There will be a need for efficiency of movement. Therefore the varying demands for strength, flexibility, power, endurance, balance and co-ordination must be met. Training for an activity will help increase efficiency.

The influence of learning

The achievement of efficient movement will involve learning. Any training will have a learning effect as time proceeds. One of the chief methods to be used in training or retraining is the activity itself, especially if once achieved it can be put to immediate use.

Steps to aid learning will include the following factors:

1. The pattern of the activity is well planned so that the activity will be performed by the patient with a minimum of effort and maximum safety.
2. The training steps are clear to the patient.
3. The pattern, once set and proved possible, is held constant.
4. The working space is well designed so that safety is ensured and undue stress is not caused. Where possible it will be related to that in which the patient will operate in the near future; for example the home situation or a simulated work space.

The activity will be demonstrated slowly as a whole so that a general concept of the activity is gained. If the activity is complex, each sequence will be shown in its order together with the words of instruction that will be used. The words should be clear, brief and simple. Once set, the form of activity and words of instruction will be kept constant. An example of the break-up of an activity is given in Appendix 2.

Some patients will have a memory of the activity and will use it in working towards a recovery. For many, particularly the heavily handicapped and the old, the task will be difficult.

Carlsoo[6] points out that a demonstration, because of its complexity and speed of movement, is difficult for even the trained eye to follow. It occurs so rapidly that the eye has not enough time to record the course of the movement of the body segments and the successive changes in the position of the joints.

Videotapes, photographs, slides, illustrations and written instructions may be useful as preliminary training measures so that the patient has a knowledge of the steps to be taken and the instructions he will receive before he attempts the task.

Warm-up

Many physiotherapists consider a warm-up of benefit for their patients. Athletes and dancers with heavy demands on strength and/or flexibility always do a preliminary warm-up before commencing strenuous work. It raises the level of arousal and the alertness of the patient as well as increasing circulation to a level close to that required for the activity.

The warm-up may consist of:

1. A gentle easing into the task itself
or
2. A general loosening or mild stretching activity gradually increasing in range and speed.

A certain amount of research has been done to discover the effects obtained from a warm-up as well as its value but the results are inconclusive.

The activity attempted

The patient attempts the activity either as a whole or in part, with or without help, depending on his ability. Manual help may be given if needed. Stretch and resistance may be used to give direction to the movement, build up strength and increase the demand on the patient.

Correct head and body alignment is important. It helps the patient gain a correct feeling of the movement and lessens the energy requirements.

Many persons, particularly when performing a new activity tend to hold their breath, thus increasing cranial and thoracic blood pressure. The pattern of breathing is altered and ab-

normal muscle work occurs. This must be checked and correct breathing control established for the activity being undertaken.

Practice, supervision, correction and praise

Success will only come through repetition and regular practice. Practice will be supervised and correction sensitively given during the treatment session so that learning can take place. The work must be well taught and well done. Praise should be given when earned. The word 'good' should be used only when the movement is correct. This will help the patient learn the feeling of an accurate movement. An incorrect response by the physiotherapist will hinder his progress. Other words of encouragement should be used and correction given if the movement is incorrect. A videotape recording of the patient's performance may be made so that both the physiotherapist and the patient can study it at their leisure and note the points where movement is difficult or incorrect.

As soon as possible, independent practice will be started and carried out regularly and frequently so that accuracy is gained. Gradually an orderly sequence will be set up. Economy of movement is established. Skill is gained.

The level of skill will depend, to a certain extent, on the natural attributes of the patient. Some people are naturally skilful in the performance of movement, others are awkward. This must be appreciated by the physiotherapist.

Speed and rhythm

For most activities there is a specific and economic rate of movement for the task. It is usually a steady rhythmic movement interspersed with regular rest intervals. Any increase or decrease in speed beyond normal limits will lead to inefficiency.

Progression

Progression should proceed as quickly as possible. An activity may be progressed by:

1. Increasing the load
2. Altering the speed of the movement
3. Increasing the number of times it is done
4. Varying the arc of the movement
5. Changing the base when appropriate.

An assured way of estimating improvement is through the use of accurate measurement and recording done at regular intervals so that an improvement, static state or regression is identified and recorded. For example, measurement may indicate changes in strength, flexibility, speed of movement, new activities achieved, a greater distance walked and so on.

Intensity

The degree of intensity of the training depends on the patient's local and general condition at any one time. It must be safe and within his exercise tolerance so that no unfavourable complications may arise. In early treatment, tolerance may be low, therefore the amount of work done may be small.

All people have an inbuilt 'braking system'. They know when they have done enough and stop.

The physiotherapist, who is aware of the patient's condition can usually judge how much can be done on a day to day basis. She will be aware of signs of change, for better or worse, in his condition. Quite quickly she will gain a good idea of his ability to work and to endure discomfort if necessary, as well as the level of his concentration period.

As soon as possible the demand will be stepped up so that the patient works at his maximum capacity or near it.

Standard of training

The standard of training to be reached will depend to a great extent on the needs of the individual patient in daily life. For example, a clerk who has an injury to the knee joint will need a much lower level of efficiency than the athlete training for a match.

The overall standard set should be just above that necessary to carry out all essential activities freely without strain and should provide a margin of safety – a reserve of strength and range.

Time of day

The time of day may be important for some patients, particularly those with pain, such as the patient with rheumatoid arthritis. If the patient is allowed to move around at his own speed for an hour or two before treatment, more will be accomplished. This could be considered a 'warm-up' period. Again treatment late in the afternoon may be less effective as the patient may be tired.

Maintenance

It is important that strength is maintained and/or gained in the uninjured parts of the body, particularly of the trunk and weight bearing limbs, during the time of rehabilitation so that damage does not occur following return to work. The patient's confidence in himself will be gained when this is stressed throughout the rehabilitation period.

If there is a delay before a patient recommences work he must be informed of the need to maintain strength and so safeguard himself against injury. Much has still to be learned about the methods of retaining strength and endurance.

An unsatisfactory performance

If difficulties occur which cannot be easily corrected, the physiotherapist must analyse the reason for the patient's difficulties including how, where and why the movement fails.

The cause may be due to:

Planning faults such as:

1. Too much may have been attempted too quickly
2. A further breakdown of the task or more preliminary training may be needed
3. The method may be unsatisfactory
4. Inadequate assistance may have been given

5. The environment of the treatment room may be unsuitable, for example, a lack of privacy in the early stage, excessive noise and/or temperature and so on.

Psychological and emotional factors such as:
1. Lack of ability by the patient to understand what is wanted
2. Poor memory
3. Poor awareness of his own body
4. Boredom and lack of interest and real effort
5. Fear of pain and his condition worsening
6. Fear of inadequacy in the outside world
7. Dislike of the physiotherapist.

Teaching faults such as:
1. Poor explanation and demonstration
2. Lack of suitable stimuli
3. Inadequate help given
4. Inadequate correction.

Other complicating factors may be:
1. Poor vision and hearing
2. Poor general health with lack of energy and motivation
3. Inflammation and other conditions of the musculoskeletal system including osteoporosis
4. Sensory loss
5. Impending litigation
6. The patient may be satisfied to be dependent or is encouraged to do so by his relatives.

A new attempt

A new attempt is made following a reassessment. More preliminary training and help may be given or the task may be replanned. With encouragement the patient tries again. He practises, progresses and succeeds.

The level of treatment

Progress may be handicapped by:

1. Too much done too soon
or
2. Too little done too slowly.

Both may be harmful to the patient.

Too much done too soon may cause pain and loss of movement and prove harmful mentally and physically to the patient.

If the patient has pain which was not there before treatment and lasts for longer than an hour after treatment and/or if movement is less than on the previous day, then the query arises as to whether too much has been done in the treatment session or whether there has been extra incidental activity outside the patient's usual routine.

It has to be accepted that all people vary slightly from day to day in their level of activity.

Too little done too slowly is more usual. It is inefficient physiotherapy and costly to both the patient and the employing authority.

A happy medium between the two must be found.

REFERENCES AND FURTHER READING

1. Anderson, T. McClurg (1951) *Human Kinetics*. London: Heinemann.
2. Astrand, P. O. & Rodahl, K. (1977) *Textbook of Work Physiology*, 2nd edn. New York: McGraw-Hill.
3. Basmajian, J. V. (Ed.) (1984) *Therapeutic Exercise*, 4th edn. Baltimore: Williams & Wilkins.
4. Broer, M. R. & Zernicke, R. F. (1979) *Efficiency of Human Movement*, 4th edn. Philadelphia: W. B. Saunders.
5. Buchwald, E. (1952) *Physical Rehabilitation for Daily Living*. New York: McGraw-Hill.
6. Carlsöö, S. (1972) *How Man Moves*. London: Heinemann.
7. De Vries, H. A. (1980) *Physiology of Exercise*, 3rd edn. Dubuque: Wm. C. Brown Company.
8. Gardiner, M. D. (1963) *The Principles of Exercise Therapy*, 3rd edn. London: Bell & Hyman.
9. Knuttgen, H. G. (Ed.) (1976) *Neuromuscular Mechanisms for Therapeutic and Conditioning Exercise*. Baltimore: University Park Press.
10. Mennell, J. (1934) *Physical Treatment by Movement, Manipulation and Massage*, 3rd edn. London: J. A. Churchill.
11. N.U.S.T.E.P. (1967) An exploratory and analytical survey of therapeutic exercise. *American Journal of Physical Medicine*, Vol 46, No. 1.
12. Rasch, P. J. & Burke, R. K. (1978) *Kinesiology and Applied Anatomy*, 6th edn. Philadelphia: Lea & Febiger.
13. Sullivan, P. E., Markos, P. D. & Minor, M. A. (1982) *An Integrated Approach to Therapeutic Exercise*. Reston: Reston Publishing Company.
14. Wells, K. F. & Luttgens, K. (1976) *Kinesiology*, 6th edn. Philadelphia: W. B. Saunders.

15

The relief of pain and reduction of oedema

Inflammation is the reaction of living tissue to injury or disease. The clinical signs of inflammation are pain, oedema, redness and heat.

PAIN

Pain, a part of the inflammatory process, is a signal of tissue damage caused by injury and/or disease. It interferes with a person's performance of his usual activities and acts as a cautionary signal calling attention to possible damage. All injuries or diseases produce a perception of pain at some stage although the physiological mechanisms underlying this phenomenon are not yet clear.[2,3,5,12]

Pain is often associated with oedema, due to the increased tension arising in the tissues as part of the inflammatory response to tissue damage. By reducing the oedema, the increased tension on the nerve endings is reduced, leading to pain reduction.

Acute pain following injury is as a rule temporary and eased or at least minimised with treatment and time. Some patients with more chronic problems such as those with rheumatoid arthritis have very varying levels of pain though some pain is usually present. Chronic pain usually causes depression, anxiety and weariness though most people come to terms with it and arrange their lives so that it causes minimal disturbance. A few patients, for example those with pain from cancer, rheumatoid arthritis, severe causalgia or an avulsion of the brachial plexus, experience long-term severe pain which can have profound effects on both mind and body.

Each pain has its own specific qualities and its level is difficult to evaluate. Attempts have been made to develop standardised questionnaires taking into account the quality, intensity, location and behaviour of the patient's reported pain.[10]

A useful method of arbitrarily grading a patient's pain is to ask the following questions:

1. How does the pain interfere with the performance of the patient's usual activities?
2. Is the pain:
    a. Minimal – is it annoying?
    b. Slight – does it interfere with some or all usual activities?
    c. Moderate – does it prevent usual activities?
    d. Severe – does it prevent usual activities and also cause distress?

Emotional response to pain

Pain is a subjective and personal experience and always unpleasant. The level of pain experienced by patients with similar conditions varies in pain perception and tolerance. For example, if a person is worried, depressed or alone, the sensation of pain is usually increased. If the same person is busy, stimulated and enjoying the situation he becomes more tolerant and less conscious of his pain. The pain level is also influenced by the patient's previous experience of pain, the initial sight of his injury or the appearance of his affected body part, the anticipated course of the injury or disease, the medical and counselling facilities available and his fear of the ultimate consequences. It is undoubtedly influenced by the culture in which he lives.

The importance of graded rest and activity in the relief of pain

The relief of pain is the key to releasing movement. If treatment is to be effective it is essential to break the pain cycle, prevent further pain and try to solve the problem of severe long-term pain.

Rest is an essential part of the healing process and the need for it must be respected. In treatment a balance must be struck between doing too much or too little by either the therapist or the patient. There is often a narrow margin between what the patient can do actively without causing or increasing pain and the therapist must watch carefully the reaction of the tissues to exercise.

It is essential that the patient and the therapist can distinguish the difference between true pain and discomfort. Discomfort following activity, as defined by Flatt,[6] is that which recedes rapidly during a rest period of one to three hours with the subsequent level of movement being held constant. This level is acceptable and allows the grading of the treatment and general activities programme to be gradually intensified.

True pain is that which persists for several hours with the level of movement reduced. It is a guide to the extent and level of the treatment that can be given by the therapist and of the activities that can be done by the patient. It must be respected. The patient must understand the importance of the balance between rest and activity. Short frequent bouts of treatment and/or activity rather than a prolonged treatment and/or activity may prevent pain occurring. If pain occurs, the body part must be rested in a suitable position and the level of activity reduced at least temporarily. A change in position from time to time may help ease the pain.

Pain and/or discomfort may also be caused by too little movement and may be eased if some movement is encouraged.

The reason for any increasing pain must be found. It may be that:

1. The condition is worsening and inflammation is increasing
2. There is inadequate blood flow to the working muscles
3. Too much has been done by the therapist and/or patient

4. The patient has poor postural and working habits
5. The patient's limb is dependent with an increase in oedema
6. There is an uncomfortable splint or bandage.

Many physiotherapy modalities, as, for example, heat, cold, transcutaneous electrical nerve stimulation (TENS), electrotherapy and manual therapy, may be used to relieve pain by breaking the pain cycle.[4,8,9,12,13,14]

OEDEMA

When tissue damage occurs, chemical substances are liberated which produce dilatation of the minute blood vessels and increase their permeability. This increased permeability allows more fluid than is normal to leak into the tissue spaces. Damage may also have occurred to the lymphatics which disrupts their capacity to drain the interstitial spaces effectively. Oedema or excess fluid in the interstitial spaces is the result and the circulation to the part is impaired.

If oedema is allowed to remain or increase, fibrosis of the subcutaneous tissues will occur and indirectly hinder the excursion of muscles, tendons, nerves and other soft tissues which normally glide freely in relation to each other. The ligaments will become softened and stretched, thereby reducing their capacity to support the joints. Pain will also increase due to increased pressure, so the patient is reluctant to move the body part. This all leads to a progressive stiffening of the joints directly involved as well as those not originally injured, which can occur very quickly (Fig. 15.1).

The relationship of the inflammatory process to the development of joint stiffness is particularly important in the hand as stiffened small joints of the hand and/or lack of mobility in the palm greatly disturbs a patient's capacity to perform many activities.

In any injury early healing with minimal scarring is of prime importance in bringing about

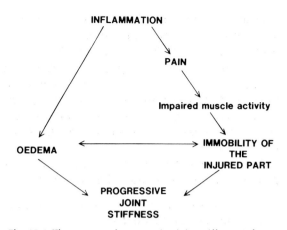

Fig. 15.1 The causes of progressive joint stiffness (*after Beasley, R. W. (1981) Hand Injuries. Philadelphia: W. B. Saunders*).

efficient early function. Therefore, measures to prevent oedema formation or reduce it if already present, should start as soon as possible so that it does not increase and become chronic.

Elevation and active exercise

On the slightest sign of oedema, elevation of the limb is essential. The atrium of the heart is the point of reference for the elevation, with the distal part of the involved extremity being positioned above the proximal part which in turn is positioned above the heart. Dependency is to be avoided but when this is not possible, as for example, when walking after an injury to the lower limb, compression can be used in the form of pressure bandages or stockings. This will help control oedema formation.

Exercise together with elevation is the key to the reduction of oedema. The pumping action of the muscles creates changes in pressure which bring about an increased flow of blood to and from the affected body part. The removal of lymph is also facilitated. At first the movements should be supervised by the therapist and their importance stressed to the patient who will continue them. They should not cause pain. As soon as possible the limb should be used freely and purposefully.

Exercise may not be immediately possible to those areas directly affected by an injury because of the need to immobilise the injured part to allow early healing to occur, for example, following a fracture. However, all free joints should be exercised regularly and frequently in as full a range as possible while awaiting healing of the damaged structure to occur.

Most patients tend to hold their injured limb in some degree of tension which can be caused by pain, fear or uncertainty. This hinders the circulation and increases the pain. The gaining of relaxation of the whole limb will increase the patient's comfort while in elevation and later will help ease pain and aid movement. The patient will appreciate the change.

Other treatments can be used by the therapist to reduce oedema. These include the use of cold, intermittant pressure pumps, interferential therapy and contrast baths.[9]

REFERENCES AND FURTHER READING

1. Beasley, R. W. (1981) *Hand Injuries.* Philadelphia: W. B. Saunders.
2. Bishop, B. (1980) Pain: Its physiology and rationale for management. Part 1. Neuro-anatomical substrate of pain. *Physical Therapy*, Vol. 60, pp. 13–20.
3. Bishop, B. (1980) Pain: Its physiology and rationale for management. Part 2. Analgesic systems of the C.N.S. *Physical Therapy*, Vol. 60, pp. 21–23.
4. Bishop, B. (1980) Pain: Its physiology and rationale for management. Part 3. Consequences of current concepts of pain mechanisms related to pain management. *Physical Therapy*, Vol. 60, pp. 24–37.
5. Bogduk, N. & Lance, J. W. (1981) Pain and pain syndromes including headache. In *Current Neurology*, Appel, S. H. (Ed.) Vol. 3, Ch. 14, pp. 377–419. New York: Wiley Medical Publication.
6. Flatt, A. E. (1974) *The Care of the Rheumatoid Hand*, 3rd edn. St Louis: C. V. Mosby.
7. Florey, H. W. (1970) Inflammation. In *General Pathology*, Florey, H. W. (Ed.), 4th edn, Chs. 2 & 3, pp. 22–123. London: Lloyd-Luke Medical.
8. Lehmann, J. F. & de Lateur, B. J. (1982) Therapeutic heat. In *Therapeutic Heat & Cold*, Lehmann, J. F. (Ed.), 3rd edn, Ch. 10, pp. 404–562. Baltimore: Williams & Wilkins.
9. Lehmann, J. F. & de Lateur, B. J. (1982) Cryotherapy. In *Therapeutic Heat & Cold*, Lehmann, J. F. (Ed.), 3rd edn, Ch. 11, pp. 563–602. Baltimore: Williams & Wilkins.
10. Melzack, R. (1975) The McGill pain questionnaire: major properties and scoring methods. *Pain*, Vol. 1, pp. 277–299.
11. Melzack, R. (Ed.) (1983) *Pain Measurement and Assessment.* New York: Raven Press.
12. Melzack, R. & Wall, P. (1982) *The Challenge of Pain.* Harmondsworth: Penguin.
13. Thorsteinsson, G. (1983) Electrical stimulation for analgesia. In *Therapeutic Electricity and Ultraviolet Radiation*, Stillwell, G. K. (Ed.), Ch. 3, pp. 109–123. Baltimore: Williams & Wilkins.
14. Wolf, S. L. (1978) Perspectives on central nervous system responsiveness to transcutaneous electrical nerve stimulation. *Physical Therapy*, Vol. 5, No. 12, pp. 1443–1449.

16

Strength, power and endurance

STRENGTH, POWER

Strength may be defined as the maximal effective force that can be actively exerted by a muscle in a specific movement. The maximal strength capacity of a normal muscle is related directly to its physiological cross-sectional area. The larger this cross-section, the greater the tension (force) the muscle is capable of producing.

Training alters the size of the muscle by increasing the size of its muscle fibres but it does not lead to an increase in the total number of muscle fibres present. An increase in the size of a muscle is called hypertrophy: a decrease in size – atrophy.

The amount of muscle tension produced is also related to the extent and synchrony of motor unit recruitment. Greater tension production occurs when many motor units in a muscle are activated simultaneously. This is under the control of the nervous system.

The tension produced by a muscle when it contracts cannot be measured directly in the physiotherapy clinic. What is actually measured when performing a 'strength' test is torque or the rotational component of the force produced by the contracting muscle in a particular movement pattern (Fig. 5.12).

Power can be defined as the rate at which a muscle can do mechanical work. It is a measure of the force which the muscle can produce and the velocity at which it shortens.

A muscle is said to develop its greatest power when its velocity of shortening is about a third of the maximum possible and the force produced is about a third of the isometric maximum that the muscle can generate.[5]

Types of strength

There are two basic types of strength:

1. Dynamic (isotonic) strength, where continuous force is exerted and motion occurs. The movement may be slow, smooth and sustained or explosive. Muscle activity may be concentric or eccentric. If the rate of movement is kept constant the muscle is said to act isokinetically.

The maximum torque that can be produced when a muscle actively shortens at different velocities can be measured continuously, using an isokinetic dynamometer for example, Cybex II, to produce an isokinetic torque curve (Fig. 5.23). The maximal torque which can be developed at some point during the movement can be read off from these curves.

Maximum isokinetic torque values at slow speeds are similar to maximal isometric torque values but as the speed of movement increases, the maximum values throughout the range of motion decrease and peak torque occurs later in the range.

2. Isometric (static) strength, where continuous force is exerted though no movement accompanies muscle tension production. The muscle contraction involved is isometric.

The maximum effective isometric strength of a muscle is found indirectly by identifying the joint angle at which peak torque production occurs (Fig. 16.1). This is taken from a series of recordings of the force produced by maximal isometric contractions performed at different joint angles.[71]

Physiological or mechanical factors predominate at different parts of the range. In general, it has been shown that isometric torque drops from the lengthened to the shortened position of a muscle due to length–tension considerations, although there are a number of exceptions to this such as biceps and brachialis, which have a peak torque reading when the elbow is at 90° flexion (Fig. 5.12), and quadriceps, where peak isometric torque occurs at about 60° flexion (Fig. 16.1).

Knowledge of isometric and isokinetic torque curves provides a practical guide to the physiotherapist when applying manual resistance during muscle strength testing and when giving exercise to patients.

Factors involved in muscle strength

Strength is a complex quality. It depends on

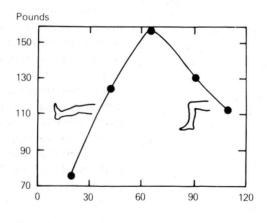

Knee extension: degrees

Fig. 16.1 Isometric torque curve of the quadriceps. *Reprinted from Physical Therapy, Vol. 39, No. 3, 1959, p. 149. With the kind permission of the American Physical Therapy Association.*

anatomical, physiological, psychological and mechanical factors. It is governed by the nervous system and can be influenced by training, the patient's motivation and his will to make an all-out effort.

Muscle strength depends on the:

1. Number and size of the motor units activated and the synchronisation of their contractions. Greater tension production occurs when many motor units are activated simultaneously
2. Type of muscle action – eccentric, concentric, isometric
3. Length of the muscle when it is stimulated to contract
4. Angle of pull of the muscle
5. Length of the lever arm involved
6. Velocity of muscle action
7. Integrity of joint and muscle structures
8. Blood supply to the muscles and joints.

Maximum active muscle tension is produced when a muscle is stimulated at its resting length. It declines as the muscle shortens or lengthens relative to this. For many muscles their maximum torque production occurs when they are at this physiological advantage, but for others, as this physiological advantage declines, mechanical factors improve so that torque is actually enhanced (Fig. 5.12). For example, the elbow flexors are at a physiological advantage when the elbow is in extension. As the elbow approaches 90° flexion, the angle of pull and leverage of the elbow flexors are such that the rotational effect of the tension produced by them is actually increased even though their tension production capacity has dropped because of change in length.

Active muscle tension is related proportionally to the number of motor units stimulated. This depends on the task. No more and no fewer motor units than those needed will be called into play. If strength is to be improved, progression of the demands made by the task on the muscle or muscle group, whether in load carried or speed of movement, is essential.

A person's build, health, age and sex will influence the amount of tension that can be produced in any one activity. Strength reaches its peak in the early twenties and from then on slowly declines. In both sexes the maximum decline will be in the trunk and leg muscles. On average the muscle strength of women is about two-thirds that of men.[5]

Gradually during a person's life a level of strength necessary for living is set up and unless circumstances alter, strength will be held at this level. The level of strength essential for daily living does not vary greatly from person to person living in similar environments. However, the level set by the person's work and recreation may differ significantly. All need a reserve of strength slightly above that necessary for all daily activities, so that stress can be met without strain and damage.

When injury or disease occurs the level of strength falls and the need to regain it becomes apparent. In planning for the development of strength each person must work on an individual plan at his own level and pace, with consideration given to his needs and to both his local and general condition.

Patients come for treatment with varying degrees of loss of strength. All have a need to regain it.

REGAINING OF STRENGTH

EARLY RE-EDUCATION OF MOVEMENT

If a free movement is impossible through injury, disease or disuse, assisted active movement must be used. The disability may consist of lack of strength of individual muscles and/or the synergist group, or may take a more generalised form. The muscles needing assistance will be in the zero to poor (0–2) grade (see Appendix 1). The assisting force should be the minimum necessary to enable the patient to initiate, move through range and control simple voluntary movement patterns. It is a necessary supplementary force only.

Measurement of disability

A muscle chart, measurement of joint range

and assessment of muscle length, as well as knowledge of the patient's abilities and needs, is made before treatment starts and rechecked regularly (Appendix 1).

Preparation of the body for treatment

If the loss of movement in a limb is severe the circulation and nutrition of the part may be impaired and the limb may be cold and blue. Pain may be present. Gentle warmth may improve the circulation to muscles and joints, ease pain and help prepare the limb for exercise. This may be needed before any measurement is done.

The maintenance of full joint range and muscle length in all affected and unaffected parts of the body will be necessary so that there is no hindrance to movement when recovery occurs. It will also help prevent deformity.

Body alignment

Often the patient's kinaesthetic sense is impaired by muscle weakness, loss of sensation or poor habits. He may have little or no appreciation of his own posture. Correct body and limb alignment is an essential factor in the gaining of accurate movement. Continuous correction will be necessary if the maximum function is to be gained as quickly as possible and deformities avoided.

The starting position

The starting position should be chosen so that the working parts are in a suitable position, usually with gravity eliminated. The body, with relevant parts bared, should be supported when necessary and the working parts clearly seen by the therapist and the patient if possible. Thus the patient's concentration is maximal and strain avoided.

The assisting force

The most usual method of treating grade zero to poor (0–2) (Appendix 1) muscles is by manual assistance provided by the physiotherapist, or, following instruction, by the patient. Assistance may also be provided by water, a polished board, supportive sling, or other mechanical means.

The physiotherapist needs to determine how to position the part, stimulate it, how best to treat it, how much to do, and how best to do it, as well as to capitalise on what has been gained.

The resistance to be overcome includes the weight of the limb, friction and possibly a contraction or spasm of the antagonist muscle.

The ability to develop maximum tension depends on adequate proprioception. The patient will be helped by the sight of the movement, the words of instruction, the placement of the physiotherapist's hands, his concentration, the emphasis on his gaining the 'feel' of the movement, together with continuous encouragement.

Manual assistance

The patient gains confidence and reassurance in working closely with the physiotherapist. In carrying out assisted movement both hands are used by the physiotherapist. They should be warm and comfortable and help the patient understand what to do. One hand will control the proximal area and apply pressure as a stimulus over the working muscle. The second hand will provide support, stretch, direction and assistance or resistance to the moving part. Both hands will be sensitive to the response of the working muscles. The physiotherapist's body should move as one with the patient's limb in the direction of the required movement and supply extra directional aid.

Stretch

Stretch is a natural stimulus to the muscle spindle. A cortical stimulation that is below threshold level when a muscle is slack may become effective when the muscle is stretched.[6,15]

Stretch should be applied at the lengthened range of the muscle or muscle group. Care should be taken not to overstretch the weakened muscle.

A quick stretch can be superimposed on the muscles in the normal lengthened position.[35]

Mechanical vibration can also be used.

Demonstration

Before any movement by the patient is attempted a clear demonstration is given. The patient will watch the demonstration and listen to the clear, brief and relevant instructions. When possible the demonstration is given first on the unaffected limb so that the patient gains a mental picture and the feel of a normal movement or contraction. This will be followed by a demonstration on the affected limb.

Initiation of movement

Initiation of movement is usually obtained in the inner part of the outer range. At first it may be just a 'flicker' of movement. The timing of stretch and of the verbal stimulus is important in obtaining a contraction.

The influence of motor learning

Undoubtedly motor learning plays a major part in early re-education. By seeing and feeling the correct movement on the affected limb knowledge is gained by patient and physiotherapist.

Practice makes the initiation easier. Biofeedback may provide both visual and auditory signals to help the patient gain a knowledge of the success of his movement. The patient develops his motor memory.

Progression

Once a contraction can be initiated, progress should proceed. This may be achieved by:

1. Initiating contractions through various parts of the range and later co-ordinating them into a movement through range

2. Transforming the assisted active movement into an assisted-resisted movement and later into a resisted movement as strength increases
3. Increasing the number of repetitions
4. Increasing the speed of movement
5. Increasing the length of the lever arm
6. Increasing the complexity and control of movement so that a pattern involving rotation is gradually set up
7. Encouraging independent work by the patient.

The use of manual resistance

Resistance will be introduced as soon as possible to increase the strength of the contraction or movement. At first it may be used in the form of an assisted-resisted movement, with the physiotherapist's hand assisting when necessary in one part of the range and then resisting in that part of the range which has greater strength. As soon as possible the total movement will be resisted.

The level of resistance given to a dynamic contraction will be graded to allow all possible movement through range to occur. When applied to an isometric contraction the level of resistance should be the strongest the body part or muscle will take and still hold steady. This hold should not be broken.

Manual resistance has many advantages. It is quick and easy to apply, it may be varied through different parts of the range and it can be directional in the building up of strength. Its application is sensitive to the response of the working muscles, helping build up the patient's and the physiotherapist's knowledge of the patient's abilities. The disadvantage of manual resistance is that it is not accurately measurable.

Patterns of movement

The patterns of movement used in daily living, work and recreation have already been discussed. The patterns and techniques initiated by Kabat and Knott called Proprioceptive Neuromuscular Facilitation (PNF) have proved most useful in the treatment of patients with muscles graded from poor to the lower levels of grade good (2–4) (Appendix 1) as well as for patients with specific muscle weakness within a total pattern.[35]

These patterns are related to functional movements. All patterns have a diagonal direction and a strong rotary component. In each pattern muscles work from a lengthened to a shortened state. Emphasis is placed on the gaining or retaining of a strong trunk.

In the use of the technique, stress is laid on maximal proprioceptive stimulation. Visual and auditory stimuli, stretch, manual resistance, hand pressure and so on are used to gain a maximal effective response. The use of manual resistance is advocated, though in the later stages of treatment, when patterns can be performed adequately, other forms of resistance should be used and the physiotherapist's strength spared.

The patterns and techniques have been well described by Knott and Voss[35] and Waddington.[68]

The techniques used in these patterns can be usefully applied to any functional activity – including those of daily living – provided that the form of the pattern has been carefully analysed so that stretch and resistance can be applied to each muscle component of the pattern, in the right direction, in the correct sequence and at the required time.

Irradiation

Within a pattern there may be muscles with varying degrees of strength. If this is present the order and synchronisation of the movement must be kept. It may be found that if resistance is given to the stronger muscles an overflow – irradiation – may occur to the weaker muscles and assist them to take part in the total movement.[5,25,35]

Trick movements

If the prime mover of the desired action is unable to produce the movement then an attempt will be made by the patient to use any available muscle to reproduce this action or one which is as nearly as possible a substitute for it. Common examples are the use of the lateral abdominals to lift the pelvis if the hip abductors are not present or graded poor or hitching of the shoulder girdle if the deltoid is weak or absent.

In early re-education the use of trick movements should be avoided as they tend to inhibit the return and use of the correct weakened muscle. They may lead to deformity. Later if normal muscle action does not occur their use may be necessary to improve function but their effect on the body's structure needs to be closely watched.

Cross education

There is some evidence that when strong exercise is given to muscles in a normal limb over a period of time, corresponding muscles in the weak limb are stimulated even if that limb is not deliberately exercised.[28] This will usually occur only if that movement is strong in the normal limb. Cross transfer of strength in normal subjects has also been reported. This concept was controversial for some time but lately seems to be increasingly accepted.

Fatigue[4]

A recovering muscle should be used to its full capacity but if it becomes fatigued, movement will become less efficient and there is no purpose in proceeding. Fatigue is a reversible phenomenon provided adequate rest is given. Treatment should move to another muscle group and return later when the fatigued muscle has recovered. It is helpful to prevent mental fatigue if work with movements requiring great concentration is alternated with easier movement within the treatment session.

Muscle imbalance

The presence of muscle imbalance must be watched as deformity can occur if full joint range and muscle length are not preserved.

There are differing opinions as to whether a muscle group which is markedly stronger than its opposing group should be exercised to gain normal strength if at the same time it will stretch still further the weaker group. However this work may improve the nutrition of the limb as a whole and may help the weaker muscle, provided the potential for improvement is there. The situation needs to be carefully watched and regularly reassessed.

General maintenance

It is important at this stage of the patient's treatment that strength and co-ordination of the whole body is maintained. The prognosis may be unknown, for some there will be improvement, for others deterioration or a static state. If a suitable task is set, the patient should be encouraged to work at it so that respiration, circulation and limb nutrition, as well as strength and joint range, may be maintained or even improved and all possible functions carried out which will help towards independence.

LATER STAGE TREATMENT

Once the muscle is able to lift the body or body part against gravity, Grade 3 (Appendix 1), the emphasis will be on independent work by the patient whenever possible. If there are difficulties in achieving a correct pattern because of muscle imbalance, manual help may still be necessary.

The aim of the physiotherapy programme will be to achieve the greatest possible strength in the shortest possible time, by requiring a maximum voluntary effort from the patient each time an exercise is done. This can only be brought about by increasing the demand on the muscle or synergist group. Success will only come through training.

Maximum strength is regulated automatically by the intensity of frequent muscular contractions. Stronger contractions act as a stimulus to gain further strength.

The main objective is to develop strength of the type and intensity that the patient needs for daily living and work. The need may be for training in dynamic or isometric strength or, as is more usual, for both. If strength in a specific task is needed the best training is the task itself. Usually the patient comes for treatment with a local or general problem rather than a difficulty in performing one specific task.

The most usual method of gaining strength at this stage is by the use of resistance in the form of a weighted boot, barbell, pulleys or springs, although in recent years there has been an increased use of isokinetic exercise machines. Greater emphasis on increasing the pace of exercising as a method of overloading the neuromuscular system is also practised. This increases power.

Some of the characteristics of the various forms of exercise used to increase strength are as follows.

Dynamic (isotonic) exercise

The term 'isotonic' exercise is often used in the literature to describe this type of programme in contrast to isometric and isokinetic exercise. Its use is not advisable – see Chapter 3.

The characteristics of such exercises are that the:

1. Movement is dynamic in nature – a shortening and/or lengthening of the muscle takes place
2. Load is moved through the available range
3. Resistance (load) applied to the moving lever is constant throughout the entire range
4. Resistance to the muscle contraction is not constant because of the modification of the lever system thereby altering torque
5. Weight that can be applied will be adapted to the weakest part of the range unless specific movement is given to a section of the range. Maximum work done is related to the ability to overcome inertia.[32]

There has been comparatively little research into the differing characteristics and use of eccentric as compared to concentric contractions in exercise programmes. Usually the muscle shortening and lengthening components of an exercise have not been separated in research methods. Some of the characteristics of eccentric exercise are that:

1. The muscle lengthens during contraction to resist the movement produced by gravity and any added weight
2. Pain appears to be more frequent in this type of exercise[66]
3. Muscular strength is lessened during the painful period
4. Greater strength is gained in eccentric than in concentric exercise in the long term but is less in the short term[5,37]
5. Strength is increased with faster contraction velocity
6. The energy cost is less.[5]

Because of the pain factor, eccentric exercise has no particular advantage over concentric exercise. Both types of muscle action are a necessary part of normal movement.

Isometric exercise[48,49,50]

The characteristics of an isometric exercise are that:

1. A contraction occurs with no visible joint movement
2. The resistance is sufficient to prevent any movement through range
3. It is related to the holding of a posture
4. It may be used to preserve and build up strength when motion is inadvisable
5. No mechanical work is done
6. It does not increase general body endurance
7. It can set a relatively high heart rate and arterial pressure
8. Learning is more difficult as the isometric 'setting' of a muscle is not a natural movement
9. Once learnt, if done against a dynamometer, it is easier and quicker to perform than dynamic exercise.

Isokinetic exercise[32,46,67]

Machines are now available which allow for the controlled movement of a body segment at a constant speed. The movement can be likened to that of an accommodating, manually-resisted movement. The characteristics of the exercise are that:

1. The movement is dynamic through the available range
2. The speed of the movement will be set and held constant throughout the range
3. The resistance throughout the range will be variable and proportional to the strength of the patient's contraction at each point in the available range
4. Pain is reported to be lessened
5. The machine can be reversed to use the antagonists
6. Muscle power can be accurately assessed
7. An objective measurement can be obtained on a print-out (Fig. 5.23)
8. The motivation of the patient is aided as he can know the result of his efforts
9. The movement does not simulate everyday movement.

Specificity of training

The type of muscle contraction given in training for strength influences the result of training. Concentric and eccentric contractions influence dynamic strength; isometric contractions – static strength.[7] All have some influence on overall strength. Training for strength in a certain part of joint range results in greatest strength increase in that part of the range in which the training has been done, though it will have some influence on overall range. When training for strength in a particular activity the best training is the activity itself.

Measurement

Before treatment starts a measurement of strength will be necessary. A muscle test should be made.

A test of a one repetition maximum (1 RM)

may be carried out for both dynamic or isometric muscle contractions. A one repetition maximum is the maximum weight that the patient can lift in a dynamic contraction through the full available range or hold in an isometric contraction in a particular part of the range. This is a test weight. Both tests may be taken in one position or in various known joint positions. Isokinetic testing may be used when the equipment is available.

The strength of the unaffected limb should also be tested so that a knowledge may be gained of the probable level of strength necessary for the patient to achieve. The balance between agonist and antagonist through range in both the normal and affected limb may give pointers for treatment.

The time of day of the test and retesting should be held constant as an afternoon test is usually superior to one taken in the morning.[31]

Motivation

If maximal strength is to be achieved the patient must work hard. An 'all out' effort will be needed.

Demand – the 'overload' principle[24,25,26,56]

The term 'overload', when used in relation to the gaining of strength by a patient, means that a muscle or synergist group works against a greater resistance than that to which it is accustomed. The resistance must be increased constantly in proportion to the maximum tested strength whether the contraction is dynamic or isometric. A demand will be placed on the muscle to produce greater tension. This is the principal factor in working for strength.

The 'overload' principle is just as important for the rehabilitation of the patient as it is for the training of an athlete. Strength will not be increased by the mere repetition of exercise of the same intensity over a period of time.[25,26,43]

The level of the load is controversial. In practice it is considered that if a muscle works either dynamically or isometrically at less than one-third ($\frac{1}{3}$) of its maximum strength, even if the number of repetitions is increased, strength will not be increased.[5,38,48]

The upper level is more difficult to assess and it will be governed to some extent by the reaction of the joints and muscles to the exercise. Many authorities consider the exercise weight level should be set around 60–70 per cent of the maximum possible.[5]

In an isometric contraction the level is set at two-thirds ($\frac{2}{3}$) the maximum the patient can hold for one to six (1–6) seconds. A dynamometer is usually used to ensure that a maximal contraction is achieved. Muller[48] suggests that a willed maximum contraction against any fixed resistance held for one second on five days weekly will significantly increase muscle strength. Considerable training may be necessary to achieve the maximum contraction.

The increase in load increases the intensity of the exercise probably by increasing proprioceptive impulses. Learning will also play a part in the ability to carry the extra load, eliminate unnecessary muscle work and gain skill.

In early rehabilitation the level of resistance may, if necessary, be kept low. However, it may be enough to help build up endurance slightly and gradually an increasing amount of resistance can be taken.

In any strength programme the 'overload' factor must be watched carefully if it is to be integrated into a total training programme.

A 'warm-up' will be necessary before the strength training begins.

Intensity and power

Intensity is concerned with the speed of the movement. Two factors – load and speed – are interdependent in creating a demand and in performing work. Just as the load is known so should the speed be known.[26,45,54]

Progressive training demands an increase so that either the same work is done in a shorter time or more work is done in the same time, or both. An increase in power is the end result in both instances.

Research has shown that exercise is speed specific. Moffroid and Whipple[45] trained two groups, one exercising concentrically at a low power output and the other concentrically at a high power output. Their findings were as follows:

1. Low power (low speed, high load) exercise produces greater increases in muscular force only at slow speeds.
2. High power (high speed, low load) exercise:
   a. Produces increases in muscular force at all speeds of contraction and below the training speed
   b. Increases muscular endurance at high speeds more than low power exercise increases muscular endurance at low speeds.

The amount of strength gained will only be increased if the level of the performance is regularly extended.

With volitional work there is an 'inbuilt' safety system – a subconscious control. A patient will not willingly allow pain or undue fatigue to occur particularly under guidance by the physiotherapist. Rest or a change of emphasis to another part of the limb or body is useful.

Hypertrophy

Many researchers have reported the development of hypertrophy in subjects involved in progressive strength development programmes. Others have reported no development of hypertrophy although strength was considerably increased.

Researchers who worked with patients have reported the development of hypertrophy when progressive resistance exercises were used in the treatment of patients.[16,40,41,72]

The starting position

When using progressive resistance exercises body stability and/or support will be needed to hold the body and the relevant parts steady and in good alignment, so that maximal movement can be performed with minimal stress and strain. For example, in quadriceps strengthening exercises, the position of sitting, with the back supported and the hip angle set at 110°–130° and the hands gripping the side of the table if necessary, provides the best position for maximal quadriceps activity.[12]

Frequency

The frequency of carrying out either dynamic or isometric 'overload' exercises will vary from 3–7 days in each week.

Repetition

Limited research has been done in this area. Most commonly a set of exercises consists of ten repetitions but the number of sets and the repetitions in the set will depend on the level of the overload. It has been found by Berger working with a 2,4,6,8, to 12 repetition maximum as between 3–9 repetitions – that is 4–8 contractions for one set.[8]

Cadence and rhythm of work

In training for strength, a steady rhythm should be set up at the speed selected with no jerking or unnecessary straining allowed. In this way a concentration of effort is possible and the probability of injury lessened.

Irradiation

With a small resistance there will be a contraction of the prime movers; with a greater resistance the synergists will contract and with even stronger resistance the antagonists will contract towards the end of the range probably to increase joint stability.

With maximal effort against a strong resistance responses will occur in the other parts of the body. Usually the head will move and other parts of the body will change their position. This is not a haphazard change. It appears as a constant and predictable response for that patient. No such movement occurs with underload exercise.[24]

The rate of increase in strength

The rate of increase in strength depends upon the initial level of strength – the less the amount of strength present initially, the faster the rate of initial improvement. As movement approaches the level of maximal performance for the muscle, the rate of improvement slows down until a final level is reached.

Skill learning

Learning, will have a marked effect on the gaining of strength by weight lifting. It is difficult to estimate the total effect that learning has in this type of programme. As skill improves unnecessary movements are eliminated and less effort will be necessary to produce the same result, so progress is made.

It is likely that a greater learning effort is necessary to gain an isometric contraction than that involved in obtaining a dynamic contraction which is a normal, known movement.

The influence of the position of the joint

The amount of strength through range that the patient has is often uneven and the force produced in a dynamic movement will change with the angle of pull of the muscle.[71] Most muscles also show a drop in strength from their elongated position to their shortened position. For example, full extension of the knee in sitting is difficult because the joint is in a disadvantageous position to produce maximal tension for both these reasons (Fig. 16.1, Fig. 5.23). This points to the need for specific training, either dynamic or isometric, through specific areas of need.

Agonist and antagonist

As the joint range alters so does the relation-ship between agonist and antagonist. There will be a point in the range of all joints where the balance of muscle pull is equal.[71]

Types of training and their relative value

Writers over many years have shown the value of progressive resistance exercises in increasing strength. The methods have varied greatly in respect to the load necessary, the intensity, speed, frequency and duration as well as the type of muscle action to be used – whether dynamic (isotonic), isometric or in special circumstances, isokinetic.

The evidence as to the most effective type of training for strength is inconclusive and controversial.

Many workers in the field have compared dynamic (isotonic) exercise with isometric exercise and have produced varied reports. Some favour isometric exercise, as the load in this type of exercise is constant, whereas the load carried in dynamic (isotonic) exercise is changing and must be set at the level of the weakest part of the range.

The level of dynamic training described varies from a two repetition maximum (2 RM) for one set; to a ten repetition maximum (10 RM) for three sets.[18] The level of isometric training described varies from fifty per cent (50%) of maximum isometric strength for five seconds to one maximum contraction daily for one second.[48,49,50] Both seem to result in a considerable increase in strength.

Usually both dynamic muscle shortening and lengthening exercises have been used. This is normal everyday movement and because the patient sees and knows the results of his work, it provides strong motivation. Isometric work done without a dynamometer is criticised as boring and lacking in stimulation. With a dynamometer the patient sees some result for his work.

Both dynamic and isometric exercises have the advantage that they can be used in a home programme with a minimum of equipment and therefore remain the most usual methods of gaining strength.

In life, muscles have different prime functions. For example, the quadriceps has the chief function of providing stability for the knee joint; others, for example, the biceps brachii, have the prime function of providing the mobility of the forearm necessary for versatile hand function. These factors may influence to some extent the type of training necessary.[69]

Isokinetic exercise has the advantage of providing an adaptable measure of resistance throughout the range as well as providing an objective measurement of work done. Its application in a general way is limited because of expense.

Much research work on the development and maintenance of strength still remains to be done.

Dynamic (Isotonic) exercise training programmes

(a) Progressive resistance training

The Delorme programme

Although exercises with dead weight and weight and pulley circuits had been used for many years[43] it was not until 1945 that a systematic programme of weight resisted measured dynamic exercises was set up by Delorme.[16] He called the system 'Progressive Resistance Exercises' (PRE). The measurement used was the 10 repetition maximum (10 RM) – the maximum weight that could be lifted 10 times through the available range at a steady natural rate without rest. A one repetition maximum (1 RM) was used as a test of progress. The weight was applied by means of a weighted boot, or barbell held in the hand.

The exercise programme passed through several changes. The system often used is that of Delorme and Watkins, 1945. It consists of three sets of:

10 lifts of $\frac{1}{2}$ 10 RM
    Rest
10 lifts of $\frac{3}{4}$ 10 RM
    Rest
10 lifts of 10 RM

This is done five times weekly with the 10 RM and 1 RM retested at weekly intervals. A rest period in a fully supported position is given between the sets.

Thus it is a system with a known load and measure of progress.[17]

The Oxford programme

Zinovieff[72] set up a programme known as the Oxford technique in which the weight is progressively reduced. It consists of 10 sets of 10 repetitions as follows:

10 lifts of the 10 RM
    Rest
10 lifts of the 10 RM minus 1 lb
    Rest
10 lifts of the 10 RM minus 2 lb and so on

for 10 sets of 10 repetitions making a total of 100 lifts to be done five times weekly. Every day at the end of the session a test is done to find if a new 10 RM is possible. If so this is used the next day. The programme is carried out for five days weekly.

The McQueen programmes

McQueen after studying the methods of body builders and of weight lifters set up two programmes.[40,41]

The 'hypertrophy' programme. This consists of three sets of the 10 repetition maximum (10 RM) for each set, with a rest between each set.

The 'power' programme. This consists of one set of the ten repetition maximum (10 RM) and then the weight is increased and the number of repetitions decreased.

For example
10 lifts of the 10 RM
    Rest
8 lifts of 8–6 RM
    Rest and so on

with the maximum weight lifted dependent on the patient's condition. This is the heaviest programme of the four.

It was found that the hypertrophy programme increased hypertrophy to a greater degree than the power programme. However, the power programme increased power to a greater degree than the hypertrophy programme.

Delorme[16] found that clinically there was a higher relapse rate in patients whose muscle strength had been restored but not muscle volume. Perhaps a suitable programme for patients should incorporate elements of both programmes.

All programmes mentioned above were said to increase strength and endurance and promote some hypertrophy.

Whatever the method chosen, care in teaching and supervising the performance is essential. The patient's body should be in a good position with the load adequate for the purpose to be served. The movement should be rhythmical and the ability present to control the speed of the movement.

Types of equipment

There are many types of equipment in general use providing resistance. They include weights, pulley and spring resistance as well as elastic belts and malleable substances such as putty. Water can be used particularly if turbulence is created.

(b) Progressive rate training

The strength of a muscle can be increased by progressively increasing the pace at which a set load is lifted over a series of training sessions. This method was devised by Hellebrandt & Houtz[26] and tested on well trained normal subjects.

A metronome is used in this procedure.

Preliminary measurements are taken on two consecutive days.

Day 1. The load that the subject can lift comfortably at a natural pace for a set number of times and no more.

Day 2. The maximum rate at which this load can now be lifted for the same set number of times.

Once these preliminary measures have been made the training programme can commence at the next treatment session. Dosage details for patients have not been reported in the literature; therefore the principles underlying the method can only be described here.

In successive training sessions:

1. The load is set for each patient and kept constant.
2. A set number of bouts of exercise each containing the same number of repetitions is used.
3. The pace is progressively increased from session to session to match the increases in the functional capacity of the muscle from day to day. Therefore the time taken to complete a training session decreases daily.
4. A rest period is given between each bout of exercise. The time of each period is kept constant.

Care must be taken when applying this method to patients and trauma due to uncontrolled momentum avoided. The movements should be kept well co-ordinated and accurate.

Isometric exercise

There does not appear to be any one system of isometric training in general use with patients.

The use of isometrics gained ground with the report of the work of Hettinger and Muller[29] because of the ease and speed of the application of the technique. The programme advocated the use of one daily contraction of six seconds' duration of two-thirds ($\frac{2}{3}$) maximum strength for five to seven days weekly. The intensity will vary with the force and the duration of the contraction.

Later work by Muller[50] advocated the use of one daily maximal contraction of one second's duration either five to seven days weekly. The maximal contraction is exerted against any immovable object. It may be used for any part of the body or through any part of the joint range. A dynamometer is used for regular testing.

It is obvious if this type of training is to be used to maximum advantage that the patient must learn to appreciate the 'feel' of the maximum contraction.

Hislop[31] reported that greater results could be obtained by two bouts of measured exercise of 15 second's duration rather than by one bout. The results were greater than those obtained by exercise for six seconds duration.

The exercise level appears to be set between 33 per cent and 75 per cent of the maximum measurable strength. Below 33 per cent no significant gains are recorded and there is no appreciable gain in exercising at 66–75 per cent of the maximum.

Many people have used and are still using isometric exercise. The method is quick, can be done at home, at work or in the treatment area. It can be used without special equipment though a measurement of progress should be made.

ENDURANCE

Endurance may be defined as the ability to continue a particular dynamic or static task accurately for a prolonged period of time. The person may be fatiguing but his ability to resist this fatigue is a measure of his endurance.

Two types of endurance are necessary:

1. Muscular endurance
2. Cardiovascular endurance.

Both are closely related.

Muscular endurance

Muscular endurance is defined as the ability of a muscle to sustain an isometric contraction or to continue dynamic contractions. It depends on the strength of the muscle involved, the localised energy stores in the muscle and the adequacy of the local circulation. Training methods which increase the blood supply to the muscles involved are necessary for the improvement of muscular endurance.

Muscular endurance is required in activities involving muscles at:

1. A local level, in which prolonged activity of the small muscles of the hand occurs as in repetitive lifting of small objects and placing them in a bag.
2. A general level, in which prolonged activity of the large muscle groups of the trunk and limbs occurs, as in repetitive heavy lifting in industry or swimming.

When an activity requires that a large percentage of the body's musculature be involved, cardiovascular endurance is required as well.

Muscular fatigue[4]

Muscular fatigue is a transient decrease in the performance capacity of muscles when they have been active for a certain period of time. The amount and rate of this decrease will vary with the type of exercise, the rate of work (power) and the individual muscle groups involved.

Muscular fatigue is usually recorded as a failure of the muscle to maintain or develop a certain expected force or power. Local factors contributing to such fatigue may include a depletion of energy producing substances necessary for continued activity or an accumulation of metabolites, such as lactate.

The level of fatigue may vary from a feeling of tiredness to complete exhaustion. Movement becomes inaccurate because muscles not primarily required for the activity are progressively recruited, thereby increasing the energy cost of the activity. The person becomes tense and more energy is required to continue working, which with time, the body is unable to meet.

Training for muscular endurance occurs as long as the task is continued to the point of fatigue.

Cardiovascular endurance

Cardiovascular endurance is defined as the capacity of the individual to maintain strenuous activity of a number of muscle groups or of the whole body for a prolonged period.[63] It depends on the overall functioning of the cardiovascular and respiratory systems and their ability to deliver oxygen anywhere it is needed in the whole body. It also depends on the body's ability to mobilise its energy stores and remove waste products. The heart's capacity to pump blood effectively is the most common limiting factor in cardiovascular endurance although it is not the only one.[54]

Endurance depends on the ready availability of oxygen to the exercising muscles as well as the presence of energy producing fuels such as carbohydrates and fats. Energy for muscle contractions is produced through biochemical processes involving the presence of oxygen (aerobic metabolism) and not requiring the presence of oxygen (anaerobic metabolism). The by-products of anaerobic metabolism accumulate and contribute to the development of fatigue.

During short bouts of work involving a few seconds the anaerobic processes play a dominant role, but if the exercise is to continue for a longer period aerobic processes play the major role.

Oxygen uptake and endurance

There are physiological limits to the amount of oxygen that can be taken up by the body as it exercises against increasing loads. This limiting level of oxygen consumption is called the maximum oxygen uptake or VO_2 max.

Aerobic capacity which is defined as the highest rate of aerobic metabolism during the performance of rhythmic dynamic muscle work that exhausts the subject within 5–10 minutes, is assessed through the measurement of the maximal oxygen uptake. Various exercise testing procedures have been described which determine a person's aerobic capacity.[2,5,18,62]

The maximal oxygen uptake is influenced by a person's age, sex and bodily dimensions. For example, after 25–30 years it steadily declines so at 70 years of age the $\dot{V}O_2$ max may be only 50 per cent of what it was at 20 years.[2]

The $\dot{V}O_2$ max, has also been shown to diminish with bed rest.[61] Therefore any rehabilitation regime after illness or injury, should include general activities to improve the patient's cardiorespiratory fitness as well as the more specific treatments aimed at his local condition.

In daily life the majority of activities are carried out at submaximal levels except for bursts of extra effort which may be required from time to time. By performing at submaximal levels only, an individual can continue an activity for a longer period of time before experiencing fatigue.

ENDURANCE TRAINING

Training for muscular endurance

The development of muscular endurance is closely related to the development of muscle strength and power. Many of the principles already discussed in the previous section on muscle strength and power, apply here as well.

Endurance does not develop unless the muscle is worked so some fatigue is present. Repetition with light work loads does not bring about an optimal improvement in muscular endurance. Therefore the patient must progressively increase the amount of work done by the muscle using the principle 'overload' which has been described previously.

In endurance training, submaximal dynamic muscle contractions from approximately 30–50 per cent of the muscle's maximal strength are useful.[38] Loads using less than 15 per cent maximal strength are useless as the stimulus placed on the muscle is not sufficiently demanding to get the desired training effect.

Isometric contractions are rarely used alone in an endurance programme although they may be used in a combined training programme when both static and dynamic endurance are needed. This may be best achieved using circuit training.

Strength is not the only factor to be considered in an endurance training programme. The task itself may be the most effective. Here multiple muscles are exercised repetitively in specific patterns, which with practice increases the patient's skill for that task. As he becomes more skillful unnecessary movements are eliminated, thereby reducing the energy cost of the task and allowing the patient to continue the task much longer.

A measurement of the work done in the training programme is necessary. The load carried, range used, the number of repetitions and the time taken should be recorded.

Motivation is necessary. The patient must understand the general purpose of the training if he is going to push himself sufficiently hard to the point of fatigue and endure some discomfort – a factor necessary if an adequate training stimulus is to be gained.

For safety reasons, modifications must be made to training programmes for those people who should avoid all-out effort. Here heart rate levels are a useful general guide. The use of a heart rate meter, or the simple taking of the patient's pulse is an easy procedure to perform. Exercise should stop when the patient's heart rate reaches the following values shown in Table 16.1.[2]

All exercise should be discontinued if the patient complains of pain in the chest, difficulty in breathing or severe fatigue.

Training for cardio-respiratory fitness

In the later stages of rehabilitation, training for cardio-respiratory fitness is often necessary to prepare the patient for return to work.

The American College of Sports Medicine has issued the following guidelines for the quantity and quality of training for developing and maintaining cardio-respiratory fitness in the healthy adult.[1]

1. Frequency of training: 3 to 5 days per week.
2. Intensity of training: 60 per cent to 90 per cent of the maximum heart rate reserve or 50 per cent to 80 per cent of maximum oxygen uptake.
3. Duration of training: 15–60 minutes of continuous aerobic activity. This is dependant on the intensity of the activity. Lower intensity activity should be conducted over a longer period of time. Lower to moderate intensity activity of longer duration is recommended for the non-athlete adult.
4. Mode of activity: any activity that uses large muscle groups, that can be maintained continuously and is aerobic in nature such as walking, running, swimming, bicycling, rowing and skiing is effective.

In general, the lower the stimuli the lower the training effect. Endurance training less than two days per week, less than 50 per cent of maximum oxygen uptake and less than 10 minutes per day is inadequate for developing and maintaining cardio-respiratory fitness in healthy adults.

Circuit training[5]

Circuit training entails a series of four to six activities, performed one after the other with a rest period between each activity. For many patients some general, as well as specific training for a task, is necessary. The activities can be planned to increase a patient's strength, endurance and flexibility and/or to improve his general condition. Aerobic or anaerobic power may be developed. In planning the programme the purpose of each activity must be considered by the physiotherapist and explained to the patient so that he is motivated to work independently.

Table 16.1

Age (years)	Upper limits (beats/min)
20–29	170
30–39	160
40–49	150
50–59	140
60 and over	130

Each proposed activity is tested and a suitable programme of diversified activities arranged taking into account the patient's local and general condition. The extent of the activity, the number of repetitions, the length of time to be taken by the activity and the rest period to follow, is determined. The higher the extent of the activity, the fewer will be the repetitions. The reverse also occurs. Often the level is set so that the period of the activity and the rest period are equal. A measurement can be made of the work done at each point in the training sequence.

Depending on the purpose, the programme is often arranged so that an activity involving large muscle groups is followed by one using smaller groups or the activity is transferred to another part of the body. Both static and dynamic activities are usually included. The programme must be done regularly.

Retesting is carried out weekly and a new level of activity set up. Once carefully taught the programme can be done in the department with minimum supervision and if the activities are suitable, used as a home programme. In this case it is helpful if a regular time is set for the patient to carry out this programme.

REFERENCES AND FURTHER READING

1. American College of Sports Medicine (1978) Position statement on the recommended quantity and quality of exercise for developing and maintaining fitness in healthy adults. *Medicine and Science in Sports*, Vol. 10, No. 3, pp. vii–x.
2. Anderson, K. L., Shephard, R. J., Denolin, H., Vannauskas, E. & Masironi, R. (1971) *Fundamentals of Exercise Testing.* Geneva: World Health Organization.
3. Asmussen, E. (1953) Positive and negative muscular work. *Acta Physiologica Scandinavica*, Vol. 28, pp. 364–382.
4. Asmussen, E. (1979) Muscle Fatigue. *Medicine and Science in Sports*, Vol. 11, No. 4, pp. 313–321.
5. Astrand, P. O. & Rodahl, K. (1977) *Textbook of Work Physiology*, 2nd edn. New York: McGraw-Hill.
6. Basmajian, J. V. (Ed) (1984) *Therapeutic Exercise*, 4th edn. Baltimore: Williams & Wilkins.
7. Berger, R. A. (1962) Comparison of static and dynamic strength increases. *Research Quarterly*, Vol. 33, No. 3, pp. 329–333.
8. Berger, R. A. (1962) Optimum repetitions for development of strength. *Research Quarterly*, Vol. 33, No. 3, pp. 334–338.
9. Clarke, D. H. (1973) Adaptations in strength and muscular endurance resulting from exercise. *Exercise and Sports Sciences Reviews*, Vol. 1, pp. 73–102.
10. Cooper, K. H. (1970) *The New Aerobics.* U.S.A.: Bantam Books.
11. Currier, D. P. (1972) Maximal isometric tension of the elbow extensors at varied positions. *Physical Therapy*, Vol. 52, No. 10, pp. 1043–1049.
12. Currier, D. P. (1977) Positioning for knee strengthening exercises. *Physical Therapy*, Vol. 57, No. 2, pp. 148–152.
13. Darcus, H. D. & Salter, N. (1955) The effect of repeated muscular exertion on muscle strength. *Journal of Physiology*, Vol. 129, pp. 325–336.
14. Delateur, B. J., Lehmann, J. & Giaconi, R. (1968) A test of the Delorme axiom. *Archives of Physical Medicine and Rehabilitation*, Vol. 49, pp. 245–248.
15. Delateur, B. J., Lehmann, J. & Giaconi, R. (1976) Mechanical work and fatigue: their roles in the development of muscle work capacity. *Archives of Physical Medicine and Rehabilitation*, Vol. 57, July, pp. 319–324.
16. Delorme, T. L. (1946) Heavy resistance exercises. *Archives of Physical Medicine*, Vol. 27, pp. 607–625.
17. Delorme, T. L. & Watkins, A. L. (1948) Technics of progressive resistance exercise. *Archives of Physical Medicine*, Vol. 29, pp. 263–273.
18. DeVries, H. A. (1980) *Physiology of Exercise*, 3rd edn. Dubuque: W. C. Brown.
19. Eccles, J. C. (1944) Investigations on muscle atrophies arising from disuse and tenotomy. *Journal of Physiology*, Vol. 103, pp. 253–266.
20. Eckert, H. (1965) A concept of force-energy in human movement. *Journal of the American Physical Therapy Association*, Vol. 45, No. 3, pp. 213–218.
21. Gilliam, T. B., Sady, S. D., Freedom, P. & Villanacci, J. (1979) Isokinetic torque levels for high school football players. *Archives of Physical Medicine and Rehabilitation*, Vol. 60, March, pp. 110–114.
22. Goslin, B. R. & Charteris, J. (1979) Isokinetic dynamometry: normative data for clinical use in lower extremity knee cases. *Scandinavian Journal of Rehabilitation Medicine*, Vol. 11, pp. 105–109.
23. Gregory, L. W. (1979) The development of aerobic capacity: a comparison of continuous and interval training. *Research Quarterly*, Vol. 50, No. 2, pp. 199–206.
24. Hellebrandt, F. A. (1958) Application of the overload principle to muscle training in man. *International Review of Physical Medicine and Rehabilitation*, October, pp. 278–283.
25. Hellebrandt, F. A. & Houtz, S. J. (1956) Mechanisms of muscle training in man. *Physical Therapy Review*, Vol. 36, No. 6, pp. 371–383.
26. Hellebrandt, F. A. & Houtz, S. J. (1958) Methods of muscle training: the influence of pacing. *Physical Therapy Review*, Vol. 38, No. 5, pp. 319–322.

27. Hellebrandt, F. A. & Waterland, J. C. (1962) Indirect learning. *American Journal of Physical Medicine*, Vol. 41, No. 2, pp. 45–55.

28. Hellebrandt, F. A., Parrish, A. M. & Houtz, S. A. (1947) Cross education. *Archives of Physical Medicine*, Vol. 28, pp. 76–85.

29. Hettinger, T. & Muller, E. A. Muskelleistung und Muskeltraining Arbeitsphysiol. 15, (1953) cited by Muller, E. A. Influence of Training and of inactivity on Muscle Strength. *Archives of Physical Medicine*, Vol. 51, 1970. pp. 449–462.

30. Hinson, M. & Rosentswieg, J. (1973) Comparative Electromyographic values of Isometric, Isotonic and Isokinetic contraction. *Research Quarterly*, Vol. 44, No. 1, pp. 71–78.

31. Hislop, H. J. (1963) Quantitative changes in human muscular strength during isometric exercise. *Journal of the American Physical Therapy Association*, Vol. 43, No. 1, pp. 21–38.

32. Hislop, H. J. & Perrine, J. J. (1967) The isokinetic concept of exercise. *Physical Therapy*, Vol. 47, No. 2, pp. 114–117.

33. International Committee for the Standardisation of Physical Fitness Tests, Larson L. A. (Ed.) (1974) *Fitness, Health and Work Capacity: International Standards for Assessment.* New York: MacMillan.

34. Johnson, B. L., Adamozyk, J. W., Tennoe, K. O. & Stømme, S. B. (1976) A comparison of concentric and eccentric muscle training. *Medicine and Science in Sports*, Vol. 8, No. 1, pp. 35–38.

35. Knott, M. & Voss, D. E. (1968) *Proprioceptive Neuromuscular Facilitation*, 2nd edn. New York: Harper and Row.

36. Knuttgen, H. G. (Ed.) (1976) *Neuromuscular Mechanisms for Therapeutic and Conditioning Exercise.* Baltimore: University Park Press.

37. Komi, P. V. & Buskirk, E. R. (1972) Effects of eccentric and concentric muscle conditioning on tension and electrical activity of human muscles. *Ergonomics*, Vol. 15, No. 4, pp. 417–434.

38. Kottke, F. J. (1971) Therapeutic Exercise. In Krusen, F. H. (Ed) *Handbook of Physical Medicine and Rehabilitation*, 2nd edn, Chapter 16, pp. 385–425. Philadelphia: W. B. Saunders.

39. Laird, C. E. & Rozier, C. K. (1979) Towards understanding the terminology of exercise mechanics. *Physical Therapy*, Vol. 59, No. 3, pp. 287–292.

40. MacQueen, I. J. (1954) Recent advances in the technique of progressive resistance exercise. *British Medical Journal*, Vol. 2, pp. 1193–1198.

41. MacQueen, I. J. (1956) The application of progressive resistance exercise in physiotherapy. *Physiotherapy*, Vol. 40, pp. 83–93.

42. McCafferty, W. B. & Horvath, S. M. (1977) Specificity of exercise and specificity of training: a subcellular review. *Research Quarterly*, Vol. 48, No. 2, pp. 358–371.

43. Mennell, J. (1934) *Physical Treatment by Movement, Manipulation, and Massage.* London: J. A. Churchill.

44. Moffroid, M. T. & Kusiak, E. T. (1975) The power struggle: definition and evaluation of power of muscular performance. *Physical Therapy*, Vol. 55, No. 10, pp. 1098–1104.

45. Moffroid, M. T. & Whipple, R. H. (1970) Specificity of speed of exercise. *Physical Therapy*, Vol. 50, No. 12, pp. 1692–1700.

46. Moffroid, M., Whipple, R. H., Hofkosh, J., Lowman, E. & Thistle, H. (1969) A study of Isokinetic exercise. *Physical Therapy*, Vol. 49, No. 7, pp. 735–746.

47. Moritani, M. A. & Devries, H. A. (1979) Neural factors versus hypertrophy in the time course of muscle strength gain. *American Journal of Physical Medicine*, Vol. 59, No. 3, pp. 115–130.

48. Muller, E. A. (1959) Training muscle strength. *Ergonomics*, Vol. 2, No. 2, pp. 218–222.

49. Muller, E. A. (1965) Physiological methods of increasing human physical work capacity. *Ergonomics*, Vol. 8, No. 4, pp. 409–424.

50. Muller, E. A. (1970) Influence of training and of inactivity on muscle strength. *Archives of Physical Medicine and Rehabilitation*, Vol. 51, pp. 449–462.

51. Murray, M. P., Baldwin, J. M., Garner, G. M., Sepic, S. S. & Downs, W. J. (1977) Maximum isometric knee flexor and extensor muscle contractions. *Physical Therapy*, Vol. 57, No. 6, pp. 637–643.

52. Perrine, J. J. & Edgerton, R. (1978) Muscle force–velocity and power – velocity relationships under isokinetic loading. *Medicine and Science in Sports*, Vol. 10, No. 3, pp. 159–166.

53. Pipes, T. V. & Wilmore, J. H. (1975) Isokinetic versus isotonic training in adult men. *Medicine and Science in Sports*, Vol. 7, No. 4, pp. 262–274.

54. Rasch, P. J. & Burke, R. K. (1978) *Kinesiology and Applied Anatomy*, 6th edn. Philadelphia: Lea and Febiger.

55. Rasch, P. J. & Morehouse, L. E. (1957) Effect of static and dynamic exercises on muscular strength and hypertrophy. *Journal of Applied Physiology*, Vol. 11, No. 1, pp. 20–34.

56. Rasch, P. J., Pierson, W. R. & Logan, G. A. (1961) The effect of isometric exercise upon the strength of antagonistic muscles. *Int. Z. Angeu. Physiol. einschl. Arbeitsphysiol*, Vol. 19, pp. 18–22.

57. Rose, S. J. & Rothstein, J. M. (1982) Muscle Mutability. Part 1 – General concepts and altered patterns of use. *Physical Therapy*, Vol. 62, No. 12, pp. 1773–1787.

58. Rosentswieg, J. & Hinson, M. M. (1972) Comparison of isometric, isotonic and isokinetic exercises by electromyography. *Archives of Physical Medicine and Rehabilitation*, Vol. 53, No. 6, pp. 249–252.

59. Rothstein, J. M. (1982) Muscle Biology. *Physical Therapy*, Vol. 62, No. 12, pp. 1823–1830.

60. Rothstein, J. M. & Rose, S. J. (1982) Muscle Mutability. Part 2 – Adaptation to drugs, metabolic factors and aging. *Physical Therapy*, Vol. 62, No. 12, pp. 1789–1798.

61. Saltin, B. B., Blomqvist, J. H., Mitchell, R. L., Johnson, J., Wildenthal, K. & Chapman, C. B. (1968) Response to submaximal and maximal exercise after bed rest and training. *Circulation*, Vol. 38 (Supp.7).

62. Shephard, R. J. (1968) Methodology of exercise tests in healthy subjects and in cardiac patient. *Canadian Medical Association Journal*, Vol. 99, pp. 354–359.

63. Simri, U. (1974) Assessment procedures for human performance. In International Committee for the standardisation of physical fitness tests, Larson L. A. (Ed.) *Fitness Health and Work Capacity: International Standards for Assessment*, Chapter 19, pp. 362–379.

64. Singh, M. & Karpovich, P. V. (1967) Effect of eccentric training of agonists on antagonistic muscles. *Journal of Applied Physiology*, Vol. 23, No. 5, pp. 742–745.

65. Singh, M. & Karpovich, P. V. (1968) Strength of forearm flexors and extensors in men and women. *Journal of Applied Physiology*, Vol. 25, No. 2, pp. 177–180.

66. Talag, T. S. (1973) Residual muscular soreness as influenced by concentric, eccentric and static contractions. *Research Quarterly*, Vol. 44, No. 4, pp. 458–469.

67. Thistle, H. C., Hislop, H. J., Moffroid, M. & Lowman, E. W. (1967) Isokinetic contraction: a new concept of resistive exercise. *Archives of Physical Medicine and Rehabilitation*, Vol. 48, pp. 279–282.

68. Waddington, P. J. (1976) Chapters 21–25. In Hollis, M. (Ed.) *Practical Exercise Therapy*. London: Blackwell Scientific.

69. Ward, J. & Fisk, G. H. (1964) The difference in response of the quadriceps and the biceps brachii muscles to isometric and isotonic exercise. *Archives of Physical Medicine and Rehabilitation*, Vol. 45, pp. 614–620.

70. Whitley, J. D. & Allan, L. G. (1971) Specificity versus generality in static strength performance. *Archives of Physical Medicine and Rehabilitation*, Aug., pp. 371–375.

71. Williams, M. & Stutzman, L. (1959) Strength variation through the range of joint motion. *Physical Therapy Review*, Vol. 39, June, pp. 145–152.

72. Zinovieff, A. N. (1951) Heavy resistance exercises. *British Journal of Physical Medicine*, June, pp. 129–133.

17
Flexibility

Flexibility may be defined as the ability of a person to move a part or parts of the body in a wide range of purposeful movements at the required speed. The range should be no less or no more than is normal for that person. This implies that movement is versatile and flows easily in all directions at varying speeds so that the demands of both dynamic movement and maintained postures may be met. It is controlled mobility and it should be considered from both general and local bodily aspects.

Flexibility of a joint depends on the type of joint, its bony integrity, the soft tissues forming an integral part of its structure and its muscular control. It will be specific to the particular joint.

In early life children are very flexible. This lessens as bony growth occurs and there is a gradual tightening of fascia and ligaments as well as the strengthening of muscles, bringing with it increasing stability. From the ages of 11–12 years flexibility increases up to early adulthood after which time there is a general decline.

Each person has a uniqueness of range in their joints with active persons being generally more mobile than inactive. Thus it is often associated with habitual activities. The extent of flexibility of one joint does not necessarily mean the same degree in other joints.

The need for flexibility varies from task to task. Injury or disease of a joint can lead to an unwanted restriction or an excess of movement which produces unnecessary stresses not only on the surrounding structures of the particular joint involved but often in those joints associated with it when performing various movements. If some restriction of range is present the physiotherapist should have a knowledge of the most important part of the range to be preserved or gained for that person.

Usually flexibility should not be gained at the expense of stability, as an unstable joint becomes prone to further injury and causes strain to joints associated with it in a movement. Bracing can be applied if stability is impossible to achieve.

The common causes of loss of joint range are:

1. Pain
2. Oedema
3. Destruction of joint structure, for example, through erosion as in arthritis or a fracture
4. Muscle, fascial or skin tightness
5. Muscle weakness or imbalance
6. Long-term habits of general and local posture.

Exercise can be used to improve flexibility because the soft tissues surrounding the joint are viscoelastic and have an inherent extensibility. These tissues include the joint capsule, ligaments, the muscles and their fascial sheaths, tendons, nerves, blood vessels, connective tissue and skin.

The muscles can be readily controlled at will to vary their tension and also have an inbuilt safety system, the stretch reflex, which provides a braking force to prevent over-stretching when active exercise is undertaken.

Where changes in bony structure of the joint impede movement, exercise cannot directly influence the regaining of flexibility. Other methods such as joint replacement surgery may be advised, after which the pysiotherapist can use exercise to aid in the improvement of soft tissue extensibility and strength so that a well-controlled movement is achieved.

The examination of joint function

Treatment will commence with a complete examination of the function of the affected joint and all other joints in the limb. For example, the shoulder, elbow and digital joints should be examined when a patient has a Colles fracture involving the wrist joint, to ensure that a loss of flexibility through disuse or associated trauma has not occurred.

The examination should include standard tests of joint range, palpation of accessory movements, muscle length and strength tests including muscle balance around the affected joints (Appendix 1). An appreciation of the quality of the restriction as the end of range is approached should also be gauged while palpating. Any pain present and the point in the range where it occurs should be noted. Functional activities are carefully tested so that faults in the pattern of movement and any slight restriction in range can be observed. The results of all tests should be recorded and further tests carried out regularly under the same conditions. Any improvement should be reported to the patient. It acts as an encouragement to him. Any decrease in range should be investigated and the cause found if possible. This should be reported and the patient's programme reviewed.

THE REGAINING OF FLEXIBILITY

The aim of physiotherapy procedures is to regain all possible normal movement in all directions at a normal speed for the activity in all the affected parts of the body. Such encouragement of normal use or function sets the basis for the return of freedom to stiff joints. There is a close relationship between normal muscle function and the achievement of full joint range of motion, as muscles cannot be restored to their full capacity if the joints they normally move are not free to do so. Therefore active movements form the major part of any flexibility programme.

The methods used to increase flexibility

basically involve frequent and regular stretching of the shortened tissues which over time will lengthen, provided the potential is there. This lengthened state is more likely to be preserved if all the muscles surrounding the joint are functioning effectively. Adequate muscle strength is essential to maintain general and local stability, to protect the joint and muscles from trauma as well as to prevent the possible development of an unstable joint. Thus, mobilising and strengthening measures must go hand in hand as increases in joint range are achieved.

The level of function to be reached should be sufficiently high to allow a margin of safety, so that unexpected stress placed on the body or its parts should not cause undue joint or muscle strain. The amount and extent of treatment that can be given to the patient at any one time will depend on the inflammatory state of his joint and/or muscle as well as the degree of pain, the presence of fatigue and his own level of activities.

Pain is a major inhibitor of movement. Therefore appropriate measures such as the use of heat, cold, massage or electrotherapy are often used as a preliminary to exercise treatment.

Active preventive measures

In the early stages of treatment, preventive measures are important so that further disability does not occur.

The prevention of loss of joint range and possible deformity is a key factor in the treatment of joint and soft tissue injuries. The following principles are important:

1. Active movements through range will start as soon as the condition allows. Where joints must be immobilised after injury, isometric muscle contractions are started as soon as possible. In this way some strength of muscle contraction and the mobility of the tissues as they glide over each other as well as the circulation to all joint structures will be maintained.

2. Positioning is important. The patient's knowledge of the maintenance of good body and joint alignment, both at rest and during activity, may prove a major factor in the prevention of trauma, loss of joint range and deformity. The patient is made aware of resting positions and good habits of movement which help preserve function as well as those to avoid. For example, prone lying may help prevent a hip flexion deformity, whereas prolonged sitting could encourage its development.

3. Free uninjured joints usually can be kept moving actively within the limits set by the injury or its treatment. It is a matter of a little activity done regularly. A few minutes of appropriate exercise on the hour is a common routine which will make rehabilitation easier.

4. Muscle length needs to be maintained. Any muscle is likely to become shortened through muscle damage with scarring, unresolved oedema or disuse. Active movements when possible or passive movements through full joint range, will help to maintain length. In particular, the normal length of two joint muscles must be carefully maintained.

5. Relaxed passive movement is used when active movement is impossible. This is a fully supported movement given by the physiotherapist in a slow smooth manner through the available range. These movements are used to maintain range, as well as to preserve a kinaesthetic sense and memory of the movement prior to active movement returning. A knowledge of the normal patterns of movement, including rotation, is essential if the physiotherapist is to perform these movements effectively. It is important that the passive movements are carefully given and that trauma, with resultant pain and oedema leading to further decrease in joint range, does not occur.

Methods of active treatment

1. Local relaxation

In the subacute stage, local relaxation is a most useful method of regaining range. A careful history and observation of the patient followed by gentle palpation will indicate areas of pain and tension. The patient, in a comfortably supported position, is made aware of the areas of major tension and the need for relaxation. One of the techniques described in Chapter 7, together with the use of massage, heat and/or cold, may prove helpful in lessening tension and relieving pain.

With skilled and sensitive handling by the physiotherapist, pain may be lessened and mobility gradually increased. The techniques of hold–relax or contract–relax[17] may also be useful at a slightly later time.

2. Progressive positional relaxation

This is a most useful method of treatment particularly for the joints of the wrist and hand. For example, in sitting the hand is placed comfortably on the opposite thigh and relaxed in that position. It is then moved gently and progressively laterally and forwards over the thigh if flexion of the wrist is needed or over the knee if both wrist and finger flexion is needed. It is drawn upwards and medially on the thigh if extension is wanted.

It can also be used in sitting, drawing the foot backwards to increase dorsiflexion.

3. Pool exercise

Exercise in water is one of the easiest and most pleasant methods of regaining range for a patient with joint pain, muscle weakness and spasm. Water acts as an assistance since gravitational forces are reduced and its buoyancy allows movement with little effort. Its warmth may ease the pain and spasm. Stabilisation of parts of the body may be needed if the movements are to be most effective in improving the range of specific joints.

As soon as possible the demands on the patient are stepped up. The programmes will include correction of head and body alignment when necessary.

Stretching exercises

To stretch may be defined as to elongate or extend in length. The objective of any stretching activity is to place stress on tightened structures so that they will increase in length. A muscle which has been stretched from a shortened position will return to the shortened position unless it is habitually used in its stretched position in order to maintain its new length. A muscle which is tense and has been relaxed also will return to its tense state unless the process of relaxation is continued or the condition which caused the tension is removed.

A preliminary 'warming up' involving the use of gentle, smooth, rhythmic movements in an easy pain-free range is helpful and necessary before beginning stretching exercises. For example, in sitting or standing, relaxation followed by a gentle shaking of the arm or a pendular arm swinging by the patient are useful preliminaries to movements of the upper limb.

Active measures to produce a stretching effect can be classified as:

1. Self-stretching. These movements consist of either prolonged or intermittent stretching.

A prolonged self-stretch consists of a slow stretching movement taken to the extreme of range, held there and then gradually released. If pain is present it may be taken to the point of pain and just beyond it, held momentarily, and then slowly relaxed. Intermittent self-stretches may be described as ballistic or 'bobbing' type movements which consist of a series of fast stretches followed by slight withdrawals. They are done to a beat or rhythm. In research carried out on these two methods, both have proved effective in gaining range.

De Vries[5] and others found no difference between the two methods when done by persons with postural tightness. Weber and Kraus[25] working with children of an average age of 8½ years with postural tightness found the bobbing method much more satisfactory than active and passive stretching. De Vries makes the point that prolonged stretching may be the safer of the two methods. It may be controlled more easily by the patient as pain would be felt before tissue damage occurred. In the ballistic method this would not be possible because of the speed of the movement.

It could be considered that there are physiological reasons for using the slow stretch. In the 'bobbing' movement the shortened muscles could respond to the quick stretch towards the end of their available range by tightening – a reflex response. In the slow stretching method against a force, the tight antagonists (the shortened muscles) will relax reciprocally as the agonists (the lengthened muscles) contract. The energy requirements for prolonged stretching are lower than for the 'bobbing' method.

2. Assisted stretching by either the patient or the physiotherapist. Assistance will be needed if the patient cannot move through range in a correct pattern. The help will be graded according to the needs of the movement. Self-help has the great advantage that the movement can be done frequently by the patient: for example, sitting, double arm flexion and extension with the fingers interlocked – a movement which can be used by patients with muscle weakness to prevent joint stiffness and muscle shortening as well as providing a sensation of movement and position.

3. Apparatus-assisted self-stretching. Reciprocal pulleys provide a useful method (Fig. 17.1a). The action will consist of a stretching movement at the end of the range with over-pressure applied by the sound limb. Rods or a towel may also be used and provide a varied, interesting and imaginative flexibility and strengthening programme (Fig. 17.1b, c, d, e).

4. Gravity-assisted self-stretching. This is a swinging movement, initiated by the muscles and then taken over by a pendular action of the limb.

5. A long general stretch. A long general stretch involving many joints, often combined with trunk movement, may give general relief and at the same time show up small areas of unexpected tightness, particularly in those joints above and below the affected one.

6. A series of general stretching exercises. A series of general stretching exercises will be useful to persons who have had an injury and are to return to manual work or sport.

Serial plasters

Serial plasters may be used to give a constant stretch to muscles and soft tissues between treatment sessions where new gains in length have been obtained through stretching activities. The serial plasters enable the new length to be maintained between treatment sessions, allowing time for the viscoelastic tissues to accommodate to the new joint position.

Strengthening exercises

The importance of and the need for strength to maintain any new position gained through stretching tightened structures has already been discussed. Methods of regaining strength have been described in Chapter 16.

Mobilising and co-ordination exercises

Co-ordination in many movements can be disturbed by joint restriction as the total number of degrees of freedom available is reduced.

A variety of interesting free exercises involving varied starting positions and changing movement patterns to involve many movements of the affected joint and related joints is most useful in a treatment programme. These exercises can be planned to provide both a mobilising and co-ordinating effect. If they incorporate some of the patient's daily activities or pleasures they are more likely to be put into regular use.

Characteristics of mobilising and co-ordination exercises

Rhythm entails a regular alternation, a rise and fall of intensity which is measured and balanced, giving a 'flow' to the movement. Some patients find this difficult and need help by counting, music or by a rhythm set by another person. A metronome is a very useful aid.

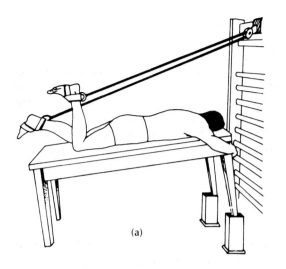

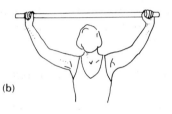

(a)

(b)

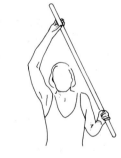

(c)

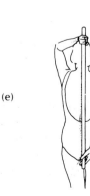

(d)

(e)

Speed in many cases is allied to rhythm and most exercises are done at a natural speed. Speed should be varied in a training programme so that the patient can cope with the many demands placed on these movements in everyday life.

Smoothness, accuracy, dexterity and precision lead to a controlled economy of effort and to skill in movement.

Contrasting movements test the ability of the patient to perform and control movements which demand sudden changes in quality. Exercises involving tensing and relaxing, resisting and yielding, pushing, stretching and pulling and the grading of lightness and heaviness are all useful.

These contrasting movements can be incorporated into longer movements where one movement effortlessly flows into the next and so on. For example, a flowing sequence of movement may start in a small range and continue on with increasing range and changes in direction, demanding good co-ordination, range, rhythm and postural control and the testing of the patient's ability to perform with ease.

Passive movements

Passive movements, used in the following ways, may prove helpful for some patients to gain flexibility.

1. A gentle stretching in a particular part of the range. The stretch is given to the tight structures. An exact appreciation of the amount of range, including rotation, normally present and its present state must be made, so that the stretch is correctly directed. This movement is capable of being stopped by the patient.

2. A thrusting movement. This is usually a quick movement carried out in the inner

Fig. 17.1 (a) Reciprocal pulleys to the knee.
(b), (c), (d), (e) Exercises for the shoulders using an arm rod.

range of the patient's movement. It cannot be stopped by the patient.

3. Traction may be given. The patient can sometimes reduce the effectiveness of the movement by opposing the pull with his muscles.

Specialised manipulative techniques using passive movements are described elsewhere by writers such as Mennell[22], Cyriax[2], Maitland[20,21] and Grieve.[9,10]

Where soft tissue changes have occurred through damage, the use of other physical modalities will be necessary in addition to passive mobilisation.

Retention of range

Once a pain-free range of normal movement and the necessary strength and co-ordination to control it is gained, function should be retained if the patient uses the function in daily life.

Excessive range

Hypermobility of one or more joints is relatively common. If excessive range of movement is controlled adequately by the muscles – as in the ballet dancer – the joint will be symptomless.

If excessive range has occurred in the absence of training, the joint will probably be unstable. There may be capsular and ligamentous laxity accompanied by poor muscular control of the joint.

The physiotherapist will aim to strengthen both agonist and antagonist muscles and so improve the control of the joint, provided the potential is there. These muscles could be considered as 'active ligaments' which need to be trained so they spring quickly into action on demand to compensate for laxity in the other restraining structures. The speed of response is important as well as the muscles resistance to fatigue.

Advice should be given on the positioning of the joint at rest and in use, so that preventable deformities are avoided.

REFERENCES AND FURTHER READING

1. Astrand, P. & Rodahl, K. (1977) *Textbook of Work Physiology*, 2nd edn. New York: McGraw Hill.
2. Cyriax, J. (1977) *Textbook of Orthopaedic Medicine, Vol. 2. Treatment by Manipulation, Massage and Injection*, 9th edn. London: Cassell.
3. Daniels, L. & Worthingham, C. (1980) *Muscle Testing*, 4th edn. Philadelphia: W. B. Saunders.
4. Daniels, L. & Worthingham, C. (1979) *Therapeutic Exercise*. Philadelphia: W. B. Saunders.
5. De Vries, H. A. (1962) Evaluation of static stretching procedures for improvement of flexibility. *Research Quarterly*, Vol 32, pp. 222–229.
6. De Vries, H. A. (1980) *Physiology of Exercise*, 3rd edn. Dubuque: W. C. Brown & Co.
7. Gardiner, M. D. (1963) *The Principles of Exercise Therapy*, 3rd edn. London: Bell & Hyman.
8. Gossman, M. R., Sahrmann, S. A. & Rose, S. J. (1982) Review of length-associated changes in muscle. *Physical Therapy*, Vol. 62, No. 12, pp. 1799–1808.
9. Grieve, G. P. (1984) *Mobilisation of the Spine*, 4th edn. Edinburgh: Churchill Livingstone.
10. Grieve, G. P. (1981) *Common Vertebral Joint Problems*. Edinburgh: Churchill Livingstone.
11. Harris, M. L. (1969) Flexibility. *Physical Therapy*, Vol. 49, No. 6, pp. 591–601.
12. Hollis, M. (1981) *Practical Exercise Therapy*, 2nd edn. Oxford: Blackwell.
13. Janda, V. (1983) *Muscle Function Testing*. London: Butterworths.
14. Johns, H. T. & Wright, V. (1962) Relative importance of various tissues in joint stiffness. *Journal of Applied Physiology*, Vol. 17, No. 5, pp. 824–828.
15. Kendall, H. O., Kendall, F. P. & Boynton, D. A. (1952) *Posture & Pain*. Baltimore: Williams & Wilkins.
16. Kendall, F. P. & McCreary, E. K. (1983) *Muscles, Testing and Function*, 3rd edn. Baltimore: Williams & Wilkins.
17. Knott, M. & Voss, D. (1968) *Proprioceptive Neuromuscular Facilitation*, 2nd edn. New York: Harper & Row.
18. Krusen, F. H., Kottke, P. J. & Elwood, P. M. (1971) *Handbook of Physical Medicine*, 2nd edn, Ch. 16. Philadelphia: W. B. Saunders.
19. Larsen, L. A. (Ed.) (1974) *Fitness, Health & Working Capacity. International Standards for Assessment*. New York: Macmillan.
20. Maitland, G. D. (1977) *Peripheral Manipulation*, 2nd edn. London: Butterworths.
21. Maitland, G. D. (1977) *Vertebral Manipulation*, 4th edn. London: Butterworths.
22. Mennell, J. (1934) *Physical Treatment by Movement, Manipulation and Massage*, 3rd edn. London: J. A. Churchill.

23. Rasch, P. J. & Burke, R. K. (1976) *Kinesiology & Applied Anatomy*, 6th edn. Philadelphia: Lea & Febiger.
24. Reid, J. C. (1977) Effects of constant & intermittent forces on range of joint motion. In *Biomechanics VA*, Komi, P. V. (Ed.), pp. 461–467. Baltimore: University Park Press.
25. Weber, S. & Kraus, H. (1949) Passive and active stretching of muscles. *Physical Therapy Review*, Vol. 29, pp. 407–410.

18

Balance

Balance may be defined as a state in which the body is in equilibrium. It depends on the body's ability to neutralise those forces such as gravity which tend to displace it further by counterforces, so the resultant of all the forces acting is zero.

When the body's equilibrium is disturbed, either by changes of position that the patient makes himself or by the application of some external force, automatic postural adjustments are made to right the body and prevent it falling. These postural adjustments are called equilibrium reactions. They may involve movements of small or large amplitude and may be elicited in any position the body may adopt. Depending on the circumstances they may serve to:

1. Keep the centre of gravity over its original base – counterpoise movements
2. Widen the base and lower the centre of gravity – protective extension reactions
3. Move the base to keep it under a moving centre of gravity – stepping and hopping reactions.

Although balance is in the main automatic, it is a trained art. The child learns it as he experiments. He falls, picks himself up and regains his balance many times over during his early years. Gradually this balance control becomes automatic. The dancer, gymnast and athlete gain a knowledge of what is possible at any one time and work to raise the level of their ability to balance. Learning, spatial judgement and level of skill all play a part in balance control.

The postural tasks of maintaining the upright position and maintaining balance, are intimately related and form the major responsibility of the postural reflex mechanism. This relationship creates a stable background which allows a wide variety of movements to be performed with agility and skill.

The conflicting requirements of stability and mobility are always present; background stability ultimately governing the amount of movement that can be done safely without a loss of balance.

The ability to maintain balance when holding a position is called static balance; the maintaining of balance while moving, dynamic balance.

The whole body is involved in every movement done in daily life, either directly as it takes part in movement or indirectly as it maintains stability to allow the limbs to move.

The shape of the body changes as it bends, turns, twists, stretches or crouches and the limbs adapt to change by moving the position of the legs or arms or both, in order to maintain balance.

In the same way the body maintains balance as the limbs move. The arms move, reach up and down, pull, push, press and withdraw. The hands catch and throw, grasp and release, manipulate and adapt to the handling of objects of various sizes, weights, shapes and textures. The legs move to allow one to walk, jump, hop and skip and use both limbs in a variety of ways.

During life, the situation for each individual is always changing and there will be few occasions in which stable equilibrium is maintained for any length of time, except when the body is at rest.

Balance will be most efficient in young adults and in the middle-aged. The very young, whose postural reflex mechanism is not yet perfected and the elderly, whose control has declined with age, will be less able to adapt to changing circumstances and are thereby the most vulnerable.

Balance may be affected by a person's build. For example, when standing, a tall slender person is in a position of greater unstable equilibrium than a stocky short-legged person, because his centre of gravity is much higher in relation to his base. An efficient postural reflex mechanism will compensate for this apparent mechanical disadvantage.

Balance can also be affected by a person's natural movement ability – one person will have the ability to change position and direction quickly and maintain balance; the less agile person may tend to stiffen and become vulnerable and falls.

A person also needs to be aware of where his body is in relation to the vertical. This requires adequate visuo-spatial perception if his balance is to be maintained.

The control of balance

The maintenance of balance is a complex ability which depends on the integrity of the:

1. Central nervous system
2. Musculo-skeletal system.

It relies on adequate:

1. Vision
2. Vestibular function
3. Proprioceptive efficiency
4. Tactile input, particularly from the feet and hands
5. Integration at different levels of the central nervous system of all stimuli from various receptors
6. Visuo-spatial perception
7. Effective muscle tone which adapts appropriately to changing circumstances
8. Muscle strength and endurance
9. Joint flexibility.

Disorders of any of these factors will influence balance ability.

When displacement of the body occurs, information primarily from the eyes, vestibular system, muscle and joint proprioceptors and tactile receptors, is registered in the central nervous system through various reflex pathways. This information ultimately influences those motor responses involved in the postural adjustments required to maintain balance.

This activity in the central nervous system automatically governs the:

1. Level of contraction necessary in the muscle groups involved
2. Velocity of muscle contraction
3. Timing involved to gain the necessary muscle co-ordination.

Visual control[16,17]

The eyes play a most important part in controlling balance. Good head and neck alignment is necessary to position the head so that the eyes can function most effectively.

The influence of the eyes on balance can be seen when a person is asked to stand on one leg, firstly with his eyes open, then with his eyes closed or when he attempts to move in the dark. In both cases balance tends to become unsteady.

The eyes give a person a picture of the environment and its hazards, distance information and a point of reference including the type of surface on which the movement will take place. They also give information on the position of the body parts at any one time and often of the difficulties and intensity of the required movement, alerting the person and allowing him to think ahead.

The more difficult the movement and the greater the intensity, precision and speed necessary for it, the greater is the importance of the eyes. In this way precise timing and control can be aided. For example, in stepping off a curb, vision and proprioception combine to ensure that the foot strikes the ground in the right place and in the right way. If the movement is too short, jarring can occur. Thus vision can provide a substitute for or augment proprioceptive information from other sources.

Vestibular control[8,12]

The vestibular system of the ear and its central connections, control balance by:

1. Influencing muscle tone particularly of the anti-gravity extensor muscles

2. Maintaining a stable visual perception when the individual moves or the environment moves
3. Directing the position and movement of the head in space.

When the vestibular system is damaged, vertigo often accompanied by giddiness and nausea may occur and balance during movement will be hard to maintain. However, the ability to stand or sit still will be much less affected.

Both vestibular and visual cues aid in the orientation of the body in space, contributing towards an individual's perception of verticality. If a person has no perception of what position is upright and what is horizontal, his ability to balance will be impaired.

Proprioceptive control

Important kinaesthetic information, arising from the muscle, tendon and joint receptors particularly in those areas involved in providing support for the body, includes that about the:

1. Current position of joints and whether they are static or moving
2. Commencement, range and duration of joint movements
3. Velocities and accelerations of the various body segments
4. Pressure and tension in the various joint structures
5. Relative lengths of the muscles involved in maintaining the position of the various joints.

The integration of these sensory impulses provides an appreciation of the position of the various parts of the body and the degree and character of the resistance offered to the movement. These kinaesthetic impulses will be integrated closely with those from the visual and vestibular systems.

Tactile control

Changing pressures primarily on the feet, buttocks and hands provide information indicating the need for body adjustment. This is particularly important when coping with any alterations of the supporting surface which may be at one moment slippery, rough, moving or still.

The feet being adaptable supporting structures play a major role in balance. They provide an adjustable base for the body to prevent overbalancing when performing a particular action by:

1. Adapting themselves to the surface on which they are placed
2. Altering their position in relation to each other by a stepping movement, to substantially alter the shape of the base.

Other factors which also have some effect on the control of balance are as follows.

Muscle tone

Problems of increased or decreased muscle tone will be dealt with in the next chapter.

Hearing[12]

Good hearing may help towards the maintenance of body balance through the person's ability to hear instructions or warnings clearly, sounds of approaching traffic and so on. Deficient hearing may be a danger, because of the risk of surprise, causing the person to be startled and confused and so fall.

Psychological factors

Psychological factors such as fear of falling leading to excessive muscle tension, over-anxiety, inattention or mental confusion, all tend to upset balance and lead to falls. This is particularly apparent in the elderly.

The psychological factors themselves may be created by some underlying neurological disturbances.

Environmental factors

Good illumination, non-slipping even surfaces, suitable clothing and footwear all help in the maintenance of balance. Accidents may be caused by poor lighting, especially if there are shadows; unsuitable clothing such as long nightdresses and dressing gowns; slippers instead of well-fitting, well-soled shoes; high heels, loose mats and unsuitable or carelessly placed furniture. Undue noise or excessive movement in the area may also prove distracting.

Disturbed balance[11,20]

Some of the factors most likely to upset balance include:

1. Impaired central balance control particularly cerebellar
2. Impaired vision
3. Muscle imbalance, particularly around the supporting joints
4. Excessively high or low muscle tone
5. Disordered movement patterns
6. Abnormal reflex activity
7. Increased body sway
8. Giddiness
9. Quick turning or extension of the head
10. Drop attacks.

Some of these factors are closely related. Other factors will include the mechanical, psychological and environmental factors previously discussed.

The assessment of balance[15]

Balance tests are functional in nature and include tests of both static and dynamic balance. Some basic or derived positions will be included as well as movement between these positions. Relevant functional activities are also tested. The patient's safety must be ensured at all times.

The test will be structured as follows.

Can the patient:

1. a. Maintain the stability of a required position on a stable base unaided?
   b. Maintain stability between the body and its parts?
   c. React to external stimuli in a reasonable time and make the necessary postural adjustments?

d. Make normal counterbalancing actions?
e. Be aided by support? If so how much is needed?
2. a. Perform a movement while maintaining body stability?
   b. Perform the movement accurately, adjusting the background if necessary and return to the original position or move to another?
   c. Vary the speed of movement and cope with acceleration or deceleration?
   d. Be helped by assistance to perform the movement?
3. Maintain balance on a moving base?
4. a. Maintain balance while meeting or exerting a force?
   b. Maintain balance while coping with a distraction or disturbance?
5. Control posture and movement in all relevant tests with the eyes open and closed?

Tests of postural reflex reactions will also be necessary.[9] These are done by displacing the patient in different starting positions and observing whether a response occurs. The quality of the response, if present, should be noted including the time it takes:

1. Before the response is actually observed after the displacing force has been applied – reaction time
2. For the movements which form the response to be completed – movement time.

If normal, postural reflex reactions may be used as a treatment medium. If abnormal reactions are present they must be inhibited and an effort made to gain a more normal reaction.

Other tests will vary according to the cause of the patient's condition and may include such tests as strength, joint flexibility and sensation.

In all tests the physiotherapist will be assessing the quality of the performance and learning something of the patient's potential and limitations.

Possible aims of treatment may be to:
1. Work towards gaining stability in positions of instability so the possibilities for and the boundaries of movement can be extended
2. Ensure the safety of the patient when moving in the treatment area and at home and work
3. Prevent further disability
4. Establish when necessary a new sense of balance when there is no possibility of achieving a normal state of balance
5. Endeavour to achieve as normal a pattern of movement as possible.

Retraining of balance

In this section some general factors related to the retraining of balance will be discussed. The effect of tone on balance will be described in the next chapter.

The gaining of relaxation

Relaxation may be needed at the start of the exercise programme so that unnecessary mental and muscle tension is reduced and accurate work done. The patient will gain confidence in the physiotherapist and in himself as he understands his abilities and disabilities and feels he is safe to move.

The encouragement of balance on a stable base

In the retraining of static balance it is hoped to gain as normal as possible integration of muscle activity to control postural sway and to provide the stability necessary for holding a sustained position. The gaining of strength and flexibility will be carried out in association with the balance training.

For all patients a functional and necessary position will be chosen; for example, sitting up in bed, sitting with legs over the bed supported or unsupported according to ability or sitting in a chair with the feet on the floor. Whatever the position the patient's safety must be ensured and appropriate stimuli provided.

In the case of the paraplegic, training will involve the development of a new sense of balance. A paraplegic patient with a complete lesion above T12 will have lost all sensation and motor power below the level of the lesion. Latissimus dorsi with its high segmental nerve supply and wide attachment to the spine and pelvis will provide the necessary sensory and motor connection between the normal upper and paralysed lower part of the body and will help the patient gain a new postural sense which will gradually become automatic.[4]

At first a mirror may be placed in front of the patient so that he may see, as well as feel, the correct or new position.

As soon as possible, single and double arm movement will be practised with the emphasis on correct movement while maintaining balance. Overall balance will be improved if a variety of movements are carried out on the base.

Within the position and as soon as possible, directional pressure may be given to the patient. The command will be 'hold – don't let me move you!' The direction of pressure may be at first on the front, then on the back of the shoulder girdle, side to side, or against rotation of the upper or total trunk. The pressure should be placed on the body slowly and smoothly, matching the mounting muscle contraction by the patient. An isometric contraction will be gained. The patient's hold should not be broken. The pressure then should be slowly relaxed. Adjustment may be slow at first.

Once some security in balance has been gained light quick taps in varying directions on the shoulder girdle may be used to test the patient's ability to react to an outside stimulus.

The patient may also be placed in a position, slightly off balance, that demands correction either consciously or automatically.

Regular practice of balance by the patient in a position of safety – in bed, on a mat or in a safe chair – should be done as soon and as often as possible.

Stability exercises demand intense concentration and may fatigue the patient both mentally and physically. Rests must be given against a support.

Progression may be achieved by the patient moving from a position of stability to one of less stability.

Balance on a moving base

Balance on a moving base, such as is needed in public transport, will be helped by practice on balance boards, a trampoline and the use of a treadmill.

Regaining of co-ordination following loss of proprioception[13,14]

A patient with a loss of proprioceptive functions, such as occurs in sensory ataxia, will tend to have unco-ordinated movement leading to balance problems. Vision, of necessity, may be used by the patient to compensate for these functions but it is important that all remaining proprioceptive functions are used.

The emphasis in exercise therapy will be on gaining an awareness of the 'feel' of a co-ordinated movement as well as improving the body's background stability.

The training programme, devised by Frenkel, for patients with sensory ataxia mainly affecting the lower limbs follows this principle and is also useful, though to a lesser degree, for patients with cerebellar ataxia.

Frenkel's exercise programme uses movement patterns aimed at improving balance and co-ordination to help provide a background for locomotion. The movements are done slowly, often to a count of four.

At first during treatment, the patient performs the movement under visual control. A mirror may be used when necessary. Accurate feedback is important. Once the movement pattern and co-ordination have improved, the patient should try to do the movements with his eyes closed. Intense concentration is essential, therefore a quiet atmosphere and frequent short rest periods are needed by the patient.

A usual programme is as follows:

Half-lying

1. Alternate hip and knee
   a. Flexion and extension
   b. Abduction and adduction with knee bent
   c. Abduction and adduction with knee extended – sliding along a board or bed surface
2. Alternate hip and knee
   a. Flexion and extension
   b. Abduction and adduction – with leg off the bed
3. One knee flexed and the heel of the same limb placed in varying positions and held there temporarily
4. One knee flexed and the heel of the same limb sliding down the tibia of the opposite leg
5. Flexion and extension of both hips and knees simultaneously
6. Reciprocal flexion and extension of the legs.

Sitting

1. The patient maintains the sitting position for a few minutes at a time then rests against a back support
2. Raising the foot and placing it in the hand of the physiotherapist while she constantly changes her hand position
3. Raising and lowering heels
4. Rising from sitting to standing.

Standing

Standing at first should be done between bars and the patient should feel secure in walking with the physiotherapist guarding him.

1. Sideways walking
2. Forward walking
3. Walking between two parallel lines
4. Performing a wide circular step turn

5. Foot placement on a tracing of footprints on the floor
6. Progress should be made to the use of steps and inclines.

The patient's safety should be ensured during standing and walking practice. Regular practice should be encouraged in positions of safety.

Regaining of balance in the presence of vertigo

Some patients with vertigo from vestibular lesions, head injuries or Ménière's disease come for a specific exercise programme to help them to accommodate to this distressing symptom of disturbed balance which is often accompanied by giddiness, nausea and a fear of falling. The patient avoids moving his head and holds it rigidly in an effort to reduce stimulating his vestibular receptors. This, in turn, also influences his balance and the movements of the whole body.

The exercise routine advocated by Cawthorne and Cooksey and described by Dix has proved valuable in helping these patients.[6,7,8] Initially the exercises should be performed in a well-supported position where the patient knows he is secure. As his tolerance of eye and head movement improves over time, less stable positions as well as larger body movements with frequent changes of direction and head position can be included. The progressive routine is as follows:

1. In bed, in a fully supported semi-recumbent position
   a. Eye movements – at first slow, then quick
      (i) Up and down
      (ii) Side to side
      (iii) Circular – clockwise and anticlockwise
      (iv) Focussing on a finger moving from 3 ft to 1 ft away from the face
   b. Head movements at first slow, then quick; later with the eyes closed
      (i) Bending forwards and backwards
      (ii) Turning from side to side
      (iii) Circling – clockwise and anticlockwise

2. Sitting
    a. and b. as above
    c. Shoulder shrugging and circling
    d. Bending forwards and picking up objects from the ground
    e. Lifting objects above the head while following with head and eyes
    f. Passing an object from one outstretched hand across the front of the body to the other hand and around behind the body
3. Standing
    a. 1.a. and b. and 2.c.
    b. Changing from the sitting to the standing position with eyes open and shut
    c. Throwing a small ball from hand to hand above eye level
    d. Throwing ball from hand to hand under the knee
    e. Change from sitting to standing and turning round in between
4. Moving about (in class)
    a. Circle round centre person who will throw a large ball and to whom it will be returned
    b. Walk across the room with eyes open and then closed
    c. Walk up and down a slope with eyes open and then closed
    d. Walk up and down steps with eyes open and then closed
    e. Any game involving stooping or stretching and aiming such things as skittles, bowls or basketball.

Loss of muscle strength and flexibility

Muscle imbalance, loss of strength and joint range, pain and oedema together with inactivity, tend to create a situation where the patient is less ready to adapt to change or disturbance. He will tend to hold his body rigid with little rotary movement, his arms are often held by his side and the normal reciprocal movements of arm and leg are absent. Co-ordination is poor. Normal postural balance reactions are reduced. Movement tends to be slow and inco-ordinated and the ability to regain balance quickly is upset. A small incident, which normally he could cope with such as tripping on uneven ground or a stone, may throw him off balance and he may fall.

Reduction of pain, regaining strength and increased range will help towards achieving good balance.

THE PREVENTION OF FALLS IN THE ELDERLY

It has been shown that postural sway increases after the age of 60. Many elderly people fall and injure themselves with the risk of falls increasing with age. Sheldon[24] working in England, carried out a study of 500 falls in elderly people varying in ages from 50−85+ and classified the falls as shown in Tables 18.1 and 18.2.

There were 171 accidental falls by 125 people. One-third of the falls occurring at home were accidental in origin. It is possible that some of these could have been prevented.

Stairs accounted for one-third of the accidental falls. The most frequent cause lay in missing the last step or group of steps and falling. Sheldon points out that a handrail

Table 18.1

Accidental falls	171
Drop-attacks	125
Trips	53
Vertigo	37
Recognisable CNS lesion	27
Head back	20
Postural hypotension	18
Weakness in leg	16
Falling out of bed or chair	10
Uncertain	23

Table 18.2

On stairs		63
Missing last step or steps	15	
Poor illumination	13	
Vertigo	12	
Various	23	
Slipping		49
Falling over unexpected objects		16
Dark		12
Various		31

easily gripped and fashioned so that the terminal part of the rail would not be reached until the feet left the staircase, would prevent some of these falls.

Loss of balance on slippery surfaces caused 49 falls, half of them on ice and snow. Many people in the survey tripped. This seemed to be directly associated with increasing age for most of the subjects were in the 75–84 group.

It was considered by the persons themselves that the cause was that they:

1. Did not lift their feet as high as they used to
2. Found recovery of balance almost impossible

3. Were more likely to trip when tired or in a hurry.

The most frequent single cause was the edge of rugs and carpets. Steps in the house, kerbstones and uneven pavements also took their toll.

Limb weakness and co-existing disease led to some falls as the person did not have sufficient strength to regain balance.

Some other falls were associated with sudden head movement such as head extension or rotation, particularly if reaching upwards. These risks increased with age.

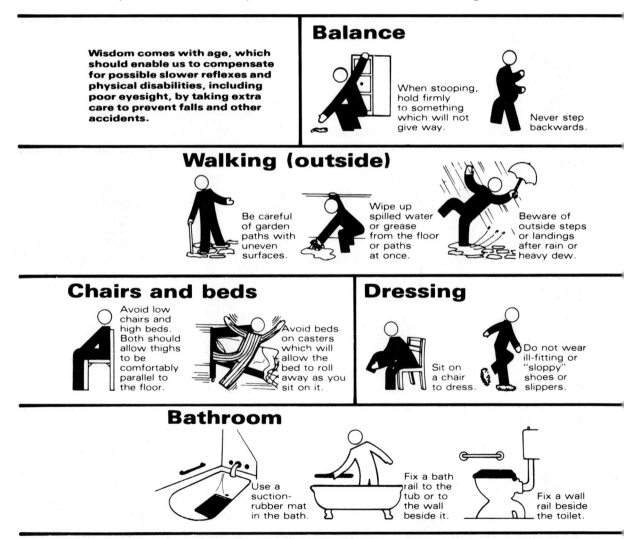

Fig. 18.1 'Home Accidents and the Senior Citizen' reproduced with permission from a brochure designed by the Queensland Government Department of Health, Division of Health Education and Information.

Many of the hazards in the home and the environment should be pointed out by the physiotherapist working in the hospital, in domiciliary care or in day centres.

The physiotherapist should pay particular attention to strengthening the intrinsic muscles of the feet, increasing the step ability of the patient and to reducing the risks caused by unsuitable shoes. The patient should be advised not to climb onto chairs. She should also warn the patient of such outdoor hazards as uneven pavements, tripping over hoses and so on.

A useful poster such as that circulated by the Queensland Department of Health, Division of Health Education and Information sets out common hazards and the precautions necessary to help prevent falls (Fig. 18.1).

The physiotherapist can improve the patient's balance and make him safer while moving, by encouraging him to take his weight correctly on his feet, turn slowly in a circle rather than abruptly, take a step backwards and then look up rather than use the vulnerable acute head extension posture and to get up slowly from lying or sitting to standing.

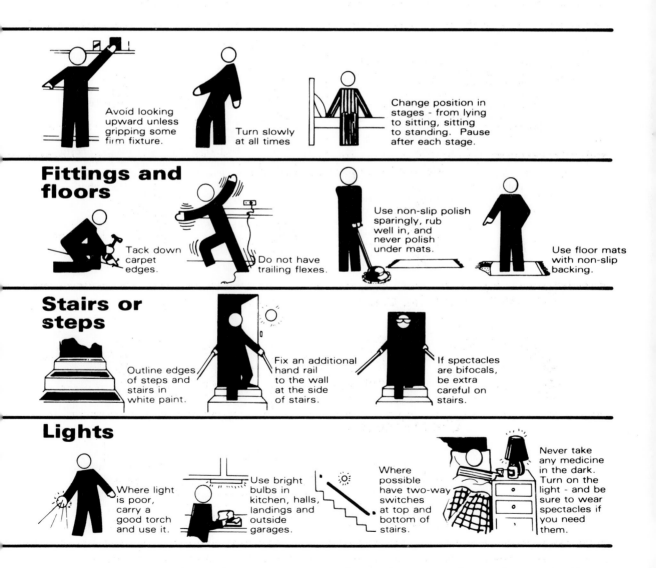

REFERENCES AND FURTHER READING

1. Begbie, G. H. (1969) The assessment of imbalance. *Physiotherapy*, Vol. 55, pp. 411–413.
2. Bobath, K. (1980) *A Neurophysiological Basis for the Treatment of Cerebral Palsy. Clinics in Developmental Medicine No. 75.* London: William Heinemann Medical.
3. Broer, M. R. & Zernicke, R. F. (1979) *Efficiency of Human Movement*, 4th edn. Philadelphia: W. B. Saunders.
4. Bromley, I. (1981) *Tetraplegia and Paraplegia*, 2nd edn. Edinburgh: Churchill Livingstone.
5. Cash, J. (1974) *Neurology for Physiotherapists.* London: Faber and Faber.
6. Cawthorne, T. (1945) The physiological basis for head exercises. *The Journal of the Chartered Society of Physiotherapy*, Vol. XXX, No. 10, pp. 106–107.
7. Cooksey, F. S. (1945) Rehabilitation in vestibular injuries. *Proceedings of the Royal Society of Medicine*, pp. 273–275.
8. Dix, M. R. (1974) Treatment of vertigo. *Physiotherapy*, Vol. 60, pp. 380–384.
9. Fiorentino, M. R. (1973) *Reflex Testing Methods for evaluating C.N.S. Development.* Springfield: Charles C. Thomas.
10. Guyton, A. C. (1981) *Textbook of Medical Physiology*, 6th edn. Philadelphia: W. B. Saunders.
11. Hasselkus, B. R. & Shambes, G. M. (1975) Aging and postural sway in women. *Journal of Gerontology*, Vol. 30, pp. 661–667.
12. Hinchcliffe, R. (Ed.) (1983) *Hearing and Balance in the Elderly.* Edinburgh: Churchill Livingstone.
13. Kottke, F. J. (1971) Therapeutic exercise. In Krusen, F. H., Kottke, F. J. & Ellwood, P. H. *Handbook of Physical Medicine and Rehabilitation*, 2nd edn. Philadelphia: W. B. Saunders.
14. Kottke, F. J. (1980) From reflex to skill: the training of coordination. *Archives of Physical Medicine and Rehabilitation*, Vol. 61, pp. 551–561.
15. Lane, R. E. (1969) Physiotherapy in the treatment of balance problems. *Physiotherapy*, Vol. 55, pp. 415–420.
16. Lee, D. N. & Lishman, J. R. (1977) Vision – the most efficient source of proprioceptive information for balance control. *Agressologie*, Vol. 13A, pp. 83–94.
17. Lee, D. N. & Lishman, R. (1977) Visual control of locomotion. *Scandinavian Journal of Psychology*, Vol. 18, pp. 224–240.
18. Metheny, E. (1952) *Body Dynamics.* New York: McGraw-Hill.
19. Murray, M. P. & Peterson, R. M. (1973) Weight distribution and weight shifting actions. *Physical Therapy*, Vol. 53, pp. 741–748.
20. Overstall, P. W., Exton Smith, A. R., Imms, F. J. & Johnson, A. L. (1977) Falls in the elderly related to postural imbalance. *British Medical Journal*, Vol. 1, pp. 261–284.
21. Rasch, P. J. & Burke, R. K. (1978) *Kinesiology and Applied Anatomy*, 6th Edn. Philadelphia: Lea and Febiger.
22. Roberts, T. D. M. (1969) The mechanics of the upright posture. *Physiotherapy*, Vol. 55, pp. 398–404.
23. Roberts, T. D. M. (1978) *Neurophysiology of Postural Mechanisms*, 2nd edn. London: Butterworths.
24. Sheldon, J. H. (1960) On the natural history of falls in old age. *British Medical Journal*, December, pp. 1685–1690.

19

Abnormal muscle tone

The ability to modulate muscle tone in a normal manner (Chapter 4) is affected by damage to the nervous system. As a result muscle tone may be excessively decreased – hypotonia or increased – hypertonia. It may also tend to fluctuate in an abnormal manner.

Hypotonia, spasticity and rigidity are the most common changes of tone seen by the physiotherapist.

In planning physiotherapy treatment, the age when damage to the nervous system occurs is important. The infant with brain damage will lack background knowledge on which to base movements and learn skills, whereas the adult already has experienced normal movement and has a memory of these movements.

HYPOTONIA

Hypotonia may be caused by an interruption to the reflex arc on the afferent, efferent or both sides. A peripheral nerve lesion affects both sides of the arc so that sensory and motor disturbances occur.

Hypotonia may also be caused by an acute infection of the anterior horn cells of the spinal cord, as in acute anterior poliomyelitis, or when the motor neuron is predominantly affected as in the Guillian Barre syndrome (acute post-infective polyneuritis). In the latter case minimal or temporary sensory disturbance also occurs.

Some degree of hypotonia is also seen in cerebellar damage, Chapter 18.

The characteristics of hypotonia arising from damage to the efferent side of the reflex arc only will be discussed in this section.

These characteristics are:

1. Muscle tenderness which may be present in the early stages
2. Muscle weakness and loss of voluntary movement
3. Diminished or absent reflexes
4. Diminished resistance to passive movement
5. Muscle wasting, circulatory and nutritional changes
6. Abnormal body and limb positions
7. Muscle imbalance with possible deformity.

The prognosis will depend on the extent of the damage.

The examination of the patient will focus on the characteristics outlined above. Observation of trunk and limb contours, tests of muscle tone and muscle strength, with particular regard for muscle imbalance in the trunk and around the joints will be made. Tests of joint movement and muscle length will be done. When possible, sitting, standing, functional activities and gait will be tested. If pain is present, only a general estimate of the patient's condition can be made.

Once the stage of tenderness is over, every effort must be made to regain all possible strength and quality of movement as well as independence for the patient.

As sensory conduction is normal, proprioceptive and cutaneous stimuli must be provided to bring about a maximum motor response and with it, an increased awareness of the limb.

Skilled manual handling provides the stimulus, guidance and assistance to aid movement. Stimulus can be provided by slow or quick stretch within normal limits and at varying speeds, together with assistance or resistance at suitable levels. Mechanical and thermal stimuli can also be used. If active movement is impossible, passive movement will be necessary to maintain full joint range and muscle length.

Repetition together with regular practice helps to bring about a greater central awareness of the required movement.

Early activity including weight bearing on the feet and/or hands, will aid recovery by allowing for maximum sensory stimuli from both the feet and the hands and the joints of the lower and upper limbs, provided the correct trunk and limb alignment is preserved.

Deformity, caused by muscle imbalance, poor posture of the limb or by gravity, must be prevented by careful attention to the position of the limbs, joint range and muscle length.

Methods of regaining strength have been discussed in detail in Chapter 16.

HYPERTONIA

Hypertonia can be described as a pathological increase in striated muscle tone due to excessive motor unit activity. There is a release or partial release of certain reflex reactions from higher control.

The condition may be caused by damage during, after, or even before birth – for example, in cerebral palsy, or by a degenerative disease such as cerebrovascular disease or by head injury.

The spasticity which may be caused by any of these three conditions will be discussed in this section.

The characteristics of hypertonia are:

1. Abnormal and hyperactive reflex activity
2. Increased resistance to passive and/or active stretch and tension on palpation
3. Abnormal asymmetry and scarcity of postures
4. Abnormal asymmetry and scarcity of patterns of movement
5. Hyperexcitability to both internal and external stimuli
6. Possible muscle weakness
7. Possible deformity.

There may be accompanying sensory defects which will disturb the ability to move effectively.

Sometimes hypertonia may follow a period of hypotonia. For example, in the patient with hemiplegia following a stroke where there may be early hypotonia due to cerebral shock. It can also be seen in the 'floppy' child with cerebral palsy.

The degree and extent of the hypertonia will vary greatly, ranging from the patient with minimal cerebral damage whose movements are functional though clumsy and slightly inco-ordinate, to the patient who is 'locked' in his own spasticity.

In the patient with severe hypertonia the posture of the body and its segments is abnormal, exaggerated, asymmetrical and stiff. There is a scarcity of postures and the patient can move very little within a posture and that movement is slow, abnormal and usually useless. Instead of the normal reciprocal action of agonist and antagonist, co-contraction may be present, with both agonist and antagonist having abnormal tone. Initiation and co-ordination of movement are deficient. Selective movements may be missing. There is difficulty in moving from one posture to another without considerable help and in moving an affected part of the body independently of the whole. There are problems of balance.

The hemiplegic patient illustrates the following pattern of spasticity. On the affected side there is depression and retraction of the shoulder girdle, flexion, adduction and internal rotation of the shoulder, flexion of the elbow, pronation of the forearm, flexion of the wrist, flexion of the fingers and flexion and adduction of the thumb. Trunk side flexion and pelvic elevation together with extension, adduction and internal rotation of the lower limb with the foot plantar flexed and inverted, are also present.

The examination of the patient

A systematic examination of the patient, with careful attention to detail, is necessary in order to determine what the patient can do and the quality of posture and movement present. The physiotherapist must also gain a knowledge of what movements are difficult, abnormal or absent.

A total analysis must be made of the abnormal postural and movement synergies, the level of abnormal tone present and what increases and decreases it. The influence of normal and abnormal reflex activity and its effect on posture and movement, is also noted.

The ability to take up, hold and adjust a posture as well as to initiate and control an effective movement against a stable though changing background, is examined.

The degree of abnormal tone present is indicated to a certain extent by the position and appearance of the body and limbs when at rest and during movement. It is tested by moving the body or limb or its segments passively through a range of movement at varying speeds and estimating whether the force required is greater or less than usual, or by asking the patient to attempt to carry out a voluntary movement.

Other factors to be considered are balance, functional abilities and disabilities, sensory loss and associated movements if present.

Assessment is a continuing process as fresh information will be gained during treatment.

The aims of treatment

Aims and treatment will be planned on the basis of continuing assessment and an appreciation of the patient's wishes and needs. These vary greatly from person to person and from time to time. They may be influenced by the age of the patient, the circumstances in which he wishes to live as well as the level of his disability and its prognosis.

The overall aim for many patients is to decrease the abnormal tone, gain as normal a postural tone as possible, re-educate more symmetrical and normal patterns of posture and movement as well as functional ability.

The excessive muscle tone leading to the abnormal motor patterns of posture and movement must be modified otherwise the abnormal becomes a habit as the patient continuously receives abnormal feedback. Normal movement with the necessary fluctuations of tone that take place continuously cannot occur with excess tone and lack of control.

There are many different approaches to physiotherapy treatment, for example those described by Bobath,[5,6,7] Brunnstrom,[8] Finnie,[13] Kabat and Knott,[16] Rood,[19] Cotton[11] and Carr and Shepherd,[9,10] but it is essential that all treatment is individually planned and its effectiveness continually reassessed.

The achievement of normal active movement is the chief factor which influences excessive tone and decreases the abnormal reflex activity. This normalisation can be aided by knowledgeable and sensitive handling by the physiotherapist and will be discussed later.

Other factors which may markedly influence tone are discussed in the following sections.

Head and neck control

The head and neck, by their influence on the distribution of muscle tone throughout the body, have a strong influence on posture and movement. An abnormal position of the head in space or lack of its control, adversely influences the posture and movement of the rest of the body. The patient must learn to hold his head steady in space in the mid-position in relation to his shoulders, so that his eyes can be used effectively.

Head and neck control in all positions is necessary to initiate normal purposeful movement. For example, in order to move from the supine position, the patient needs to bring his head, shoulders and chest forwards; in prone, to lift his head, shoulders and chest in extension or in sitting or standing to control and hold his head erect ready to move.

Balance

Nearly every movement requires that the whole body is balanced if accuracy is to be gained. Most patients with hypertonia, even the mildly disabled, have a disturbance of balance.

The ability to balance gives the patient security, as well as gaining and maintaining symmetry of posture so that accurate movement can be achieved and excessive tone decreased. Without adequate balance the patient will be unable to adjust to his changing centre of gravity, so he dare not move. His responses will be slow or absent and the insecurity induced and the inefficiency of general and local postures and movement will greatly increase tone.

Efforts must be made to increase balance without increasing tone. Tilting movements of the head and body, encouragement of automatic movements which will demand correction, can be carried out and controlled by either the physiotherapist or the patient. The patient's correction may be automatic or voluntary. These movements have been well described by Bobath.[6]

The regaining of balance can be achieved either by adjusting the head and/or body on its base or by adjusting the base. The regaining of balance has been discussed in Chapter 18.

Rotation

Rotation is present and plays a part in almost every movement a person does, for example, rolling, turning, reaching for an object and walking. It is often absent or deficient in the movements attempted by a patient with hypertonia. It must be encouraged. It helps break up the abnormal straight pattern. It can be initiated for example, by rotation of the head on the neck, the neck on the shoulder girdle and the head, neck and shoulder girdle on the trunk. These movements can often be incorporated with rotation of the proximal joints of the limbs.

Rotation is an 'unlocking' factor which helps free the trunk and the proximal joints and thus breaks the abnormal pattern. It also tends to normalise tone and encourage normal movement.

A few gentle rhythmical rotary movements of the head, neck and trunk and of the proximal joints of the limbs are useful, whether given passively, or when possible, assisted actively. They may be started in a small but gradually increasing range as resistance to the movement lessens. They may be carried out in lying to aid rolling or in sitting when balance and weight shifting will be automatically encouraged.

The patterns used in the technique *Proprioceptive Neuromuscular Facilitation*,[16] with their strong emphasis on rotation, are useful to help break up the abnormal synergies present, provided they can be given without causing excessive tone. Often they can be used passively or assisted actively with the stretch and resistance omitted.

Bilateral and reciprocal movement

Bilateral and bilateral reciprocal movements of the limbs are encouraged. There are many of these movements used in daily life. Most have a strong rotary component. They can help gain head and trunk control and balance. They aid co-ordination. In the infant they can be seen in the creeping and crawling patterns. They also are helpful to the hemiplegic patient who may tend to ignore his affected side. These reciprocal movements draw attention to the affected side and may help to provide a correct pattern of feeling and movement. They may be started passively and as soon as possible become guided assisted active and/or active movements.

Early weight bearing

Weight bearing should start as soon as possible. The child in prone may bear weight on his forearms and the hemiplegic patient may be helped to gain extension of his elbow through weight bearing on the affected forearm and whole hand.

Early practice in sitting, with the weight evenly distributed on the buttocks and on both feet, and in standing, with the heel of the affected limb down and the weight evenly distributed between the two feet, is necessary and helpful. Weight transference of the body in many positions will aid balance and accuracy of movement.

Relaxation and self help

Often the patient is doubly handicapped, firstly by the neurological damage and secondly by his reaction to his disability. He is anxious and afraid for the future thereby becoming generally more tense. The hypertonicity already present is increased. He must learn to appreciate how he can help himself by a calm and co-operative approach to living and treatment. General relaxation will help. Local relaxation of the spastic muscles, either totally or partially, may also be practised and achieved.

The patient can help himself considerably if he learns to appreciate the changing levels of his own tone and feels and sees the postures and movements which help correct, reduce or increase it. He can be aided by the use of feedback from electronic devices which monitor and record his ability to relax or move, if he is trained in their use.

This relaxation can be helped by the calm but concerned approach of the physiotherapist as reflected in her general sensitivity, her voice, the use of her hands and the confidence she inspires in the patient and his relatives.

All the factors already discussed may play an important part in helping to achieve a change in tone, posture and movement. Many of them will be dependent on the skilful and sensitive handling of the physiotherapist.

Skilled and sensitive handling

Help will be needed by the patient in attempting to gain a more normal pattern of movement, so that tone is decreased and further excessive tone is not built up. Passive movement is usually necessary at first so that the change from the abnormal posture can be made as smoothly as possible and without undue effort on the part of the patient which would increase tone. The necessary close interplay between physiotherapist and patient has been discussed in Chapter 11.

Sensitive handling is necessary. The passive movement should start proximally and be slow and rhythmical so that tone is kept to a minimum. It can appear almost as a moulding movement as the contour of the body and its parts changes its shape.

These passive movements are not passive stretching of individual joints and muscles, as the stretch involved would increase the spasticity. Correction must be made around the total pattern, by easing the patient into a new and more normal position or movement. For example, the abnormal pattern of shoulder girdle depression and adduction which hinders shoulder movement, may be changed to the normal elevation and abduction and so help free the shoulder to move forward.

A change of the total pattern may not always be possible immediately. Gentle rhythmical rocking movements to help gain control of the proximal parts of the new patterns may prove helpful to allow adjustment to occur.

In providing this input, the physiotherapist must know and feel where and when to block, where to help, when to vary speed, hold steady or anticipate action.[18] Time may be needed to allow the adjustment to occur.

At first the physiotherapist provides the control, support, assistance, guidance, sequence and timing of the movement into the new posture, as well as setting the direction, extent and speed of the new movement. She is giving a sensory message to the patient. She aims not only to lessen the original abnormal excessive tone present but also to inhibit the extra tone and unnecessary movements, which can be caused when a person with normal movement attempts a new activity. Assistance should be adequate but the minimal necessary to bring about the desired result.

In this close interaction between patient and physiotherapist, both will feel the necessary adjustment to the new posture occurring.

The Bobaths[5,6,7] consider the key points of control in moving into a new position, are the head, neck, trunk, shoulder girdle and pelvis and the proximal joints of the limbs.

At some time and place during the easing into the new position, the physiotherapist may feel the patient assisting and sensitively reduces her help, while at the same time anticipating difficulties and keeping control of the total synergy and the body symmetry so that accuracy of the movement is ensured.

Time may be needed to settle into the new posture.

Every attempt at active movement should be encouraged provided that increased excessive tone of the rest of the body is not caused. Active movement and normal automatic reactions is what is wanted. They will be the chief factors in normalising tone and lessening the influence of the abnormal reflex patterns.

As the movement proceeds the patient learns to appreciate the differences in tone that are occurring. This will be the guiding factor to both patient and physiotherapist as they work together to gain more efficient movement.

Dynamic posture – mobility

Posture is a mobile and changing function. Progress is achieved by movement from one position to another and by carrying out movements on these positions. Positions of advantage, whether controlled by the patient or physiotherapist, are those in which tension is minimal and the limbs given greater freedom to move. They are not a series of more or less static positions.

For accurate voluntary movement, posture, balance, flexibility and movement are linked. Normal muscle tone forms the background.

Each movement has its own particular components – a synergy carried out with correct sequence and timing. For every movement there will be a changing postural background which provides the stability, the balance and the adjustments necessary for quality of movement to be gained.

Direction and speed are regulated to the degree appropriate to the particular activity.

Preparation must be made for each movement done by the patient and there will be a time of readiness for the movement to occur. While his posture is more normal, every effort should be made by the physiotherapist to encourage movement to proceed without increasing tone abnormally. For example, the side lying position with the under leg straight and upper one flexed is usually a position of minimum tone. If toys are placed in front of a child in this position he may reach for them spontaneously. His attention is focussed on the toys rather than the movement. The adult in side lying with the affected shoulder girdle controlled may reach forward in a normal movement. A self-generated sensory input is achieved. Total body reactions to the movement must be watched and control provided if needed.

Movement usually occurs because the patient is stimulated to move. The stimulation must be given but strictly controlled so that facilitation is gained but an excessive increase in tone is not caused.

The child's movements usually follow along developmental lines. For example, the infant is helped to roll from supine to prone and later to crawl with reciprocal action, if the preparation is adequate. The older child and adult are helped when necessary, to move from lying to sitting to standing. These are essential postures from which many movements take place. Each new movement achieved makes use of the improvement already gained and gradually provides another step along the way to independence.

A number of different positions, if controlled, allow versatility of movement to occur. Very slowly as control grows and experience of different positions and movements is achieved, more normal patterns of movement will be set up.

Many controlled positions from which movements can be facilitated are shown by Finnie,[13] Bobath[6] and Rood.[19]

Further progression is achieved when a pattern of extension is broken by flexion of one or more joints; for example, in flexing the knee with the hip in extension, as is necessary at the start of the 'swing' phase in walking.

The physiotherapist must watch and feel for success or failure during treatment. If success occurs she must decide on the next step to be taken; if failure occurs she must analyse when, where and why the movement failed.

Functional activities of daily living

As soon as possible, training or retraining in the activities of daily living should be attempted. The patient's own active participation and initiative rather than the therapist's handling skill can now be used to advantage.[10] The patient is taught how to guide his own movements through, for example, his speech.[11] Increased skill is attained by practice coupled with adequate feedback. Once achieved these activities can be put into daily use and a step along the road to independence has been taken.

Positions of rest

Care must be taken to ensure that the positions taken up during rest are helpful and do not reinforce the pattern of spasticity. For example, the head of the hemiplegic patient should be slightly flexed away from the hemiplegic side, the arm brought forward and supported on a pillow and the leg supported so that it does not roll outward at the hip.

Home programme

A home programme is most important for both the child and the adult in regaining more normal movement. As soon as possible one must be started with guidance from the physiotherapist. The parents of the child can be helped to provide twenty four hour care and make life easier for the child and for themselves.

Both parents, with guidance from the physiotherapist, can learn to help the disabled child greatly by gaining knowledge of methods of handling the child and of postures and movements to use and avoid. They can be encouraged to provide suitable and interesting experiences for him and so aid his movement and his enjoyment of life. They are the child's chief therapists. Finnie's work[13] is of great help to parents and to physiotherapists. Relatives of adult patients can also be guided by the physiotherapist in ways to encourage the patient to move.[9,10] Bobath's work[6] provides further guidance.

The adult in many cases can do much to help himself if the learns positions to use at rest and during movement and the positions and movements to avoid.

Early independence

All people desire independence. Some people, particularly the aged, do not want a long period of hospitalisation or attendance at hospital. They feel it may jeopardise their lifestyle for either living in their own homes or living with relatives. They want short term rehabilitation to enable them to move safely and to achieve independence in the activities of daily life. They are prepared to accept a certain level of disability. Their wishes must be respected and every effort made so that they can leave hospital for their home as soon as possible. Two or three home visits by the physiotherapist may help them greatly.

Further problems

Sensory loss

Sensory loss is a grave handicap to the patient and greatly increases treatment difficulties.

A child who is disabled by his spasticity will be unable to move out into his environment, act upon it and benefit from the sensory experiences it provides. He will be even more disabled if he has accompanying sensory deficits. Sensory experiences need to be provided and the environment brought to him so he can benefit from the stimulation and learn.

Sensory loss in an adult who was previously functioning normally, can produce movement disability as well, though in this case the physiotherapist can capitalise on the patient's memory of previously learned movements. The eyes must be used to supplement any proprioceptive or tactile sensory loss.

Muscle weakness

Once the excessive tone is lessened and movement occurs, muscle weakness may become obvious. The problem of strengthening is difficult and the normal facilitating techniques must be used with caution. The use of basic functional activities must be encouraged to help increase strength.

Associated movements

Associated movements may occur. They are defined as automatic modifications of posture in response to effort in another part of the body.[22]

In the presence of the already excessive tone the body over-reacts and there may be considerable increase in the already abnormal patterns of spasticity.

Deformities

Deformities may occur because of the more or less 'fixed' spastic pattern and the abnormal habits of movement of trunk and limbs. Usually with care, they can be prevented, by retaining full joint range and muscle length.

Progress

Progress will be slow and the level of ability to be reached difficult to predict, as the changes to be made are often complex and difficult. Each new achievement will provide a stimulus to the patient to continue.

REFERENCES AND FURTHER READING

1. Basmajian, J. V. (1977) Motor Learning and Control: A Working Hypothesis. *Archives of Physical Medicine and Rehabilitation*, Vol. 58, pp. 38–41.
2. Basmajian, J. V. & De Luca, C. J. (1985) *Muscles Alive,* 5th edn. Baltimore: Williams & Wilkins.
3. Bishop, B. (1977) Spasticity – its physiology and management. Parts 1–4. *Physical Therapy*, Vol. 57, No. 4, pp. 371–401.
4. Bishop, B. (1982) Neural Plasticity, Part 4. Lesion induced reorganization of the C.N.S. *Physical Therapy*, Vol. 62, No. 10, pp. 1442–1451.
5. Bobath, B. (1971) *Abnormal Postural Reflex Activity Caused by Brain Lesions.* London: William Heinemann.
6. Bobath, B. (1978) *Adult Hemiplegia. Evaluation and Treatment*, 2nd edn. London: William Heinemann.
7. Bobath, K. (1980) *A Neurological Basis for the Treatment of Cerebral Palsy.* London: William Heinemann Medical.
8. Brunnstrom, S. (1970) *Movement therapy in Hemiplegia.* New York: Harper & Row.
9. Carr, J. H. & Shepherd, R. B. (1980) *Physiotherapy in Disorders of the Brain.* London: William Heinemann Medical.
10. Carr, J. H. & Shepherd, R. B. (1982) *A motor relearning programme for stroke.* London: Heinemann
11. Cotton, E. & Kinsman, R. (1983) *Conductive Education for Adult Hemiplegia.* Edinburgh: Churchill Livingstone.
12. Craik, R. L. (1982) Clinical correlates of neural plasticity. *Physical Therapy*, Vol. 62, No. 10, pp. 1452–1462.
13. Finnie, N. R. (1974) *Handling the Cerebral Palsied Child at Home*, 2nd edn. London: William Heinemann Medical.
14. Holt, K. S. (1965) *Assessment of Cerebral Palsy.* London: Lloyd-Luke Medical.
15. Illis, L. S., Sedgwick, E. M. & Glanville, H. J. (1982) *Rehabilitation of the Neurological Patient.* Oxford: Blackwell Scientific.
16. Knott, M. & Voss, D. E. (1973) *Proprioceptive Neuromuscular Facilitation*, 2nd edn. New York: Harper and Row.
17. Lance, J. W. & McLeod, J. G. (1981) *A Physiological Approach to Clinical Neurology*, 3rd edn. London: Butterworths.
18. Seamans, S. (1967) The Bobath concept in treatment of neurological disorders. *American Journal of Physical Medicine*, Vol. 46, pp. 900–956.
19. Stockmeyer, S. A. (1967) An interpretation of the approach of Rood to the treatment of neuromuscular dysfunction. *American Journal of Physical Medicine*, Vol. 46, pp. 732–785.
20. Sullivan, P. E., Markos, P. D. and Minor, M. A. (1982) *An Integrated Approach to Therapeutic Exercise.* Reston: Reston Publishing.
21. Umphred, D. A. (Ed.) (1985) *Neurological Rehabilitation.* St. Louis: C. V. Mosby.
22. Walton, J. N. (1977) *Brain's Diseases of the Nervous System.* Oxford: Oxford University Press.
23. Wyke, B. (1976) Neurological mechanisms in spasticity. *Physiotherapy*, Vol. 62, pp. 316–319.

20

The trunk and neck with special reference to lifting and breathing

THE SPINE

The structure of the spine[15,23,28]

The spine functions as:
1. A support for the head, upper limbs and thorax, transferring this weight via the pelvis to the lower limbs
2. The body axis – the centre for movement
3. A protection for the spinal cord from direct injury.

It is made up of 33 vertebrae, stacked one on top of the other. Between the sacrum (5 fused vertebrae) which is the fixed part of the vertebral column and the base of the skull, are 24 movable parts. These are the 5 lumbar, 12 thoracic and 7 cervical vertebrae. The remaining 4 fused vertebrae go to make up the coccyx.

Each vertebra is composed of:

1. A weight bearing part – the vertebral body.

2. A part that protects the spinal cord – the vertebral arch. Each arch is crossed above and below by a spinal nerve.

3. Three levers to which muscles are attached. These are the spinous process and the right and left transverse processes.

4. Four projections which guide and at the same time restrict movement – the superior and inferior articular processes. The superior processes face:

a. Backward and upward in the cervical region

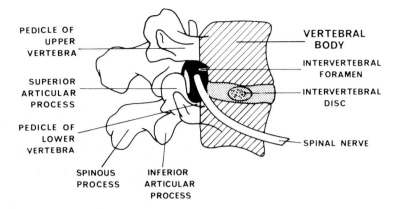

Fig. 20.1 A motion segment of two vertebrae stacked one on top of the other. The anterior weight bearing part is shaded.

b. Backward and laterally in the thoracic region

c. Backward and medially in the lumbar region.

The inferior articular processes conversely face in the opposite direction in each region.

Two adjoining vertebrae and their intervening soft tissues make up a 'motion segment' which is the basic mechanical unit of the spine (Fig. 20.1).

The spinal nerves which are formed by the union of the ventral and dorsal roots (Fig. 3.11) emerge through the intervertebral foramina which are formed by the:

1. Pedicles of adjacent vertebrae – above and below
2. Intervertebral disc as well as parts of the two vertebral bodies it unites – in the front
3. Two articular processes and the capsules uniting them.

The relationship between the segments of the spinal cord and the emergence of the corresponding nerve root is shown in Figure 20.2.

The spine forms an integral part of the trunk and neck. In the trunk it carries the thoracic cage and its contents as well as the weight of the abdominal contents. The latter may vary depending on the state of the individual, as for example, during pregnancy or where there is gross obesity.

At its base, the sacrum forms part of the bony basin of the trunk, the pelvis. Therefore, should the position of the pelvis be altered in any way, the sacrum must also be altered and accordingly, the shape of the spine. In the neck, the spine supports the weight of the head. It also contributes towards carrying the weight of the shoulder girdle and upper limbs.

Many natural movements involving the trunk are really composite movements of the trunk and hip joints. These movements serve to extend the reach of the arms and the legs, as for example, in stretching forward to pick up an object.

The bony framework of the trunk, namely the spine, thoracic cage and pelvis, encloses two inflatable cavities which contain organs vital to life. These intra-thoracic and intra-abdominal cavities are separated from each other by the diaphragm. Through muscular activity, pressure inside both these cavities can be altered.

The supportive role of the spine

The spine may be visualised as the supporting pillar of the trunk. Most of this support comes from the anterior part of this pillar made up of alternating vertebral bodies and their intervertebral discs (Fig. 20.1). The intervertebral discs account for about one-third of the total length of the column.

The size of the vertebrae increases moving down the spine from the atlas to the fifth

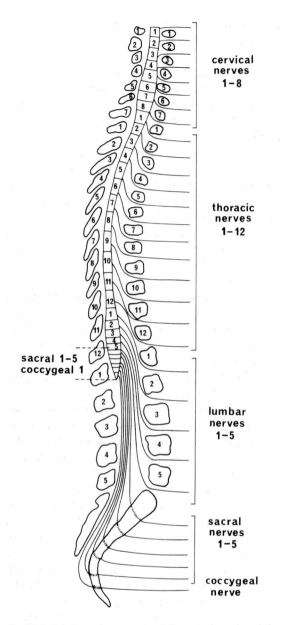

cervical
nerves
1-8

thoracic
nerves
1-12

sacral 1-5
coccygeal 1

lumbar
nerves
1-5

sacral
nerves
1-5

coccygeal
nerve

Fig. 20.2 Relation of segments of the spinal cord and the spinal nerves to the vertebral column. *Reproduced with kind permission from Barr, M. L. (1979) The Human Nervous System – an Anatomical Viewpoint, 3rd edn. Harper and Row, p. 51.*

lumbar vertebra. This design reflects the increasing amount of superimposed body weight the lower vertebrae have to support, for while the cervical vertebrae only have to support the weight of the head, the lumbar

vertebrae have the weight of the head, upper limbs and upper trunk to carry.

The intervertebral discs are designed to act like 'shock absorbers' for various compressive forces. The amount of compression placed on a disc can vary depending on the following:

1. The effect of gravity on the mass of the body in the position being considered. For example, gravity will have different leverage effects when the trunk is flexed at various angles during lifting, as compared to upright standing.

2. Changes in the state of motion of the body as occurs when there is a sudden change in acceleration or change in direction. An example of the former would be landing after a jump from a height.

3. The effect of the contractions of the muscles of the trunk. When muscles whose fibres run parallel to the spine contract, they tend to compress the vertebrae closer together and consequently compress the disc.[27]

Intradiscal pressure has been measured for the lumbar region (third lumbar disc) in living subjects during a number of activities.[18,19,20,21] Using these pressure measurements it is possible to calculate the approximate load on the lower lumbar discs (Table 20.1).

Table 20.1 Approximate loads on the L3-disc in a 70 kg subject during various activities (after Nachemson 1975).[18]

Activity	Load (kg)
Lying supine, in traction (30 kg)	10
Lying supine	30
Standing	70
Walking	85
Twisting	90
Bending sideways	95
Upright sitting, no support	100
Coughing	110
Jumping	110
Straining	120
Laughing	120
Bending forward 20°	120
Bilateral straight leg raising, supine	120
Prone lying, active back extension	150
Sit up exercise from supine with knees bent	180
Lifting of 20 kg, back straight, knees bent	210
Lifting of 20 kg, back bent, knees straight	340

The inherent mobility of the spine has to be controlled if it is to perform its important supportive role satisfactorily. Such stability is provided by:

1. Muscles, through their alternative 'give and take' activity. The muscles, under the control of the central nervous system, provide active support, in contrast to the passive support given by the ligaments. This variable co-contraction forms part of the background postural righting activity which automatically occurs if the upright position is to be maintained and the head, neck and trunk are to remain correctly aligned one to the other.

Proprioceptive information from the many joints and muscles related to the spine ensures that any necessary postural adjustments can be made from time to time.

2. Ligaments, which bind the individual vertebrae and their intervening discs together. The ligaments constrain the movements of the spine by providing a counterbalancing force through their development of passive tension as they become stretched.

Movements of the spine

The vertebrae above the sacrum are linked together by intervertebral discs and various ligaments – some long and some short – to form a flexible tube[6] which serves to protect the spinal cord from direct injury. In the upright position this 'tube' appears vertical and straight when viewed from behind. When viewed from the side, it forms a series of primary and secondary curves.

These spinal curves can alter their shape depending on the movement being performed. Sometimes there may be even a complete reversal of the shape of the curve as occurs in the lumbar spine during flexion and extension.

The presence of these curves allows the spine to withstand greater compressive forces when the person is upright than if it were just a straight sustaining rod alone.[15]

The movements of the spine are:

1. Flexion and extension

2. Lateral flexion to the right and left
3. Axial rotation.

Most spinal movements are often a combination of movements from each of the three groups above rather than the pure movement alone. For example, lateral flexion is accompanied by some axial rotation.

The gross movements of flexion, extension, lateral flexion and rotation are really composite movements, being the sum total of all the movements taking place between each vertebra and its neighbour. The shape and direction of the articular facets in the different regions of the spine contribute towards guiding and limiting motion.

Therefore, most:

1. Flexion, occurs in the cervical and upper thoracic spine.
2. Extension, occurs in the cervical as well as the lumbar spine, particularly the lumbo-sacral junction. Extension in the thoracic spine is mechanically limited by the spinous processes.
3. Lateral flexion, occurs in the cervical spine. This section has the greatest mobility, although the lumbar spine allows some lateral bending in its upper section. In the thoracic region, this movement is limited by the ribs.
4. Axial rotation, occurs in the cervical spine, particularly the atlanto-axial joint, as well as in the upper thoracic region. The ability to rotate diminishes from the occiput downwards.

The neck is the most mobile region and much of this mobility is achieved by movements at the atlanto-occipital (nodding the head), and atlantoaxial (axial rotation) joints. The upper cervical joints are richly supplied with sensory receptors accounting, in part, for the importance of neck position in the control of muscle tone throughout the body.

Muscles controlling the spine

Many muscles contribute towards producing and controlling the movements of the spine. A great number of these muscles attach to the skull and the spine itself, although some important groups such as the abdominals, do not.

The muscles concerned may have the following properties.

1. They may vary considerably in length. Some may be very short, spanning one joint only; others may span many joints thereby having a more widespread influence.

2. They may be superficial or deep. In general, the deeper muscles are shorter. The longer, more superficial muscles tend to provide a coarse adjustment, whereas the shorter deep muscles provide for fine adjustment.

3. They have lines of pull at varying distances from the joints they influence. The leverage of the deeper muscles will tend to be less because of this factor.

The muscles producing spinal movements exist in bilateral pairs. They are generally placed in a plane anterior or posterior to the spine, although some, namely quadratus lumborum and psoas major, are placed laterally.[15]

Sometimes both muscles in each pair contract at the same time with the same intensity, producing a 'pure' flexion or extension movement. Asymmetry of movement occurs, if these 'pure' movements are attempted with one member of the pair being weaker than the other. Similarly, if one member of a pair is tighter than its partner, an asymmetrical deformity may be apparent.

Often both members of each pair contract independently of each other to perform quite a different movement. For example, when both the right and left sternocleidomastoid muscles act against gravity, the head is drawn forwards, so helping the deep flexor muscles to flex the cervical column. When only one of the pair contracts, it tilts the head towards the shoulder of the same side and also rotates the head so as to carry the face towards the opposite side.

Different members of pairs of muscles on both sides of the body can co-operate with one another to produce asymmetrical movements. For example, axial rotation of the trunk towards the right is actively brought about by the simultaneous contraction of the left external oblique and right internal oblique muscles as well as by other muscles.

A special type of 'pairing' of muscles relates to the control of pelvic tilting.

When the pelvis tilts anteriorly, the lumbar curve is increased. This is counterbalanced by the contraction of the extensor muscles of the hip. When these muscles contract they tend to tilt the pelvis posteriorly. In this movement they can be actively aided by the abdominals so both the hip extensors and the abdominals create a force couple to tilt the pelvis backwards (Fig. 20.3) and thereby flatten the lumbar spine.

The activity of muscles controlling the spine has been studied electromyographically in a number of activities including:

1. Upright standing[3,14]
2. Sitting[2]
3. During flexion and extension of the trunk from the standing position, as occurs during lifting[12,17]
4. Exercises such as sit-ups and straight leg raising in supine[7,10]
5. Coughing and other straining activities.[11]

In some cases, electromyographic studies have been done concurrently with taking measures of pressure in the intervertebral discs, intra-abdominal pressure and intra-thoracic pressure.[1]

Muscle activity during flexion and extension from standing

The activity of the various muscles during flexion and extension of the spine from the standing position is of particular interest because of its practical importance in relation to lifting.

When bending forwards, two major factors contribute towards supporting the spine.

1. Tension in the structures behind the spine which act to prevent it from collapsing forward. This is produced:

a. Actively, by the contraction of the erector spinae muscles which control the

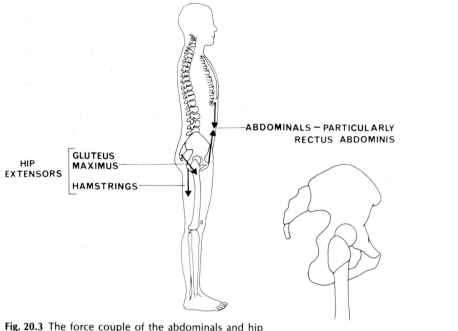

HIP
EXTENSORS
GLUTEUS
MAXIMUS
HAMSTRINGS

ABDOMINALS — PARTICULARLY
RECTUS ABDOMINIS

(i)   (ii)

Fig. 20.3 The force couple of the abdominals and hip extensors rotate the pelvis backwards around the axis through the two hip joints from position (i) to position (ii). There is also an accompanying flattening of the lumbar spine which is not shown in the diagram.

flexion movement being brought about by gravity. This contraction of the muscles which run parallel to the spine also leads to greater compression forces being placed on the intervertebral discs, particularly those of the lumbar spine. Electromyographic studies have shown that as full flexion is reached, the activity in the erector spinae muscles abruptly ceases, so that at full flexion the spine is being supported from behind by the passive tension provided by the ligaments alone.[12] Therefore at full flexion, the spine is vulnerable because one of its posterior support mechanisms – active control by the muscles – shuts down.

When the trunk is again raised from the fully flexed position, the movement is initiated by the hip extensors, which become activated before the back extensors.[12]

b. Passively, by the increasing tension building up in the posterior ligaments as they become more stretched as full flexion is approached. During trunk flexion, there is a transfer of tension from muscular to ligamentous support.

2. Compression forces which act to cushion the spine from beneath when it is flexed, helping to relieve some of the considerable pressure on the intervertebral discs. The cushioning effect comes about by a 'reflex' response in which various trunk muscles are activated to:

a. Fix the rib cage
b. Restrain and compress the abdominal contents.

This mechanism comes into action when weights are being lifted. The glottis is closed and strong activity of the diaphragm, combined with that of the abdominals, particularly the obliques and transversus abdominus, and the muscles of the pelvic floor, increase the pressure within the intra-abdominal and intra-thoracic cavities. This in turn relieves some of the compression forces on the spine itself, particularly the lumbar discs, by providing support from beneath.[9,17]

This protective mechanism is only active for a short period of time. Its effect is lessened when another breath has to be taken. It also leads to some important temporary cardio-vascular changes namely:

1. Cerebrovascular hypertension
2. Decrease in venous return
3. Decrease in pulmonary blood flow
4. Increase in pulmonary vascular resistance.[15]

LIFTING

Good lifting is a skill which all should develop. This is particularly so for those involved in occupations where regular lifting makes the lumbar spine more vulnerable to damage, as for example, the mother lifting her young child, the worker in industry and the physiotherapist.[8,16,26]

Although good design and organisation of the work-place in the home or on the factory floor may help reduce the need for lifting or lessen the extent of the lift, it is a task that cannot be completely avoided in normal life. Education is necessary so that a person does not lift those loads alone which are too heavy or cumbersome for him to manage safely. He should seek the aid of another person or a lifting machine.

Many activities involve applying a force to an object in order to move it. The object may be light or heavy and have a regular or irregular shape.

The object is either pulled or pushed in a horizontal or as in the case of lifting, in a vertical direction. For example, the task of lifting a box from the floor and placing it on a high shelf above eye level can be considered as a 'pulling' movement from the floor to chest level and a 'pushing' movement from there on.[4]

During lifting, the object has to be held and supported at the same time the vertical motion is taking place, otherwise the lift will

not be effective. This is also true when the object has to be carried from place to place. Therefore it is important that the hands are placed in such a position as to provide an upwards force to counteract the weight of the object acting downwards.

The manner in which the lifting task is performed can place unnecessary anatomical

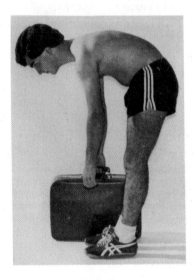

a

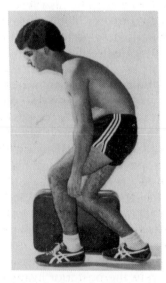

b

Fig. 20.4 a. Straining the back. b. Lifting using strong leg muscles. Use of a handle enables the hand to apply an upwards force to aid lifting.

and physiological stresses on the individual. The lumbar spine is particularly vulnerable when the body bends forwards with the knees extended even when no weight is being carried. The leverage effect of the body weight plus any additional load is greatly increased so the back extensors need to provide a much greater counter force to the combined weight of the head, arms and trunk and the object being lifted. The leverage effect of this combined weight can be reduced if the person crouches down to the object by bending the knees (Fig. 20.4).

Lifting, like every other movement, should be performed economically, demanding the least possible amount of energy. A large amount of energy is required to lift the person's body weight as well as the additional weight but with care this can be minimised. For example, holding any additional weight as close to the body as possible over the centre of the base of support, also reduces the need for muscle activity to sustain the posture, thereby reducing the need for energy.[16]

Principles of lifting[4,24]

Lifting an object from the floor (Fig. 20.5)

1. Foot placement is important. The person should stand close to the object being lifted. The base should be of a comfortable width with the feet placed to the best advantage for that particular lift. Floor surfaces should provide adequate friction for a safe lift.

2. The back is protected if the person lowers his body into a crouching position rather than bending forward with the knees straight, for reasons discussed earlier. It is not necessary to hold the back stiffly – some flexion of the spine will occur. To preserve energy and lessen the strain on the joints of the lower limbs it is important to crouch only as far as is necessary and no further, as this will reduce the distance through which the combined load has to be lifted later.

3. The hands should firmly grasp the object with the fingers widely spaced so as much of the hand as possible is in contact with it.

The object's weight is thereby more evenly distributed so unnecessary discomfort caused by undue pressure on the lifter's hands is avoided. The hands should be placed under the object to provide the upwards force. Support in the horizontal direction may be provided by the forearms and arms when required to keep a large object such as a bag of groceries steady (Fig. 20.6).

4. The strong muscles of the lower limbs provide the force to raise the combined weight of the body and the object. While the upward motion is taking place the object is held as close as possible to the body.

To place the object on the floor again, the powerful muscles of the lower limbs are used to control the downward motion as the body assumes the crouch position again.

Lifting an object from a shelf[4] (Fig. 20.7)

Attempts to lift objects from a height should not be made without help unless the object is relatively light. Many of the principles already discussed also apply here.

Before lifting, the feet are placed one in front of the other in a stride position, with the body weight over the forward limb. As the object is lifted down, the body weight shifts to the hind limb. In this way good body alignment is maintained and undue extension of the lumbar spine is avoided during the lift.

Lifting patients

Methods of lifting patients have been described in the Chartered Society of Physiotherapy booklet *Handling the Handicapped*.[8]

When lifting a patient, the physiotherapist must always consider the patient's disability, his size and his weight. A physiotherapist should never lift excessive loads and should seek help when lifting a patient whenever needed or possible.

When a 'helper' is necessary, the physiotherapist and the helper should be matched so that both can perform the activity with minimal effort.

The patient should also know exactly what

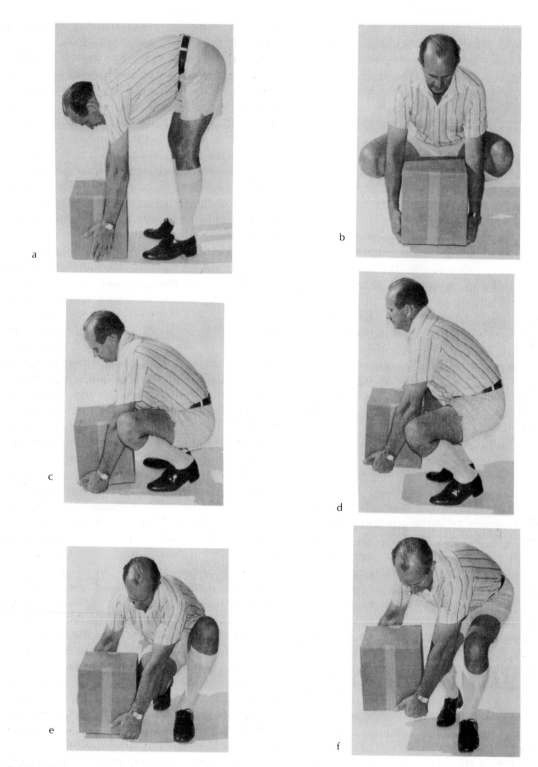

Fig. 20.5 Lifting an object from the floor. a. Incorrect lifting, as it strains the back. Note that the hand position also does not contribute to the upwards force. b to f show two ways of approaching the object so the strong leg muscles rather than the back are used to provide force for the lift.

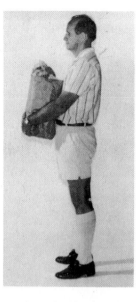

Fig. 20.6 Carrying a bag of groceries. Note that the weight is held close to the body keeping the combined centre of gravity over the base.

is expected of him as he may be able to assist, thereby reducing the load on the physiotherapist.

MOVEMENTS OF BREATHING[5,13,22]

Movements of the thoracic cage bring about inspiration and expiration. Air is drawn into the lungs by rib movement. Through muscle action the thorax can be expanded in its:

1. Antero-posterior diameter – in the upper thorax.
2. Transverse diameter – in the lower thorax.
3. Vertical diameter – by the descent of the dome of the diaphragm. Contraction of the diaphragm also contributes towards movements of the ribs in an upwards and outwards direction, thereby increasing the transverse diameter as well.[25]

The mechanics of respiration vary with age and sex. Respiration in females is predominantly upper thoracic and in children, predominantly abdominal. In adult males it is mixed, being both upper and lower thoracic.

In the elderly, breathing tends to become lower thoracic or even abdominal.[15]

For efficient respiration the joints of the thorax need to be mobile and the muscles involved should possess adequate strength to cope with the demands of a wide variety of situations as the lungs respond to every movement of the thoracic cage.

Both the lungs and the chest wall possess the property of elasticity – they recoil back to their original shape once the forces which changed their shape have been removed. A good example of this occurs during the breathing cycle when the muscles rhythmically contract and relax to produce air flow. When the muscles relax the chest and lungs resume their original form.

The shape of the thorax also varies depending on the activity being performed at the time, which in turn will have an effect on lung function. The lungs may be compressed or expanded. For example, when pushing an object the rib cage tends to flatten due to the action of serratus anterior. This tends to restrict the vital capacity. Pulling on the other hand, does not do this. Here the action of latissimus dorsi causes the rib cage to deepen.[27]

In the resting mid-position, i.e. the functional residual capacity, a balance exists, so that should the lungs need to be inflated, activity of the inspiratory muscles will be required. The functional residual capacity is the amount of air remaining in the lungs at the end of a normal respiration (Fig. 20.8).

Should the lungs need to be further deflated from the resting mid-position, activity of the expiratory muscles will be necessary. In both cases, once the 'deforming' muscles relax, the lungs and chest wall will recoil to their original resting position again.

The volume of air being moved and the rate at which it is being moved influences the amount of activity present in those muscle groups responsible for the inspiratory and expiratory phases of the breathing cycle.

During quiet breathing, only the inspiratory muscles show much activity. The diaphragm, which is the major muscle of inspiration, is

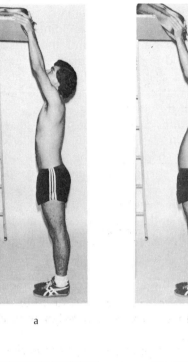

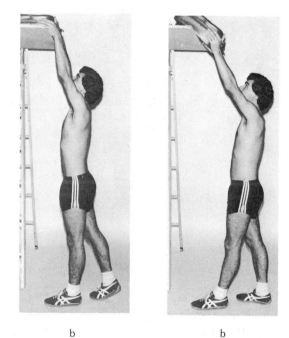

a   a   b   b

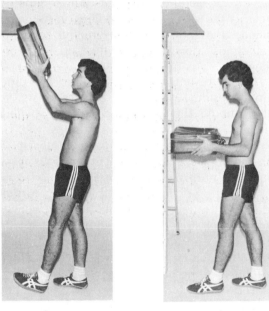

b   b

Fig. 20.7 Lifting a light object from a height. In a, note that poor foot placement leads to poor balance and consequent strain on the lower back. In b, note that the weight transfer from one foot to the other enables better balance thereby helping to bring the object down from the shelf without strain.

the most active of all. When it contracts, its dome descends about 1.5 cm, pushing against the abdominal viscera and causing the lower ribs to move in an upwards and outwards direction. By its action, the diaphragm contributes to $\frac{2}{3}$ tidal volume in sitting and standing and $\frac{3}{4}$ tidal volume in supine lying. The amount of air that moves into the lungs with each inspiration or moves out with each expiration is called the 'tidal volume' (Fig. 20.8).

The function of the intercostals is still controversial. The external intercostals and the intercartilagenous portions of the internal intercostals, as well as the scalenes, may contribute to normal quiet inspiration in some people.

When the inspiratory muscles relax, the elastic recoil of the lung and thoracic cage supplies the necessary force for expiration in normal circumstances. The abdominals which are the primary muscles of expiration are inactive in quiet breathing.

During deep breathing at a faster rate, the vertical movement of the diaphragm is now about 10 cm on inspiration. There is some extension of the spine, as well as an upwards

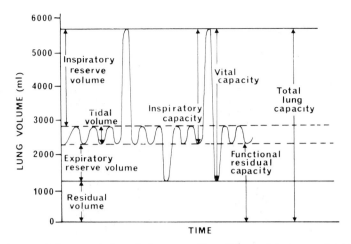

Fig. 20.8 Diagram showing respiratory excursions during normal breathing and during maximal inspiration and maximal expiration. *Reproduced with kind permission from Guyton, A. C. (1976) Textbook of Medical Physiology, 5th edn. Philadelphia: W. B. Saunders Co. p. 521.*

movement of the thoracic cage. Accessory muscles come into play including the back extensors and the sternocleidomastoids. At high rates of ventilation, the abdominal muscles are activated in expiration.

The mechanics of breathing can be altered by the position of the body. For example in:

1. Supine lying, the diaphragm is pushed upwards by the abdominal contents, thereby making inspiration more difficult.
2. Side lying, the diaphragm is pushed upwards into the thoracic cavity far more on the supporting side. This contributes towards making the lower lung on the supporting side less efficient.[15]

Coughing

The cough reflex is important for survival as it assists in keeping the airways clear. The sequence of movements involved in coughing is as follows.

After a deep inspiration the glottis is closed. Vigorous contractions of many expiratory muscles particularly of the abdominals follow leading to an increase of intrathoracic pressure.

This pressure is released when the glottis suddenly opens causing an explosive rush of air out of the lungs, carrying with it mucus and any foreign material.

The strong contraction of the abdominal muscles in coughing also causes an increase in intra-abdominal pressure, which in turn leads to an increase in the contraction of the sphincters of the pelvic floor. A similar response also occurs when laughing, speaking and in weightlifting as described earlier in this chapter.

REFERENCES AND FURTHER READING.

1. Andersson, B. J. G., Örtengren, R. & Nachemson, A. (1977) Intradiskal pressure, intra-abdominal pressure and myo-electric back muscle activity related to posture and loading. *Clinical Orthopaedics and Related Research*, Vol. 129, pp. 156–164.
2. Andersson, B. J. G., Örtengren, R., Nachemson, A. L., Elfstrom, G. & Broman, H. (1975) The sitting posture: an electromyographic and discometric study. *Orthopaedic Clinics of North America*, Vol. 6, No. 1, pp. 105–120.
3. Basmajian, J. V. & De Luca, C. J. (1985) *Muscles Alive*, 5th edn. Baltimore: Williams & Wilkins.
4. Broer, M. R. & Zernicke, R. F. (1979) *Efficiency of Human Movement*, 4th edn. Philadelphia: W. B. Saunders.
5. Campbell, E. J. M., Agostini, E. & Newsom-Davis, J.

(1970) *The Respiratory Muscles – Mechanics and Neural Control*, 2nd edn. London: Lloyd-Luke, Medical.

6. Carlsöö, S. (1972) *How Man Moves*. London: Heinemann.

7. Carman, D. J., Blanton, P. L. & Biggs, N. L. (1972) Electromyographic study of the anterolateral abdominal musculature utilising indwelling electrodes. *American Journal of Physical Medicine*, Vol. 51, pp. 113–129.

8. Chartered Society of Physiotherapy (1980) *Handling the Handicapped*, 2nd edn. Cambridge: Woodhead-Faulkener.

9. Farfan, H. F. (1975) Muscular mechanism of the lumbar spine and the position of power and efficiency. *Orthopaedic Clinics of North America*, Vol. 6, No. 1, pp. 135–144.

10. Flint, M. M. (1965) Abdominal muscle involvement during the performance of various forms of sit-up exercise. *American Journal of Physical Medicine*, Vol. 44, No. 5, pp. 224–234.

11. Floyd, W. F. & Silver, P. H. S. (1950) Electromyographic study of patterns of activity of the anterior abdominal wall muscles in man. *Journal of Anatomy*, Vol. 84, pp. 132–145.

12. Floyd, W. F. & Silver, P. H. S. (1955) The function of the Erectores spinae muscles in certain movements and postures in Man. *Journal of Physiology*, Vol. 129, pp. 184–203.

13. Guyton, A. C. (1981) *Textbook of Medical Physiology*, 6th edn. Philadelphia: W. B. Saunders.

14. Joseph, J. (1960) *Man's Posture: Electromyographic Studies*. Springfield: Charles C. Thomas.

15. Kapandji, I. A. (1974) *The Physiology of the Joints – Volume 3 – The Trunk and the Vertebral Column*. Edinburgh: Churchill Livingstone.

16. Metheny, E. (1952) *Body Dynamics*. New York: McGraw-Hill.

17. Morris, J. M., Lucas, D. B. & Bresler, B. (1961) Role of the trunk in stability of the spine. *The Journal of Bone and Joint Surgery*, Vol. 43A, No. 3, pp. 327–351.

18. Nachemson, A. (1975) Towards a better understanding of low-back pain: a review of the mechanics of the lumbar disc. *Rheumatology and Rehabilitation*, Vol. 14, pp. 129–143.

19. Nachemson, A. L. (1976) The lumbar spine: an orthopaedic challenge. *Spine*, Vol. 1, No. 1, pp. 59–71.

20. Nachemson, A. & Morris, J. M. (1964) In vivo measurements of intradiscal pressure. *The Journal of Bone and Joint Surgery*, Vol. 46A, No. 5, pp. 1077–1092.

21. Nachemson, A. & Elfstrom, G. (1970) Intravital dynamic pressure measurements in lumbar discs. *Scandinavian Journal of Rehabilitation Medicine Supplement No. 1*.

22. Rankin, J. & Dempsey, J. A. (1967) Respiratory muscles and the mechanisms of breathing. *American Journal of Physical Medicine*, Vol. 46, No. 1, pp. 198–240.

23. Steindler, A. (1955) *Kinesiology of the human body*. Springfield: Charles C. Thomas.

24. Strachan, A. (1979) Back care in industry. *Physiotherapy*, Vol. 65, No. 8, pp. 249–251.

25. Thacker, E. W. (1973) *Postural Drainage and Respiratory Control*, 3rd edn. Lloyd-Luke Medical.

26. Tichauer, E. R. (1978) *The biomechanical basis of ergonomics*. New York: John Wiley & Sons.

27. Troup, J. D. G. (1979) Biomechanics of the vertebral column. *Physiotherapy*, Vol. 65, No. 8, pp. 238–244.

28. Williams, P. L. & Warwick, R. (Eds) (1980) *Gray's Anatomy*, 36th edn. Edinburgh: Churchill Livingstone.

21

The function of the upper extremity with special reference to the hand

The hand is the active extremity of the upper limb. It is a mobile and tactile organ. Its actions are extended and reinforced and much of its skill made possible by the rest of the upper limb as well as the positioning of the head, neck and trunk. Each joint adds to the versatility, precision and possibilities for skilled movements. The shoulder is the most mobile joint of the body and, with the shoulder girdle, elbow and forearm, carries and supports the hand and provides a wide range of movement. The trunk may still further increase the reach of the upper limb. This allows the hand to move into the environment, to carry objects to and from the body and to perform essential hygiene. The elbow joint can shorten or lengthen the limb and together with the co-ordinated movement of rotation in the shoulder and forearm, allows the hand to carry food to the mouth and places the hand in the most favourable position for any possible action.

Wrist, forearm and hand actions blend together, with the wrist carrying and supporting the hand and greatly influencing the accuracy and strength of the hand by the co-ordination of its movements with those of the metacarpophalangeal joints and the fingers and thumb.

The position of the wrist and forearm is a key factor in achieving efficient hand function. The wrist:

1. Carries and supports the hand and any object it is holding
2. Positions the hand in space
3. Is the main site for change between the hand and the upper extremity
4. Acting with the forearm, strategically positions and stabilises the hand so that the required movement of the fingers can be carried out to the greatest advantage as regards strength and skill
5. Modifies hand alignment
6. By its mobility, increases the scope of hand function.

The wrist position controls the posture of the metacarpophalangeal joints, the metacarpophalangeal joints control the proximal interphalangeal joints and finally the distal interphalangeal joints. In each instance, increased active or passive extension of the proximal joints increases the flexion of the next joint distally in the chain and vice versa because of the extrinsic tendon length (Fig. 3.18). Nearly all movements of the hand require specific and changing wrist action.

The radio-carpal and the radio-ulnar joints combine in an appropriate position to provide the necessary mobility, stability and strength to ensure that adequate positioning and movement are achieved. Their positions are constantly altering as they adapt to the changing circumstances demanded by the actions of the hand, whose movements are closely linked with those of the rest of the arm.

The hand is a structure of great versatility (Fig. 21.1). It changes its shape continuously; it can vary its strength from light touch to a firm grip; it can grasp objects of different sizes and weights and work at changing speeds. The rate of movement may vary from slow to rapid, with control of direction and intensity.

Generally speaking, most hand movements towards the body are done with the wrist flexed to varying degrees and radially deviated and those away from the body are carried out with the wrist extended and ulnar deviated. It is considered by Tubiana[21] that more hand movements are done in flexion than in extension, that is, towards rather than away from the body.

The hand at rest

The hand in repose or during sleep rests in a balanced position with impulses to the hand reduced. Wood Jones[23] describes the position in sitting as that in which the hand lies somewhat pronated, the wrist slightly flexed and the palm hollowed from side to side as well as in its length. The fingers are progressively flexed at the metacarpophalangeal and the interphalangeal joints. The index finger is more extended than the other fingers and slightly ulnar deviated. The little finger is the most bent and is radially deviated. The thumb lies in a position midway between flexion and extension and is slightly adducted and opposed. The normal transverse and longitudinal arches are preserved.

The hand is in a state of rest with all muscles in a state of balanced tone and no part on stretch (Fig. 21.2). Rank[18] points out that the position of the hand at rest depends on the position of the wrist. By passive flexion and extension the degree of flexion of each finger is altered, though its relationship to the neighbouring fingers remains the same. The rest position is described by Napier[15] as being midway between the power and pinch grip and the hand 'beautiful in its tranquillity'. In standing upright the arm is in a relaxed position hanging loosely by the side. The hand is half pronated with the palmar surface facing the thigh. The four ulnar fingers are slightly flexed. The palmar surface of the thumb faces in the direction of the ulna or faces posteriorly. The characteristic posture is mainly provided by the weight of the arm and the passive elements in muscles, tendons and ligaments.

THE ARCHITECTURE OF THE HAND

The skill and the variety of movements which are carried out by the hand are only possible

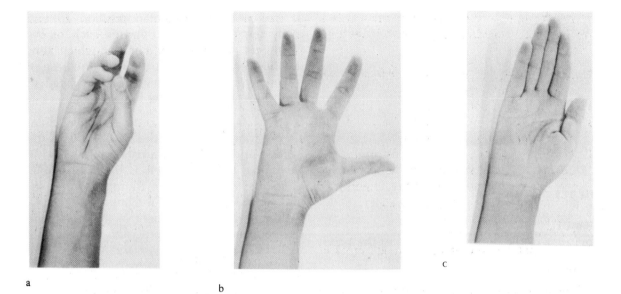

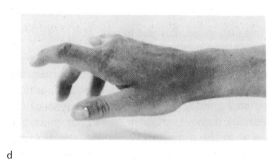

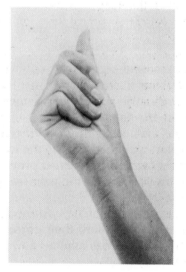

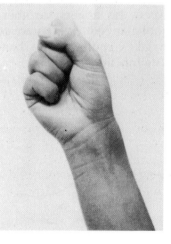

Fig. 21.1 The changing shape of the hand. (a) Opposition, (b) Fingers stretched, (c) Fingers together, (d) Independent finger movement, (e and f) Finger flexion to the palm.

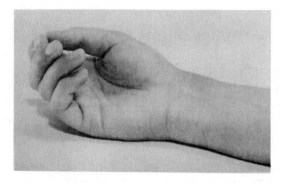

Fig. 21.2 The hand at rest.

because of the bony architecture of the hand, the muscles which control movements and its strong sensory supply.

The arches of the hand

The bony architecture of the hand is based on a series of arches. These are:

1. Two transverse arches
   (i) The carpal arch formed by the carpal bones. It is concave in shape and has little movement.
   (ii) The metacarpal arch formed by the metacarpal heads. It has the capacity to widen and flatten and so provide much of the mobility of the palm of the hand (Fig. 21.3).
2. The longitudinal arches formed by the metacarpal bones and their corresponding phalanges. They can assume a wide variety of shapes.

3. The oblique arches of opposition, formed by the thumb as it opposes each of the fingers. This creates a gutter which runs obliquely across the palm from the base of the hypothenar eminence to the head of the second metacarpal bone.

The arched hand has a central stable element or keystone formed by the rigid shafts of the second and third metacarpals firmly based in the carpal bones, as well as the very mobile elements formed by the thumb and the 4th and 5th metacarpals and the fingers (Fig. 21.4).

In general the movement of the radial side of the hand provides precision and stability and the ulnar side power and stability. The whole hand, which is normally concave, can vary greatly in shape and is capable of wide stretch.

The metacarpophalangeal joints

The metacarpophalangeal joints have a wide range of active movement, which includes flexion and extension, abduction and adduction, and greatly influence the function of the fingers. A passive rotation can occur in association with the active movements, for example in gripping. In turn, their function is influenced by the position of the wrist and the length of long extrinsic muscles. The wide web between the fingers together with the metacarpophalangeal joint movements of abduction gives width to the hand and so increases its functional abilities.

(a)   (b)

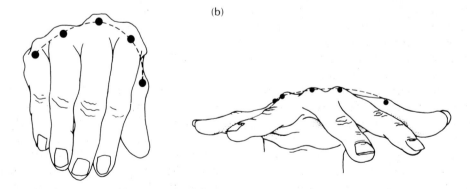

Fig. 21.3 The metacarpal arch is very versatile, being able to (a) arch and (b) widen and flatten.

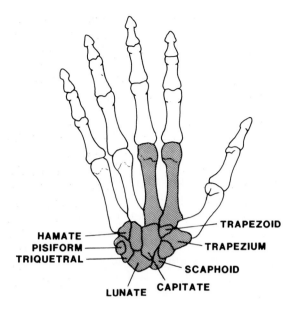

Fig. 21.4 The fixed element of the hand is shaded in this diagram.

The interphalangeal joints

The interphalangeal joints allow the movements of flexion and extension. They are stable laterally and play a major part in most hand functions.

The thumb

The thumb is the most important digit of the hand. It is used in virtually all hand activities and constitutes an active half of the prehensive hand, playing a part in both power and precision grips. Its movements, its versatility and its stability are concerned in almost all skilled movements of the hand. It is controlled by nine muscles, five intrinsic and four extrinsic, which add to the versatility of its function.[12] Opposition, which is an essential function of the hand, increases the cup shape of the hand and adds precision, strength and stability to the grip. The width of the web between the thumb and index finger influences to a great degree the overall span of the hand.

The hypothenar eminence

The hypothenar eminence provides the mobile, ulnar eminence of the hand. The muscles are not unlike those of the thumb although their movements are smaller, simpler and easier to isolate. Their prime function is to help bring about opposition between the thumb and the little finger and together with the three lateral metacarpals help to produce the cupping action of the hand and provide much of the strength of its gripping action.

The balance of movement in the hand

The function of the hand and its freedom from deformity depends on the following four factors:

1. The integrity and mobility of the arches forming the structure of the hand. If the joints and ligaments are damaged, the muscle balance is disturbed as normal movement is impossible on an abnormal and perhaps unstable structure.
2. The delicate kinaesthetic balance between the extrinsic flexors and extensors of the fingers and between the relevant extrinsic and intrinsic muscles of the hand. If this balance is disturbed stress will be placed on ligaments and joints.
3. The integrity of the wrist and the muscles moving it and working over it.
4. The ability of the central nervous system to activate and control the mobility, strength, skill and versatility necessary for efficient movement.

All are interdependent.

THE FUNCTIONING HAND

Hands can be of many types, shapes and sizes and fulfil many different functions. They will be influenced by a person's lifestyle. Firstly, there is the person who does not use them for any specialised purpose except that of daily living. Secondly, there is the manual worker whose hands have lessened mobility but are strong and have gained a thick durable protective skin on the palm and fingers. Thirdly, there is the person who uses his hands in a skilled and specialised way such as the musician, the artist and the typist. These varied functions must be considered by the physiotherapist in her treatment of patients. She, herself, helps the patient by the skilled use of her hands.

The hand in daily life

The activities of the hand in daily life vary enormously and the whole of the upper extremity is usually involved with the range of movement of all joints of the arm changing constantly in their relationship, one with the other. Many activities use both arms though their actions may be different.

The hands play a major part in the lives of most people in such essential activities as, for example, eating and drinking and personal hygiene such as toilet and bathing activities. Most of these activities can be handled by a one-handed person if necessary.

In the activities of daily work the duties vary greatly from those of the housewife caring for children, cooking and looking after a house, the manual labourer handling a spade, the skilled artisan working with tools, the secretary using pen and typewriter, to those of the highly skilled, such as the sculptor, watchmaker, dentist, nurse and physiotherapist to illustrate just a few of the variations in skills essential to individual groups of people.

The sportsman using sporting equipment uses many different grips. In most sports there is less concern for finer precision movements than for grosser movements such as grasping a racquet or ball. The shape of the grip depends on the shape and size of the object grasped as well as the purposes of the action.

Major functions of the hand

The five major functions of the hand are:

1. Manipulation
2. Sensation and touch
3. Stabilisation – a means of support
4. Protection
5. Expression and communication.

1. The hand and manipulation

Good hand function is based on three main areas in which work is involved: (i) dexterity; (ii) strength; (iii) stability. The movements of the hand are used for prehension and mobility at the end of a mobile arm. Sometimes the hand acts as a fixed non-prehensile end on a mobile arm. It can function either dynamically or statically. Its function as a whole is the sum of many sub-movements. These movements may be used to explore an object, involve actions such as gripping and carrying as well as provide dexterity and maintain stability. The strength of the hand will usually vary according to the sex of the person, the position of the wrist and muscular strength.

Hand movements may also be free and non-manipulative in which no external object is directly involved, such as opening and closing, cupping, gripping or clawing or they may involve skilled independent finger movements. They may be used as a stretch after rest, to relieve tension or to form a wide range of expressive gestures.

Another classification divides movements into three major types:

(i) Slow to rapid movements with control of direction, intensity and rate, for example, in writing or sewing.
(ii) Ballistic movements, for example, typing or playing the piano.
(iii) Fixations or co-contractions, for example, the positions which allow movement to proceed.

There have been many attempts to classify movements in which work is involved. Napier[15] classifies movement into two main areas, namely, (i) prehension; (ii) non-prehension.

Prehension may be defined as all the functions put into play when an object is gripped by the hand.

(i) A prehensile movement is a cortically controlled action in which an object which is either free or fixed, seen and/or touched, is held in a gripping or pinching action partly or wholly in the compass of the hand.

(ii) A non-prehensile movement is one which may involve the whole hand, fingers or a finger but in which no object is grasped or held. The movement may be a pushing one such as pushing an object, a finger-lifting one such as playing the piano or the movements of the gloved and skilled fingers of the puppeteer.

Prehensile movement

In any prehensile movement five main factors are involved:

(i) The intent to grip the object – a cortical involvement.

(ii) An appreciation by sight and/or memory to give the direction and distance of an object – a spatial awareness – and in many cases the shape and texture of the object. The choice of the pattern of movement is thus pre-selected. In the unsighted person, memory, exploration and palpation take the place of sight and the sense of touch and memory are highly developed.

(iii) The mechanism of the grasp and grip necessary to hold and support the object firmly, which provides stability.

(iv) The pattern, strength and accuracy of the grip which is governed to a great extent by the function to which the object is to be put.

(v) The release.

The initial opening of the fingers is an intuitive action governed by the intention to grasp. This movement will be shaped by the intended grasp. The basic shape and size of the initial grasp is created at the metacarpophalangeal joints. The hand form may enlarge or decrease from its resting position according to the size of the object. The initial touch moves to palpation and manipulation in order to gain more information and so modify the initial grasp. The level of contact increases the

appreciation of the object and establishes the flexed grip position of the metacarpophalangeal and interphalangeal joints to a greater or lesser degree. The accuracy of the grip will depend firstly on the sensory function of the fingers, especially of their pulp, and of the palm, if relevant. The nail supports the pulp and provides a rigid and protective backing. Secondly, it depends on the sense of muscular effort made to grip and then support the object.

The pattern of the total movement, which may involve the use of the whole upper extremity, will be shaped and regulated to a great extent by the function to which the object gripped will be used as well as on the size, shape, texture and temperature of the object being gripped. Normal sensory activity is essential. The mobility of the palm plays a major part in effective hand use.

The release

When the purpose of the action has been fulfilled the object is released and replaced. To do this, the hand muscles gradually relax their hold and the fingers then actively extend, though usually they do not fully extend.[6,16]

Thus the hand goes through a dynamic phase in grasping and gripping, a static phase in holding and a later phase of gradually relaxing the finger flexors slightly to be followed by an active dynamic extension stage as the fingers finally extend and release occurs.

Types of grips

Napier[15] has suggested that prehensile movement can be broadly divided into two main types:

(i) The power grip
(ii) The precision grip

with several other less common grips also available, namely:

(iii) The hook grip

(iv) The key grip
(v) The scissor grip.

Different types of grip may be applied when using the same object for different purposes.

(i) The power grip

Napier describes the power grip as one in which the object is held in a clamp formed by the partly flexed fingers and often a wide area of the palm, with counter pressure applied by the stable adducted thumb at the metacarpophalangeal and carpometacarpal joints, lying more or less in the plane of the palm, which acts as a buttress. The hand conforms to the size and shape of the object. All four fingers are more or less flexed and ulnar deviated and laterally rotated with each finger accommodating to the position so that force can be applied and the pressure of the object resisted. As the four fingers conform to the grip, phalangeal rotations, abduction and adduction may be required according to the shape gripped. The grip on large objects depends on adequate opening of the hand.

The wrist is in ulnar deviation and in a mid position between flexion and extension. Strength and power are the chief requirements in this grip with the whole hand involved, particularly the hypothenar eminence and the little and ring fingers which help to lock the object into the hand. The metacarpal bones supply much of the stability of the grip (Fig. 21.5a).

The hand will adapt to the position in which it can most ably carry out a movement with accuracy and with constant pressure maintained in order to achieve the desired result. Stability of the joints is a major need in this grip. For very heavy activities the hand is used to grip the object and the power involved to carry out the activity is provided by the shoulder and to a lesser degree by the elbow, wrist and the trunk.

(ii) The pinch or precision grip

The pinch or precision grip demands more exact control of the finger and thumb positions than in the power grip. The pinch grip is carried out between the terminal opposing pulp part of the thumb and that of one or more of the fingers. The object is held relatively lightly and manipulated between the thumb and related finger or fingers. The sensory surface of the digits is employed to the greatest advantage. The thumb is in a position of opposition. It is abducted and medially rotated at the carpometacarpal and metacarpophalangeal joints. It is held stable and forms one jaw of a clamp with the opposing side formed in part or whole by the flexor surface of the terminal joint of the finger or fingers. The wrist is markedly dorsiflexed and held midway between ulnar and radial deviation. Delicacy and accuracy are essential factors in this grip with power a secondary consideration.

With small objects the grip may involve the:

a. Thumb and the index finger
b. Thumb and the index and middle finger – a tripod grip (Fig. 21.5b)
c. Thumb and all fingers – this is used where larger objects are involved (Fig. 21.5c).

When large flat objects are grasped, the posture of the hand will depend on that grip which provides a suitable span and still ensures stability. The hand spreads out to encompass the object, the fingers are flexed and abducted at the metacarpophalangeal joints in order to increase the span of the hand and to produce a degree of axial rotation of the digits.

Many activities show elements of both power and precision grips. In Figure 21.5d the left hand is in a power grip and the right hand is using a precision grip to unscrew the lid. The right hand commences with a power grip and gradually assumes a precision grip later in the action sequence as the bottle lid becomes looser.

(iii) The hook grip

In this grip only the fingers are involved. An object, such as a bag or a light case, is held

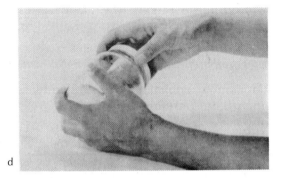

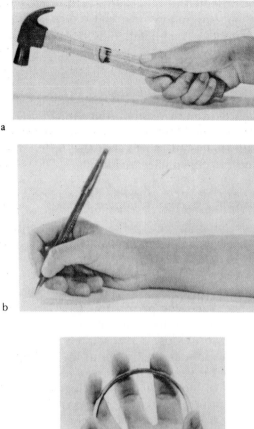

a

b

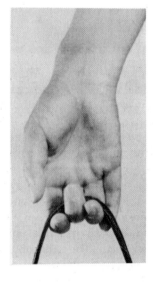

d

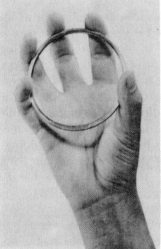

c

e

Fig. 21.5 Types of prehension. (a) A power grip, (b & c) Precision grips, (d) A power and precision grip, (e) The hook grip.

as if in a hook by the extrinsic flexors of the fingers. There is a flattening of the palm. No thumb movement and little muscle strength are involved (Fig. 21.5e).

Other grips less commonly used are:

(iv) The key or lateral grip

In the lateral grip an object such as a key is held between the pulp of the terminal joint of the adducted thumb and lateral side of the terminal joint of the index finger.

(v) The scissor grip

In this grip a object such as a cigarette is held between the sides of the terminal phalanx and sometimes part of the middle phalanx of the index and middle finger. The thumb is not involved in this action. This may be a useful grip for a patient with a grossly disabled hand.

The supinated hand

The hand in supination provides two types of support. It is positioned:

a. To receive an object placed in the palm, for example, to receive coins

or

b. With the fingers flattened to a varying degree by the weight of the object resting either on the total palmar surface or on the finger tips with the palm hollowed.

2. The hand and sensation and touch

The hand is the most highly developed sensory organ and the chief organ of touch in the body. It has a large area of representation in the sensorimotor cortex (Fig. 4.5). An intact sensory system plays an essential part in directing the motor system controlling hand movement.

Touch can be defined as the laying on of the hand so as to gain contact and to feel by means of the tactile system.

The hand has an essential exploring and testing function. The thumb, index and middle fingers are the primary fingers of exploration. They usually work with the eyes or with memory and sound, though the object may or may not be seen. When the object is sighted the hand reaches out, adapting its shape to the expected grasp. At first the contact of the object with the skin is superficial, providing cutaneous sensory information, then the contact increases in depth as the hand feels, explores and grasps the object, providing deep cutaneous impulses from the pulp of the fingers and the palm and proprioceptive sensory impulses from the muscles and joints to the cortex. A picture of the object is formed. The shape, surface, dimensions, weight, density, texture and temperature are learned and the pattern, size, shape and strength of the grip is determined which will be altered according to the demands of the movement. In the blind the manual recognition of an object is most highly developed. The hand has been called a second eye.[18]

Touch of one's own body

Touch is used to explore one's total body, to help carry out essential hygiene, to localise an area of pain and to rub and ease it. It can be a form of personal reassurance.

Touch as a person to person contact

Touch can be a social gesture used as a means of intimate communication from person to person. It forms an important part in interpersonal relationships which is appreciated both by the one being touched and the toucher. For some people touching is a spontaneous gesture, for others its use is laboured and self-conscious; a few seldom use it, may dislike and be defensive about it.

It can be used to reassure and comfort a person, to give the feeling that he is not alone, to nurture, soothe, congratulate, stimulate a person to action, to stir the senses and excite sexually. For example, it can be seen in the holding of the hand of the ill to give support, in the hand of the mother as she comforts her child, in the holding of the hand to guide and the handshake of welcome or farewell. The touch of the hand can also be inhibiting because of its limpness and impersonality.

Touch plays an important part in health care. Here the toucher has a licence to use touch as a medium of treatment. It is expected by the patient and may have diagnostic or therapeutic significance in its use to influence body systems.

3. The hand and stability

The provision of stability and support are two important functions of the hand. The ability to stabilise a joint or several joints to prevent unwanted motion is an important element in gaining efficient movement. It may involve the holding of an object with the hold modified according to the texture, shape and weight of the object.

In bilateral movement, often one hand aids in maintaining stability of an object while the other hand, acting at the end of a mobile arm, carries out a skilled movement. For example, in writing, the non-dominant hand stabilises the paper while the dominant hand uses the pen.

Both arms may act together as transmitters of force through the hands, for example, in lifting the body from sitting to standing.

4. The hand and protection

The nervous system of the skin and subcutaneous tissues play an important part in protecting the hand against trauma, such as burns or lacerations. The hand in full supination may act to protect the face against an approaching object or in fisted form, to fight back.

5. The hand and gestures

(i) The hand as an accompaniment to speech

The spoken word makes up only a part of human communication. It may be balanced or enhanced by movement of the hands and even the whole arm, which act closely with the eyes and facial movement. The whole body may give emphasis to their action.

Quintillean AD 80[17] describes the use of the hands so–'other portions of the body merely help the speaker, whereas the hands may almost be said to speak. Do we not use them to demand, promise, summon, dismiss, threaten, supplicate, express aversion or fear, question or deny? Do we not use them to indicate joy, sorrow, hesitation, confession, penitence, measure, quantity, number and time? Have they not the power to excite and prohibit, to express approval, wonder or shame? Do they not take the place of adverbs and pronouns when we point at places and things? In fact, though the people and nations of the earth speak in a multitude of tongues, they share in common the universal language of the hands.'

In daily life the hands are exposed constantly and so are free to move. Thus they provide a rich silent language capable of communicating ideas, emotions and attitudes both unconsciously and consciously. They are a means of expression which supplement and emphasise the spoken word by their gestures and even by their stillness.

Each person has his own repertoire of gestures which is gradually built up and which involves conscious and subconscious patterns of movement. Most can be considered as a spontaneous response, a reflection of the individual's attitudes, feelings and emotions. The gestures may indicate joy, sorrow, anger or even the physical state of the person, for example, the hand pointing to an area of pain.

Each gesture forms a pattern in space – a picture in the air – a physical expression of a

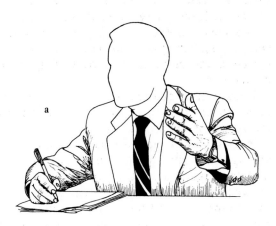

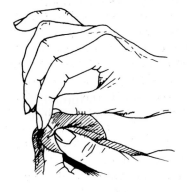

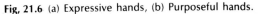

Fig, 21.6 (a) Expressive hands, (b) Purposeful hands.

mental concept. It carries a message to the receiver even though it may be delivered and received subconsciously (Fig. 21.6).

(ii) Conscious gestures of the hand used as either accompaniment to speech or without speech

These are consciously learned gestures used, for example:

a. By actors in a conscious effort to emphasise, supplement and illustrate speech
  and
b. Without speech, for example, the coded language of the deaf and dumb.

THE PATIENT WITH A DISABLED HAND

Many people experience hand disabilities either through trauma to bone, muscle, nerve, blood vessels, skin and other soft tissues, a combination of some of these or through a neurological or systemic disease such as cerebrovascular accident or rheumatoid arthritis (Fig. 21.7). The prognosis in the case of the heavily handicapped person is often unpredictable, particularly in those with a crippling or long-term disease. Much will depend on the patient and his urge for independence or to do a particular task. Even a minor injury may prove to have a serious effect on the patient, particularly if his work is skilled and the injury is to his dominant hand.

The finer the hand control needed, the more difficult rehabilitation may become because of the structural complexity of the hand, the number of joints and muscles involved and the versatility of movement necessary for daily life.

Many patients with a hand disability can become emotionally disturbed. They fear the extent of the disability, in both the short and the long term.

THE REGAINING OF HAND FUNCTION

Exercise therapy, together with advice, plays

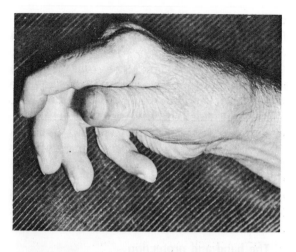

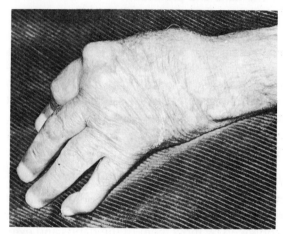

Fig. 21.7 The rheumatoid hand.

an important part in regaining the function of the hand. It is based on a careful examination of the patient's disability and needs. It will be used in conjunction with other essential measures to prevent and reduce oedema and pain which are the enemies of movement. All the functions discussed earlier in the chapter should be incorporated into the treatment if they are needed. The more relevant and varied the exercise treatment, the more versatile hand function should become.

The examination

In reading the patient's medical history, the nature of the disability and an adequate and detailed knowledge of treatment procedures, completed or anticipated, must be gained. Any precautions set out must be strictly observed by both the physiotherapist and the patient so that early healing with minimal scarring can be achieved and no harm done. This rule is particularly important following tendon or nerve repair or an injury such as a burn.

A careful and detailed assessment is necessary; it follows the format described in Chapter 13. Both hands and arms are examined and compared. In particular, tests of function related to the lifestyle of the patient are examined. Only in this way can the physiotherapist gain a clear knowledge of the problems and abilities of the patient.

Preventive measures

Exercise therapy will be made easier and more effective and some secondary disabilities may be prevented if the patient is knowledgeable about his condition, if he knows what to do to help himself, what to avoid and the important part he plays in his treatment. The relief of pain and prevention of oedema, particularly of the small joints of the fingers, is of major importance (Fig. 15.1). Instructions in early care of the hand will be given by both the doctor and the physiotherapist. The whole arm is considered.

Suitable positions and simple exercises are taught which can be practiced without trauma by the patient. For example, a patient with a Colles fracture of the wrist should exercise his fingers regularly during the day and take his arm out of the sling to exercise his shoulder and elbow. Once out of the sling the patient should move his arm freely in all directions. This will prevent the restriction of movement and the pain and oedema which can occur following this injury.

The patient with a nerve injury is warned of the dangers of burns and trauma particularly to the insensitive area of the hand. The patient with rheumatoid arthritis is shown positions of advantage and those to avoid which may lead to excessive trauma or to deformity.

The regaining of function

The most satisfactory position for early treatment of a patient with a hand disability is with the patient sitting with his hands resting comfortably on a treatment table. His head, neck and shoulders should be relaxed and positioned so that the essential co-ordination between the rotation of head, neck, shoulder and forearm with the hand is made possible. He should watch the movement. This essential eye–hand co-ordination should be trained throughout treatment. It is a natural feature of good movement.

In the early stages of treatment, active movement and the encouragement of light functional activities are the methods of choice. If this is not possible, assisted active movements will be necessary. Other physiotherapy methods to reduce pain and oedema may be essential features of treatment at this stage.

Movements of individual fingers and active or assisted movements of the finger joints should be started as soon as possible as these joints stiffen quickly, particularly if oedema is present. Pain-free active stretch of the hand is used when possible.

In re-educating the gripping movements of the hand, support and direction should be provided when giving assistance to movement, as sensory input often has been reduced by damage and/or inactivity.

For example, on attempting to re-educate the gripping action of the hand, the wrist must be stabilised in a position of advantage for the metacarpophalangeal joints and the finger flexors, that is, in 30°–40° of extension and 10°–15° of ulnar deviation. This is done, if possible, by the patient; if not, by the therapist. The direction of the movement of gripping is carefully patterned so that normal joint movement, the line of muscle pull and the arches of the hand are preserved. The patient's finger movements are directed downwards for the index finger and downwards and obliquely for the three ulnar fingers. The stabilisation given on the palm by the therapist is proximal to the metacarpophalangeal joints and obliquely placed to follow 'the gutter' of the palm. A light directional stimulus by the physiotherapist is placed on the flexor surface of the patient's finger tips and the instruction is given to press on and squeeze the physiotherapist's fingers as she guides the finger movement towards the palm.

Particular attention should be paid to preserve the mobility of the metacarpophalangeal joints so that efficient finger movements are encouraged. The maintenance of or the gaining of the width of the palm and of the webs between the fingers and that between the index and thumb are important so that the hand maintains its ability to change its shape, cup, flatten and widen. It is also important that the strength and mobility of the thumb and little finger are preserved.

Massage is particularly useful at an early stage. Apart from its useful soothing effect, it has a mobilising effect on the soft tissues of the hand, particularly of the palm, and by its changing light and deep pressures, helps to bring about a greater awareness of the part and so aids movement. It may also help to desensitise sensitive areas as well as ones disadvantaged by lack of use. Skin care and the mobilisation of any scar are important procedures. The use of massage with a suitable lubricant will help improve the skin condition and, as well, may loosen the adhesions caused by the scar and help improve the cosmetic appearance of the hand.

Bilateral movement provides a strong stimulus both in setting a pattern and in strengthening the hand. Cross-education can occur. Normally the dominant hand is the stronger of the two. Both are stronger when working together. Symmetrical and asymmetrical work can be attempted.

Early resisted exercises to strengthen the muscles are given manually at first by the physiotherapist who can direct and govern the movement in any part of the range. When the pattern of movement is correct a soft ball of a suitable size can be carried by the patient and used often and regularly. Elastic bands, hand grips and the use of a dynamometer to increase strength and soft blocks to stretch the web between the fingers, are often useful. Bouncing putty, if used imaginatively, can provide great versatility of movement and increase strength as it is stretched, compressed, flattened and moulded into various shapes and sizes.

Both prehensile and non-prehensile movements should be practised to add versatility. Gripping is a necessary action for all patients. Skilled individual finger movements are particularly useful for pianists and typists. All functions including expressive gestures must be encouraged.

Exercise opportunities can be devised for most patients so that the muscles are used in their varied functions and combinations and the versatility inherent in the hand is developed. Varying degrees of strength, mobility, precision, dexterity and co-ordination as well as effective stabilisation are needed, with the emphasis changing according to the patient's wants. As soon as possible known functional activities in such areas as personal hygiene, work and recreation are introduced.

Release of the fingers is a difficulty for some patients with neurological problems and efforts to gain relaxation of the flexors and active extension will be favourably influenced by the position of the patient's total body, especially the head, neck, shoulder girdle, shoulder and elbow.

A constant watch by the therapist is essential to ensure that the patient is using his affected hand as normally as possible and not nursing it and that bilateral movements are achieved.

Much of the success of treatment will depend on the patient's interest and desire to use his hand as much as possible and for him to devise useful and interesting opportunities for its use. The use of a known skill may prove helpful. The therapist's imaginative use of various objects and interesting planning, and her consideration, warmth and interest will help towards this end.

Pain following treatment should not occur though sometimes some discomfort during treatment may occur. With skill and judgment by the physiotherapist this should be minimal and short lived. If it continues for more than one hour, too much has been done and movement may be handicapped in the short or long term.[9]

The retraining of sensory function

Just as movement can be aided by retraining, so to a certain extent can sensory function. In the early stages of treatment, sensation may be dull because of immobilisation, oedema, pain, lack of movement and altered soft tissue and skin condition. This usually corrects itself quickly and automatically as movement improves.

A patient with a recovering nerve lesion, in which sensation is returning though still poor, may gain by sensory training. The patient needs to work with his eyes opened and then closed. At first objects are placed in his hand that are relatively easy to recognise. Training progresses to objects of different shapes, textures and temperatures and the patient is asked to recognise and/or describe objects that he cannot see. In addition, joint position, light and deep pressure and the localisation of touch need to be re-educated. The brain will gradually respond more efficiently to limited sensory function as learning takes place and with it movement will improve.

Home practice

Regular and conscientious home practice is essential for recovery. It should be started as soon as possible and a programme set up which emphasises the everyday activities needed in daily living or for a specific purpose. It should be of interest to the patient and checked and changed regularly. Practice leading to versatility of action is usually no problem for a motivated housewife whose duties are diverse. For others, movements such as those used at work are helpful, if possible. Known hobbies, particularly those involving bilateral movements, are most useful for all patients. For example, one patient may gain a wide variety of movements

playing card games, another in attempting to play the piano. Others may enjoy activities such as gardening or carpentry if the condition of the hand allows them.

Passive movements and stretching

Passive movements are necessary to maintain joint range and full muscle length when active or assisted movements are not possible. They should be given with great care so that the correct line of movement is preserved. Observation of the line of movement in the patient's normal hand will illustrate the degree and line the passive movements should take. They should not cause pain which persists when the stretch is released, although some discomfort may sometimes be felt during stretch. The joints proximal to that being passively moved must be stabilised in such a position that the passive movement can be adequately localised and directionally accurate.

Trauma from inadvisable and poorly given passive movements can cause joint damage with subsequent inflammation, oedema and pain. The use of stimuli, correctly applied to the moving surface, will often encourage a joint movement that is impossible without it. The linking together by a comfortable band of a mobile finger to the one next to it that has a restriction of movement, is often useful in encouraging movement in a correct pattern. The patient is in control of this movement.

When a contracture is present the use of traction splinting to maintain and increase range and encourage movement or slow stretching by daily applied serial plasters or a splint may prove helpful. Active movements, if possible, should follow to hold the degree of stretch gained by the stretching process.

The recording and reporting of progress

Regular records of range, strength and of essential functional activities achieved, should be kept. Photographic records of hand positions are useful, particularly for long-term patients such as those with rheumatoid arthritis (Fig. 21.7).

REFERENCES AND FURTHER READING

1. Backhouse, K. M. (1968) Functional anatomy of the hand. *Physiotherapy*, Vol. 54, pp. 114–117.
2. Basmajian, J. V. & De Luca, C. J. (1985) *Muscles Alive,* 5th edn. Baltimore: Williams & Wilkins.
3. Beasley, R. W. (1981) *Hand Injuries*. Philadelphia: W. B. Saunders.
4. Bendz, P. (1974) Systematization of the grip of the hand in relation to finger motor systems. *Scandinavian Journal of Rehabilitation Medicine*, Vol. 6, pp. 158–165.
5. Bendz, P. (1980) The motor balance of the fingers of the open hand. *Scandinavian Journal of Rehabilitation Medicine*, Vol. 12, pp. 115–121.
6. Bendz, P. (1980) Motor balance in formation and release of the extension grip. *Scandinavian Journal of Rehabilitation Medicine*, Vol. 12, pp. 155–160.
7. Cone, J. C. P. & Hueston, J. T. (1981) Psychological aspects of hand injury. In *The Hand, Vol. 1,* Tubiana, R. (Ed.). Philadelphia: W. B. Saunders.
8. Flatt, A. E. (1972) *The Care of Minor Hand Injuries*, 3rd edn. St Louis: C. V. Mosby.
9. Flatt, A. E. (1974) *The Care of the Rheumatoid Hand*, 3rd edn. St Louis: C. V. Mosby.
10. Gordon, G. (Ed.) (1978) *Active Touch – the Mechanism of Recognition of Objects by Manipulation: a multi-disciplinary approach.* Oxford: Pergamon Press.
11. Hunter, J. M., Schneider, L. H., Mackin, E. J. & Callahan, A. D. (1984) *Rehabilitation of the Hand*, 2nd edn. St Louis: C. V. Mosby.
12. Kapandji, I. A. (1982) *The Physiology of the Joints, Volume 1 — Upper Limb*, 5th edn. Edinburgh: Churchill Livingstone.
13. Long, C. (1968) Intrinsic–extrinsic muscle control of the fingers. *The Journal of Bone and Joint Surgery,* Vol. 50A, pp. 973–976.
14. Long, C., Conrad, P. W., Hall, E. A. & Furler, S. L. (1970) Intrinsic–extrinsic muscle control of the hand in power grip and precision handling. *The Journal of Bone and Joint Surgery*, Vol. 52A, pp. 853–867.
15. Napier, J. R. (1956) The prehensile movements of the human hand. *The Journal of Bone and Joint Surgery*, Vol. 38B, pp. 902–913.
16. Perry, J. (1978) Normal upper extremity kinesiology. *Physical Therapy*, Vol. 58, pp. 265–278.
17. Quintillian, M. F. (AD 80) Institutio Oratoria XI, 33, pp. 85–87. In *Loeb Classical Library*, Butler, H. E. (Tr.) Vol. 4, p. 289.
18. Rank, B. K., Wakefield, A. R. & Hueston, J. T. (1968) *Surgery of Repair as applied in Hand Injuries*. Edinburgh: E. & S. Livingstone.
19. Sunderland, S. (1944) The significance of hypothenar elevation in movements of opposition of the thumb. *Australian & New Zealand Journal of Surgery*, Vol. XIII, pp. 155–156.
20. Sunderland, S. (1944) Voluntary movements and the deceptive action of muscles in peripheral nerve lesions. *Australian & New Zealand Journal of Surgery*, Vol. XIII, pp. 160–182.
21. Tubiana, R. (1981) Architecture and functions of the hand. In *The Hand, Vol. 1*, Tubiana, R. (Ed.). Philadelphia: W. B. Saunders.
22. Williams, P. L. & Warwick, R. (1980) *Gray's Anatomy*, 36th edn. Edinburgh: Churchill Livingstone.
23. Wood Jones, F. (1941) *The principles of anatomy as seen in the hand*. London: Baillière, Tindall and Co.
24. Wynn Parry, C. B. (1981) *Rehabilitation of the Hand*, 4th edn. London: Butterworths.

22

The function of the lower extremity with particular reference to gait

The term gait means the manner of walking; locomotion means the act of moving from place to place. Walking incorporates both concepts.

The lower limbs are essentially weight-bearing structures whose major function is to maintain stability and balance, support the body weight, propel the body forward and provide the essential movements necessary for locomotion. They also carry out a wide range of activities which involve shortening, lengthening or extending the reach of the body. They take part in the many activities of work and play, for example, in crouching, running, jumping, kneeling, kicking and pedalling to name just a few.

Walking and its modifications such as running are an essential part of our daily life. Walking is a smooth, highly co-ordinated rhythmical, undulating, reciprocal movement by which the body moves step by step in the required direction at the necessary speed. It is usually done with a purpose, to reach a certain place at a certain time or it can be done for the sheer pleasure of the activity itself. One of the chief attributes of normal gait is the wide range of safe and comparatively comfortable walking speeds available. Speed is variable as a person hurries, hesitates, stops or starts.

Walking is a learned process. The infant

struggles to gain balance and take a few uncertain steps. It is some years before the activity takes on a mature form. The adult walks almost automatically. Each person walks in an uniquely personal manner, one that in many cases is easily identified.

All gaits have certain common characteristics. The lower extremities provide the major action in walking with additional involvement of the head, trunk and arms. There is a two-sided interaction of the body.

The movement of walking is a highly co-ordinated series of events in which balance is being constantly challenged and regained continuously. This action is controlled by the central nervous system with postural reflex activity playing an important part. The major afferent stimuli are provided by tactile impulses from the sole of the foot and proprioceptive impulses from the lower limbs, trunk and neck.

The essentials necessary for normal walking are that:

1. The body can stand upright and bear weight evenly on both lower limbs
2. The body can alternately maintain weight on one limb while bringing the other forward
3. The movements necessary for walking, including those of the trunk and arms, are present and can be co-ordinated.

In walking, each lower limb goes through a stance and swing phase. A step consists of the activity occurring between the heel contact of one extremity and the subsequent

STANCE PHASE

heel-strike   mid-stance   push-off

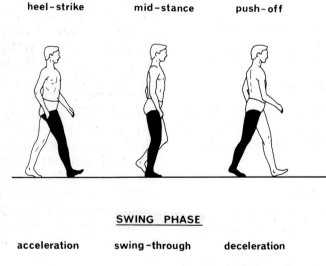

SWING PHASE

acceleration   swing-through   deceleration

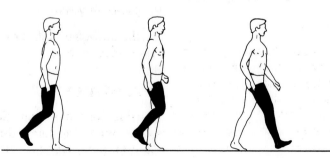

Fig. 22.1 The gait cycle.

heel contact of the other extremity (Fig.22.1).

A *gait cycle* consists of a step each by the right and left lower limbs: that is through both the stance and the swing phases and a return to their original relationship at the beginning of the cycle.

The relative duration of the two phases depends on the speed of the walk. In normal walking approximately 50–60 steps are taken per minute. The stance phase constitutes 60 per cent of the cycle and the swing phase 40 per cent.[1,24] These two periods overlap, so that both feet are on the ground together – a period of double support – for about 25 per cent of the cycle. Figure 22.1 also illustrates the interaction of the stance and swing phases of a single forward step.

There are six major determinants related to the hip, knee and ankle function during walking. These are:

1. Pelvic rotation
2. Pelvic tilt
3. Knee motion during the support phase
4. Foot and ankle motion
5. Knee motion during the swing phase and
6. Lateral motion of the pelvis.[1,26]

Throughout the movement of walking, the head and trunk are held erect and there are co-ordinated movements of the trunk and arms.

The stance or support phase

This phase provides the stability of the gait and is necesary if an accurate swing phase is to take place.

It can be divided into the following stages.

1. Heel-strike

This is a position of double support with the heel of the leading stance foot and the toes of the following foot both on the ground.

On the stance (leading) limb, the hip is flexed to approximately 30°–35°, the knee is extended with the foot at a right angle to the leg and the heel in contact with the floor. The body weight is behind the forward leg.

2. Mid-stance – foot flat on the floor

The body is carried forward over the standing limb with the hip extending and the foot gradually placed firmly on the floor. The knee is in slight flexion when walking on level ground. This is a stable position.

3. Push-off

The heel is raised and as the body moves forward over the stance limb, the hip is hyper-extended and in internal rotation and adduction. The knee is extended. This is the end of the stance phase and the beginning of the swing phase.

The swing phase

1. Acceleration

On the swinging limb the heel rises still further and there is strong contact between the toes particularly the big toe and the ground, to propel the body forward. Forward momentum is provided by ground reaction to the push-off action. The hip flexes and moves into external rotation. This rotation is carried down to the knee and foot. The pelvis rotates forward 6°–8° on the hip of the supporting limb at the time of toe-off. This is necessary to effectively lengthen the limb and so allow a forward step to be taken in the direction of the movement. The pelvis also drops approximately 5° as weight is taken on the opposite stance limb. Flexion of the hip and knee are necessary for the swinging limb to clear the ground as it moves forward.

2. Swing through

As the swinging limb moves forward it passes the stance limb.

3. Deceleration

The hip becomes more flexed and the knee is extended. The foot is in a neutral position. As the heel touches the ground the foot gradually moves into plantar flexion by the controlling action of the dorsiflexors. The whole momentum slows down as the limb moves into the stance phase again. Thus all movements of the lower limb function smoothly together in a finely coordinated movement to achieve a step.

The muscle activity of the lower limb in walking

The muscle activity at the hip, knee and ankle is summarised by Perry (1974) in Figures 22.2, 22.3 and 22.4.

The dense shading indicates concentric or shortening muscle action; the light shading eccentric or lengthening muscle action.

The hip

In the stance phase, following heel strike, the gluteus maximus and the hamstrings contract concentrically to extend the hip. The hip continues to extend past the midstance position. The extent of this extension is regulated by eccentric action of the hip flexors.

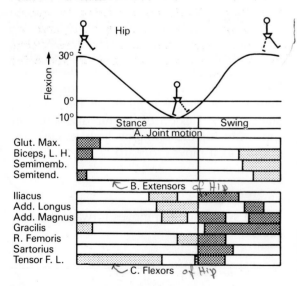

Fig. 22.2 Hip action. A. Range of hip motion during gait cycle. B. Hip extensor activity. C. Hip flexor activity. *Reproduced with kind permission from Perry, J. (1974) Kinesiology of Lower Extremity Bracing. Clinical Orthopaedics and Related Research, Vol. 102, p. 24.*

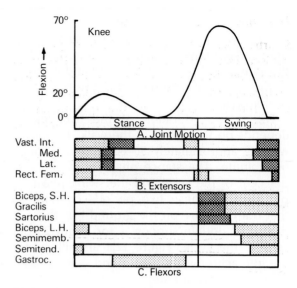

Fig. 22.3 Knee action. A. Range of knee motion during gait cycle. B. Quadriceps activity. C. Knee flexor activity. *Reproduced with kind permission from Perry, J. (1974) Kinesiology of Lower Extremity Bracing. Clinical Orthopaedics and Related Research, Vol. 102, p. 25.*

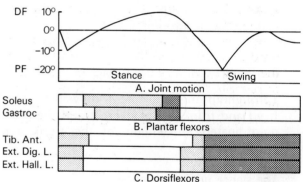

Fig. 22.4 Ankle action. A. Range of ankle motion during gait cycle. B. Plantar flexor activity. C. Dorsiflexor activity. *Reproduced with kind permission from Perry, J. (1974) Kinesiology of Lower Extremity Bracing. Clinical Orthopaedics and Related Research, Vol. 102, p. 26.*

Tensor fascia lata serves as a hip abductor through most of the stance phase thereby contributing to lateral stability.

In the early swing phase, the hip flexors act strongly and concentrically to flex the hip and so carry the limb forward. In the later part of the swing phase the hip extensors, gluteus maximus and the hamstrings, act eccentrically to decelerate this action of hip flexion.

The knee

Shortly after heel strike, there is some knee flexion. The rate and degree of this flexion is controlled by the eccentric activity of the quadriceps muscle. This is followed soon after by concentric activity of the quadriceps to extend the knee. Quadriceps activity then falls off as mid-stance is approached.

During the early swing phase, active knee flexion is necessary to lift the leg to allow for sufficient foot clearance. At mid-swing this is now not necessary and the knee extends with a pendular type action, momentum carrying the leg forward. Knee extension is restrained during deceleration by eccentric hamstring activity.

The ankle

The dorsiflexors are active at heel strike and immediately afterwards, working eccentrically to control the lowering of the foot to the ground. Dorsiflexor activity falls off as the foot is fully placed on the ground.

At mid-stance, as the body is moved forward over the supporting surface of the foot, the plantar flexors work strongly eccentrically to restrain the forward movement of the tibia on the foot.

Once the toes leave the ground the dorsiflexors become active, holding the ankle in mid-position. This activity continues throughout the swing phase.

The action of the trunk, shoulder girdle and arm

In normal walking as the pelvis rotates forward it causes a rotation of the lower trunk. The upper trunk, shoulder girdle and arm rotate forward in a compensatory movement in the opposite direction to the forward movement of the pelvis. This action keeps the body facing forward without movement of the head occurring. Reciprocal movements of the upper and lower limbs occur – the right upper limb swings forward with the left lower limb and vice versa.

The displacement of the centre of gravity

In order that walking should be economically performed the centre of gravity must be kept as near to the mid-line and the level of the second sacral vertebra as possible.

As the body moves forward a 'bobbing' movement occurs with the body undergoing a vertical displacement at each step. There is also a lateral displacement of the body at each step as the weight is moved from one limb to the other. The two displacements are approximately equal and the centre of gravity traces a sinusoidal curve in both directions; the longer the step the greater the displacement. In normal gait the average displacement would cover approximately a 5 cm (2 inch) square.

The line of the walk

The average person usually walks with about 7.5 cm (3 inches) between each foot. The direction of the steps and the inner borders of the feet should deviate as little as possible from the straight line, Fig. 22.5. In this way the movement will be as economical as possible. If the base is widened, a swaying movement will occur which is uneconomical and unattractive. There may be in-toeing or out-toeing. An elderly person usually uses an out-toeing gait.

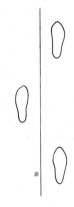

Fig. 22.5 The line of the walk.

The speed of walking

Speed can be increased or slowed. It can be increased by:

1. Lengthening the step
2. Increasing the pace
3. Lengthening the distance covered in the same time
4. Decreasing the time in which the same distance is covered.

With speed, the body tends to come forward at the ankle; the pelvis, trunk and arm movements are all increased and the arms tend to flex at the elbow. The feet tend to become parallel to the line of the walk and face directly forward. More force is exerted and the muscle work of walking is greatly increased. This is energy consuming.

The economy of movement

Provided that the various systems of the body involved in movement are normal, the economy of movement will depend on factors such as posture and balance, the position of the centre of gravity, the accuracy of the pattern of walking and its rhythm and the general lack of tension. It may be influenced to some degree by footwear.

Running

In running, the movement is quickened and the stride is lengthened. The period of double support is eliminated and there is a period of no support between the time the back foot exerts its force and is lifted from the ground, to the time the forward foot strikes the ground. The force of the push-off is greater and the runner lands usually on the ball of his foot. The body remains upright although the line of gravity falls outside the base. The movement of the upper limbs with elbows flexed is quickened and co-ordinated with the lower limb movements, helping to propel the body forward.

Walking backwards

This is an activity that many old people and patients find difficult, yet it is necessary for all people to do, for example, in opening the door towards one. Short steps with the head and body held erect are necessary in order that balance is maintained, otherwise the person becomes vulnerable to falling.

Walking up and down an incline[4]

When walking up an incline, the body must adjust and lean forward at the ankles in order to keep the body balanced over the feet. If the person bends forward from the waist extra muscular effort is necessary, back strain may occur and the action is unsightly. In walking down an incline the body must lean backwards at the ankle.

Walking up and down stairs[4]

Steps of stairs will vary in width, height or breadth; they may have a hand rail on one or both sides or none at all. The usual height of a step is 10–15 cm (4–6 inches) though the bottom step is often higher.

In ascending stairs, the supporting or back leg takes the weight of the body thereby contributing to lifting of the pelvis on the side of the moving or forward leg. The body is held in alignment leaning forward at the supporting ankle, so the centre of gravity is moved forward. The moving or front leg is lifted high with flexion at the hip and knee joints and dorsiflexion at the ankle joint, and the whole foot, when possible, is placed on the step above.

The back leg then becomes the moving leg and moves past onto the step beyond. The movement of the two lower limbs is co-ordinated so the back one starts to rise and move forwards as the front one straightens.

In descending the stairs, the body weight is held back over the supporting leg to avoid the body falling forward. The moving leg is lowered towards the step below as the back leg slowly flexes and the heel rises to allow the moving leg to reach the step below.

A hand rail is usually used by the disabled or elderly to ensure safety.

The energy used in stair climbing is greater than in walking up an incline and in ascending stairs greater than in descending them.

ABNORMAL GAIT

The correction of gait is one of the most frequent exercise treatments given by the physiotherapist. The most common disabilities involving an alteration in the normal pattern of walking are those of musculoskeletal or neurological origin. The abnormality of gait may vary from a slight disorder of one joint to gross inco-ordination of movement. A limp and/or pain may be present. If the abnormal gait is allowed to persist, further trauma will occur to the affected limb. Excessive stress will be placed on the unaffected limb and, in time, postural deviation of the trunk may occur.

The assessment of gait

The assessment of gait includes a careful examination of gait patterns, certain weight bearing tests and tests of muscle strength and endurance, joint range and muscle length, balance, co-ordination and sensation when relevant. If pain is present, its cause, extent, severity and what increases or decreases it must be investigated.

All tests are carried out with the patient suitably clad so that the body alignment can be clearly seen. Standing and walking are done with shoes on and off. The feet are examined for flexibility and strength, particularly of the intrinsic muscles. Painful pressure areas, corns or any other abnormality which could handicap the gait are noted and treated when possible. Shoes are also examined for their suitability and 'tell-tale' signs of abnormal wear.

It is essential to identify the prime cause of the gait problems and the secondary effects it has on the gait and the life style of the patient.

Observation of the gait problem is difficult because of the speed of the movement and the complexity of the pattern but a general impression can be gained of the posture and gait pattern.

Following this, systematic observations are made of the joint and muscle actions of the standing and swing phases of the lower limbs together with those of the trunk and upper limbs. The result is subjective but when used in conjunction with the other tests outlined earlier, provides a useful and practical basis for analysis and planning.

If the patient is heavily handicapped and rehabilitation is likely to be long term, methods of recording such as the use of videotapes, serial still photographs, movement notation, force plates and electromyography all help in the analysis of the disability and provide a record of progress. Pain must be eased as soon as possible if satisfactory tests are to be carried out and gait correction made.

The analysis of gait is usually simple if only one joint is involved but it is often difficult if the disability is severe especially if bad habits of walking are already established.

A number of questions need to be asked and answered by the physiotherapist when examining the patient's gait.

1. *The stability and balance of the stance*
   Can the patient:
   a. Stand upright with the body weight evenly distributed between the feet?
   b. Stand upright and bear weight accurately on either foot and lift the opposite limb off the ground without abnormal body sway or excessive dropping of the pelvis on the unsupported side?
   c. Bring the limb forward in a normal manner and transfer weight from one limb to the other without losing balance?

2. *Step ability*

Can the patient maintain:

a. The correct width of the path of movement and direction of steps?

b. The inner border of his feet in a straight line or is there in-toeing or out-toeing?

c. An even stance phase without hurrying off one limb?

d. Consistency of step and the ability to change pace and step suddenly?

and

e. Is the foot flexible and the step versatile enough to accommodate to changing surfaces and to turning?

3. *Gait efficiency*

a. Is the gait safe or is it vulnerable to internal and external forces?

b. Is the gait rhythmical and efficient or laboured and energy consuming?

c. Can the pattern be maintained with changing speed?

d. Can the direction be quickly adjusted to meet the patient's needs and those of the environment?

e. What is the distance walked in a set line? Is this distance adequate to meet his needs or does he tire?

f. Can the patient walk up and down inclines and steps?

g. Does the patient complain of pain on walking and/or increased pain after walking?

4. *The head, trunk and arms*

a. Is the head, trunk and arm pattern normal and can it change with changing circumstances?

b. Is there flexibility and rhythm of movement or is the trunk held rigidly with the arms motionless and reinforcing the immobility?

The six major determinants of gait

Throughout the examination, the presence, efficiency or absence of any or all of the six major determinants of gait is assessed carefully. The interdependence and co-ordination of their actions within the total walking pattern, as well as the interdependence of the pelvis, hip and knee, and knee, ankle and foot – with the knee forming an important linking and supporting structure – is also carefully studied.

THE CORRECTION OF GAIT

In the light of the physiotherapist's knowledge of normal gait and all the factors tested, a total analysis is made of the patient's problems and a progressive exercise programme is set up.

The exercise programme will be geared to provide correction of, or compensation for, the disability. Many patients have disabilities that can be completely corrected. If only one element of the six determinants is affected permanently the total pattern may be able to accommodate to the loss quite quickly, by exaggerating the action of another determinant, as the number of joints taking part in the gait allow for considerable versatility. If more than one determinant is involved, the emphasis in gait training will be on providing the most economical and attractive gait possible.

Attempts at full correction before the necessary elements are present or nearly so, are useless and frustrating to the patient. The patient will become tense with the effort. At this stage the aim should be to provide the best possible gait and improve it gradually as the potential grows.

Strengthening and mobilising exercises together with balance training and the encouragement of rhythmic rotary trunk movements are usually necessary. Movements used when testing the ability to weight bear may become exercises, when necessary, in the programme.

It is essential that the patient gains the knowledge, the image and the feeling of a correct posture and walking pattern. Specific corrections will be made by the physiotherapist to help him to achieve this. At this stage good demonstrations and instructions become most important.

The patient should stand upright looking straight ahead and not down at his feet. The use of a mirror may help him see his faults, correct them and so gain an appreciation of the image and feeling of the correction. Counting or music may help to establish the rhythm so necessary if a normal gait is to be achieved. As the arm movements are automatic, this can often be achieved if emphasis is placed on relaxation of the arms in the walking programme, rather than on the need to swing them.

A treadmill is a very useful piece of equipment in gait training. It gives the patient an incentive to work against an even resistance. The speed of walking can be quickened or slowed. Its use improves weight bearing, step ability, balance and endurance and gives the patient and physiotherapist a measurement of achievement. It is independent work usually enjoyed by the patient.

Walking up inclines and stairs as well as a variety of surfaces will be introduced as soon as possible. A regular record of walking progress is kept.

Safety

The dangers to the patient of slippery surfaces, loose mats, polish on the floor, the wearing of slippers and worn, ill-fitting shoes are stressed. The condition of the ferrules on the walking stick or crutches needs to be watched by both physiotherapist and patient.

Joint reaction

The reaction of the joints to the gait training programme is carefully monitored so that trauma, with pain, does not slow down progress.

Aids to walking

An aid to walking may prove helpful for some patients. The type of aid used depends on the extent of the patient's disability, his general condition and age. Suitable footwear is essential. The aid may be temporary or permanent. Three types will be briefly discussed.

1. Adjustable parallel bars

Parallel bars are a useful aid in the preparation of the patient for any type of walking. The height of the bars should be adjusted so that the patient's elbows, with his hands holding the bars, are in slight flexion. This is the position in which the upper limbs can press down on to the stick or crutches when they are used later. The bars help to take some of the patient's weight and he is more confident as he feels safer and better balanced when taking a step. Stance, balance, transfer of weight and steps are practised. At first the patient is guarded carefully by the physiotherapist. As soon as he can work safely he will use the bars independently. The type of gait used depends on whether the patient is to progress to walking independently or walking with the aid of a stick or crutches.

2. Sticks (canes)[3]

Sticks (canes) are most useful aids. One or two sticks may be used. A stick helps promote safety, reduces stress on a painful weight bearing joint and so lessens pain. It reinforces the available muscle strength by lessening the weight to be carried on one or both lower limbs.

The stick must be of the correct length and have an adequate, preferably suction ferrule. With the patient standing and his hand holding the stick, the elbow should be in a slight degree of flexion.

The stick is usually held in the opposite hand to the weak leg and moves forward with it. Another pattern used can be stick, disabled leg then the other leg. Sometimes it can be held on the same side when the leg is severely disabled where it acts almost like a brace. The pattern in this case is stick and disabled leg moving forward together and then the other leg follows.

3. Crutches

Crutches are usually used by a patient with a disability of one or both lower limbs which makes it difficult for him to balance or inadvisable for him to bear weight on an affected limb and for whom other aids are inadequate. Axillary crutches are most commonly used.

The energy demands of crutch walking, particularly for the heavily handicapped patient are heavy.

Preparation for crutch walking includes:

1. A test of muscle strength and joint range
2. An exercise programme to develop strength in the muscle groups necessary for crutch walking
3. Instruction in how to stand and balance on the crutches before taking a step
4. Teaching the type of gait to be used.

The measurement of crutches

The length of the crutches and the height of the hand-pieces are the important factors in measuring a patient for crutches. The measurement is best done, when possible, with the patient with shoes on, standing in bars or against a wall. Shoulder pads and ferrules should be on the crutches. The hand-pieces should be set with the elbows in slight flexion. Adjustable crutches are useful at first for a heavily handicapped patient.

There are many ways of measuring a patient in bed for crutches. The easiest and one of the most useful ways of gaining an estimate of crutch length is for the bed patient to have his shoes on and the physiotherapist to use an adjustable crutch for measuring. Whatever the method, the crutches often need some adjustment when the patient is standing.

The patient practises standing with and moving the crutches before gait training is started. He must be carefully guarded until he becomes adequate in crutch use so that he does not fall. The patient should be advised not to take weight on the axilla because of the risk of radial nerve palsy.

Crutch gait

The five most common crutch gaits are:

1. *Four-point alternate crutch gait*
   Crutch-leg sequence:
   a. Right crutch
   b. Left leg
   c. Left crutch
   d. Right leg.

This is a safe but slow gait as there are always three points of support on the floor. It is a useful gait to use in crowds or in a limited space.

2. *Two-point alternate crutch gait*
   Crutch-leg sequence:
   a. Right crutch and left leg together
   b. Left crutch and right leg together.

This is a speeding up of the four point gait and demands greater balance.

3. *Three-point crutch gait*
   Crutch-leg sequence:
   a. Both crutches and the weaker leg
   b. The stronger leg.

Both crutches and the weaker leg are moved forward while the stronger leg maintains balance. It is usually used when one lower extremity is unable to take any weight or only partial weight.

4. *Swing-to crutch gait*
   Crutch-body sequence:
   a. Both crutches are lifted and placed on the ground in front of the body
   b. The body swings forwards to the crutches.

5. *Swing-through crutch gait*
   Crutch-body sequence:
   a. Both crutches are lifted and placed on the ground in front of the body
   b. The body swings through past the crutches so the feet are ahead of the crutches.

Walking forwards and sideways, stepping backwards, turning, and if possible walking up and down inclines and using steps are prac-tised, as they are necessary activities of daily life.

The manner in which the patient copes with stairs will depend on his disability, the degree of bracing or the type of lower limb prosthesis prescribed.

When possible a hand rail is used. In going upstairs the unaffected leg leads and then the other leg moves up to it. The affected leg leads in descending the stairs.

Stair climbing for the heavily handicapped patient is discussed in considerable detail by Deaver and Brown,[8] Buchwald[6] and Bromley.[5]

A set of graded training steps with hand rails and with the step heights varying from 5 cm, 10 cm, 15 cm (2–4–6 inches), is most useful in a physiotherapy department.

REFERENCES AND FURTHER READING

1. Anderson, M. H., Bechtol, C. O. & Sollars, R. E. (1959) *Clinical Prosthetics for Physicians and Therapists.* Springfield: Charles C. Thomas.
2. Basmajian, J. V. & De Luca, C. J. (1985) *Muscles Alive,* 5th edn. Baltimore: Williams & Wilkins.
3. Blount, W. P. (1956) Don't throw away the cane. *The Journal of Bone and Joint Surgery,* Vol. 38A, pp. 695–708.
4. Broer, M. R. & Zernicke, R. F. (1979) *Efficiency of Human Movement,* 4th edn. Philadephia: W. B. Saunders.
5. Bromley, I. (1981) *Tetraplegia and Paraplegia,* 2nd edn. Edinburgh: Churchill Livingstone.
6. Buchwald, E. (1952) *Physical Rehabilitation for Daily Living.* New York: McGraw-Hill.
7. Carlsöö, S. (1972) *How Man Moves.* London: William Heinemann.
8. Deaver, G. G. & Brown, M. E. (1945) *The Challenge of Crutches.* Studies in Rehabilitation, No. 2, New York, Institute for the Crippled and Disabled Print Shop.
9. Ducroquet, R. J. et P. (1965) *La Marche et les Boiteries.* Paris: Masson et Cie.
10. Grieve, D. W. (1969) The assessment of gait. *Physiotherapy,* Vol. 55, pp. 452–460.
11. Gronley, J. K. & Perry, J. (1984) Gait Analysis Techniques. *Physical Therapy,* Vol. 64, No. 12, pp. 1831–1838.
12. Holt, K. S. (1965) *Assessment of Cerebral Palsy.* London: Lloyd-Luke, Medical.
13. Hughes, J. (1976) Human Locomotion. In *The Advance in Orthotics,* Murdoch, G. (Ed.) pp. 57–73. London: Edward Arnold.
14. Hughes, J. & Jacobs, N. (1979) Normal human locomotion. *Prosthetics and Orthotics International,* Vol. 3, pp. 4–12.
15. Inman, V. T. (1966) Human locomotion. *Canadian Medical Association Journal,* Vol. 94, pp. 1047–1054.
16. Joseph, J. (1964) The activity of some muscles in Locomotion. *Physiotherapy,* Vol. 50, pp. 180–183.
17. Kennedy, P. E. (1964) Locomotion and gait. The physiotherapist's assessment. *Physiotherapy,* Vol. 50, pp. 191–193.
18. Klopsteg, P. E. & Wilson, P. D. (1954) *Human Limbs and Their Substitutes.* New York: McGraw-Hill.
19. Le Veau, B. (1977) *Williams and Lissner – Biomechanics of Human Motion,* 2nd edn. Philadelphia: W. B. Saunders.
20. Morton, D. J. & Fuller, D. D. (1952) *Human Locomotion and Body Form.* Baltimore: Williams and Wilkins.
21. Murray, M. P., Drought, A. B. & Kory, R. C. (1964) Walking patterns of normal men. *The Journal of Bone and Joint Surgery,* Vol. 46A, No. 2, pp. 335–360.
22. Murray, M. P., Kory, R. C., Clarkson, B. A. & Sepic, S. B. (1966) Comparison of free and fast speed walking patterns of normal men. *American Journal of Physical Medicine,* Vol. 45, No. 1, pp. 8–24.
23. Napier, J. (1967) The antiquity of human walking. *Scientific American,* Vol. 216, No. 4, pp. 56–67.
24. Perry, J. (1967) The mechanics of walking. *Physical Therapy,* Vol. 47, pp. 778–801.
25. Perry, J. (1974) Kinesiology of lower extremity bracing. *Clinical Orthopaedics and Related Research,* No. 102, pp. 18–31.
26. Saunders, J. B., Inman, V. T. & Eberhart, H. D. (1953) The major determinants in normal and pathological gait. *The Journal of Bone and Joint Surgery,* Vol. 35A, pp. 543–558.
27. Sutherland, D. H., Olshen, R., Cooper, L., Savio, L. Y. & Woo, S. Y. (1980) The development of mature gait. *The Journal of Bone and Joint Surgery,* Vol. 62A, pp. 336–353.

Appendix 1

Tests and measurements

THE USE OF TESTS

A test, when used in physiotherapy, is a means of assessing the ability of the patient in some form of physical activity or the present potential for movement. There is a need for the use of accurate tests and measurements and their recording in the initial examination and continuing treatment of the patient. They give some objective evidence of the extent and quality of the patient's abilities and disabilities. Only in this way can accurate data be provided rather than dependence being placed on clinical impressions alone.

The purpose of the test, in the main, will be to:

1. Establish and record an initial and continuing record of the patient's abilities and disabilities, his progress, static state or regression
2. Aid in making a diagnosis and establishing a prognosis
3. Help in the analysis of the patient's movement problems
4. Aid in the formulation of a progressive treatment plan
5. Gauge the efficiency of both the overall plan and its worth in specific areas of need
6. Aid in the planning for independence in living and work situations
7. Help motivate the patient.

The tests should be:

1. Carefully selected for the patient, being

relevant, valid, reliable and recognised standardised procedures, where possible
2. Carried out efficiently in a reasonable time
3. Useful to the patient, therapist and team.

The results should be:

1. Clearly recorded, dated, signed and filed
2. Understood and evaluated by the physiotherapist and other team members
3. Used as an aid to planning for present and future needs and goals.

MUSCLE TESTING – MANUAL, ISOMETRIC AND ISOKINETIC

Manual muscle testing

A manual muscle test is a test of the voluntary muscle strength of individual muscles in their function as prime movers.

The test may be used to:

1. Provide an initial and ongoing record of the muscle strength or weakness
2. Aid diagnosis
3. Determine the level and extent of a nerve lesion.

A continuing record will aid prognosis and planning of treatment and for many patients act as a motivator. It is not a satisfactory test for upper motor neuron disability.

Three factors are considered in the assessment of muscle strength. These are the:

1. Ability of the muscle to contract
2. Ability or inability of the muscle to move through range
3. Amount of resistance which can be given to the working muscle.

PHYSIOTHERAPY DEPARTMENT

MUSCLE CHART

0 Zero—no contraction
1 Trace—Flicker
2 Poor—Active movement gravity eliminated
3 Fair— Active movement against gravity
4 Good—Active movement against gravity + some resistance
5 Normal — Normal strength
3-5 Through available joint range

Name: _ _ _ _ _ _ _ _ _ _ _ _ _

Date of Birth: _ _ _ _ _ _ _ _

Ward: _ _ _ _ _   Chart Number: _ _ _ _ _ _ _

LEFT							TRUNK AND LOWER LIMB		RIGHT					
							EXAMINER'S INITIALS:							
							DATE:							
						Neck	Flexors	Sternocleidomastoid						
							Extensor group							
						Trunk	Flexors	Rectus abdominis T_6-T_{12}						
							Rt. ext. obl.	Lt. ext. obl. T_7 – T_{12}						
							Lt. int. obl.	Rt. int. obl. T_7 – L_1						
							Extensors	Thoracic group						
								Lumbar group							
							Pelvic elev.	Quad. lumborum T_1 – L_3						

Fig. A.1 Part of a muscle chart for the trunk and lower limb.

Requirements for testing are:

1. Knowledge of muscle and joint structure, nerve supply and function
2. Knowledge of test procedures and grading
3. The ability to observe, handle and palpate accurately and sensitively
4. The ability to recognise muscle substitution – 'trick' movement.

Grading

The six gradings used will give a record of the muscle state.[1,3]

Zero	Z	O	No contraction
Trace	T	1	Flicker or trace of contraction
Poor	P	2	Active movement through full range with gravity eliminated
Fair	F	3	Active movement through full range against gravity
Good	G	4	Active movement through full range against gravity and some resistance
Normal	N	5	Normal strength.

Figures, letters or words indicate the grade on the chart. Figures are most usually used. If words are used they should accurately describe the grading.

Grade 3 is an objective test – all others are subjective. A grade 5 muscle should be able to carry out all its functions as prime mover, stabiliser, antagonist and so on.

The physiotherapist must judge what is normal for the patient. This may be done by making comparisons with the unaffected side. If both sides are affected, comparisons will need to be made against what would be expected for a person of the same build and occupation.

Although much of this test is subjective, it has proved a valid and useful method when carried out by an experienced and careful physiotherapist.[1]

Preparation for testing

1. The room should be warm, light and quiet and contain a firm examination table which can be approached from both sides.

2. The patient should be:
   a. Given an explanation of the reason for the test and his part in assisting in it
   b. Suitably dressed so that all parts of the body including the unaffected limbs can be seen
   c. Made comfortable in a correctly aligned and well supported position so that, if possible, he can see the test area.
3. The physiotherapist should:
   a. Have previously read the patient's medical history and questioned the patient about his problems
   b. Observe posture, body and limb contours, muscle wasting, as well as any reinforcement posture taken up during testing.

A series of quick unilateral and bilateral tests may prove useful to give the physiotherapist an idea of overall function before the full testing begins.

Test positions

A general rule is that when possible, tests for Grades 0–2 will be made with the supported part moving in a horizontal plane, i.e. with the effect of gravity eliminated. A trace or flicker of movement will be determined by observation and palpation of the muscle tendon and muscle belly. Tests for Grades 3–5 will be made against gravity.

Technique

1. Adequate fixation should be ensured by:
   a. The use of the patient's body weight
   b. His working muscles
   c. Firm manual fixation by the physiotherapist's hand just proximal to the joint being moved.
2. All joints should be tested through their available range either by active movement when possible or by passive movements.
   A movement by the patient against gravity (Grade 3) provides a quick screening test for possible strength or weakness.

3. The resistance may be given through the range of movement by the physiotherapist's hand. It should be smooth, adjustable and its line directly opposite to the line of pull of the muscle tendon. If given in a shortened position, it should be given smoothly as strength is built up.
4. Trick movements (substitution movements) should be eliminated.
5. All possible tests should be carried out in one position before moving the patient to another position.
6. The patient should be given an appreciation of his strength as well as his weakness by working from his strong to his weak muscles and by changing from one test demanding intense concentration to an easier one.
7. The result should be memorised as the test proceeds and recorded during the rest period for the patient.
8. The patient should not be fatigued nor should attempts be made to gain an accurate test in the presence of pain.
9. On completion of the test, the muscle chart should be signed, dated and filed. Regular retesting should be carried out at the appropriate time.
10. The note space at the bottom of most charts can be used to indicate such problems as restrictions in starting positions, loss of range and pain.

Test positions and procedures have been well set out by Daniels and Worthingham[1] and are internationally used. Kendall and McCreary[2] shows excellent photographs of tests and contains much helpful and interesting information.

Isometric (static) strength tests

The strength of an isometric contraction may be recorded using a spring balance or dynamometer. Three maximal contractions will be made at one minute intervals and the mean value taken and recorded. For motivational reasons it is useful if the dial of the dynamometer can be seen by the patient.

Isokinetic testing

Sophisticated equipment is available which measures torque changes throughout range of movement at different speeds of muscle contraction. Such equipment provides objective data related to muscle strength and power.

TESTS OF MUSCLE LENGTH

These important tests are comprehensively described in Kendall and McCreary[8] and Janda.[7]

MEASUREMENT AND RECORDING OF JOINT RANGE

The aim of measuring joint range is to obtain information which can be used to establish:
1. A measurement and recording of active and passive joint range and of painfree and painful arcs of movement within the range
2. A standard of average joint range for persons of varying build, age and sex and so aid in the design, planning and placement of equipment for living and work.

Equipment

The most commonly used equipment is a goniometer. The most usual type consists of a clearly marked protractor numbered 0°–180° in each direction, with two arms of approximately 12–16 inches attached in the centre – one is a stationary arm and the other a moving arm. It is usually made of clear plastic or metal, both of which can be easily cleaned. The type of goniometer used should be standardised throughout the hospital. Types are shown in Figure A.2. A smaller one for the hand is most useful.

Some movements do not lend themselves readily to measurement by a goniometer. Other simple methods can be used to record progress, such as:
1. A tape measure, which can be used to measure the distance between anatomical land-

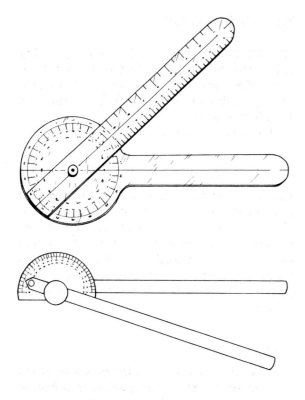

Fig. A.2 Two types of hand held goniometer.

marks and how these alter in relation to each other during movement.

2. Tracings. These are particularly useful for the hand. They are quickly prepared and are visually effective.

Measurement

In articles covering much of the history and literature on joint measurement, Moore[10,11] gives a review of different methods of measuring.

The most useful method of measuring and recording is set out in the booklet '*Joint Measurement*' produced by the American Academy of Orthopaedic Surgeons.[9] Normal range of motion, standard zero positions, methods of measurement and recording of range, together with relevant diagrams are given. This standard has been widely accepted in many countries.

Reliability

Moore states that many tests have been made to prove the reliability of measurement by the goniometer. They have indicated that in the hands of careful operators this is a reliable test instrument.[11,12]

Technique of measurement

1. The procedure and its purpose should be clearly explained to the patient.
2. The relevant parts of the body should be bared.
3. The position of the part being examined should be stable and in the standard position of zero, which is usually the extended position of the limb or as near zero as possible.
4. If pain is present, the starting position may have to be modified and the test given in the most comfortable position possible and with gentle handling.
5. When possible, the motion should be compared with the opposite limb or side.
6. The movement can be active or passive. If possible both are used. Any difference between these movements should be recorded.
7. The movement should be carried out slowly. Both limbs may be used to aid movement, improve stability or to prevent trick movements.
8. The correct placement of the goniometer is important. In practice, it is extremely difficult to find a fixed point through range from which to measure. In many joints the axis of movement alters as the movement proceeds. Moore considers there is no specific landmark which could be accurately called an axis of motion. She suggests that, if the stationary arm of the goniometer is placed parallel to the longitudinal axis of the fixed part of the limb and the moving part of the goniometer parallel to the longitudinal axis of the moving part, then the axis of motion will fall where the two intersect and will automatically localise in the approximately correct

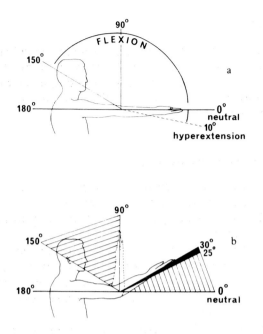

Fig. A.3 A pictorial method of recording joint range and any abnormalities. a. Full range of joint motion of the elbow joint. b. Arc of painfree movement – is from 30°–90°; arc of painful motion 25°–30°. Striped parts of the arc indicate lack of movement in those parts of the range.

position.[11,12] This point cannot be decided until the completion of the movement.

9. The patient should complete the range before measuring commences.
10. The goniometer should be placed along the lateral side of the limb in the appropriate position and should not press on the limb in any way.
11. Several readings need to be taken. The average of these readings should be recorded.
12. Joint range and the range of pain should be clearly recorded (Fig. A.3). The result in numerals, diagrams or both should be signed, dated and filed.
13. Re-testing should be done at regular intervals so that progress, static state or regression can be detected.

More sophisticated testing can be done using an electrogoniometer. This provides a measurement and records of the sequence and extent of joint motion.

TESTS OF SENSATION

The procedures to be used in sensory testing are explained to the patient who should be comfortable and relaxed before testing begins. During testing his eyes should be closed or a blindfold may be used.

The tests are as follows:

Touch and pressure

Loss of sensation to light touch is tested with a wisp of cotton wool stroked lightly over the skin of the area of suspected loss. This should be moved from the area of minimal loss to that of the suspected total loss. Deeper painless touch can be tested with tip of a finger. The patient is asked to say what he feels and where he feels it.

Pain

Pain is tested with the point of a pin gently applied to the skin. The patient is asked to distinguish between the point and head of the pin by reporting whether the sensation felt is sharp or blunt.

Temperature

Temperature appreciation is tested with two test tubes, preferably metal, one filled with hot water and the other with cold, placed against the skin surface. The tubes must be dry on the outside. The patient will be asked to identify whether the temperature is hot or cold. The tests should not follow each other too quickly.

Joint position sense

A test of joint position is given by the physiotherapist passively moving the joint into various positions and then asking the patient to identify the position. The patient may be asked to describe the position or imitate it using the other side of the body. Movement sense may be tested by asking the patient in which direction the movement being used for testing takes place.

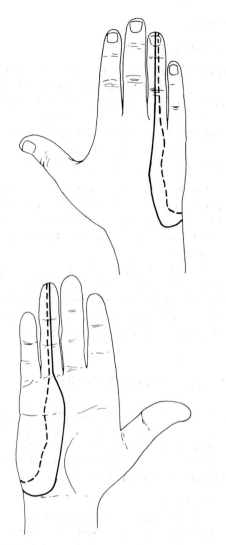

Fig. A.4 Method of recording sensory loss, in this case for an ulnar nerve lesion. The solid line indicates the affected area; the broken line delineates the area of complete sensory loss as compared to partial sensory loss.

Placement of the physiotherapist's own hands is important during this test. For example, in testing the hand, it should be grasped on the radial and ulnar sides when being moved into flexion and extension and not on the back or front of the palm or fingers, as the patient may more readily identify the direction of the movement by cutaneous input.

Stereognosis – a test of handling

A test of the patient's ability to recognise objects by their shape, size and texture is done by placing a familiar object, at first large and later small, in the blindfolded patient's hand and asking him to identify it and/or describe its form. The objects are chosen to suit the age of the patient. The actual handling process by the patient, i.e. whether he moves the object to seek out sensory cues, is carefully watched.

Recording

A record of the location of impairment or loss of the different sensory modalities tested can be made on a diagram of the body part (Fig. A.4). A full report is made of loss of various sensory modalities and location of impairment.

Dermatome chart

A knowledge of the dermatomes helps in testing in many cases (Fig. A.5).

A TEST OF THE ACTIVITIES OF DAILY LIFE

This test forms a vital part of the testing procedures for the heavily handicapped patient. It is primarily a test of the patient's abilities as well as an indication of his disabilities. The purpose of the test is to establish:

1. The level of the patient's functional ability for daily living, together with the accuracy and speed of the performance
2. The functions he is unable to do or performs poorly
3. His needs and motivation to achieve independence in daily living, social and recreational activities
4. His potential for independence
5. A basic plan, with him, for near and far goals
6. A record of the patient's progress, static state or regression

7. Possible future needs for aids or modification of his living and working environment to make living easier and safer
8. To help him think constructively about his abilities and motivate him to move towards independence.

Buchwald Lawton[17,18] was one of the pioneers in the field of functional testing and training for heavily handicapped patients. She outlined the patient's need for independence in daily living, set up a chart and a method of grading as well as methods of training for independence. She based her chart on three areas of need:

1. Self care
2. Ambulation, elevation and travelling
3. Hand activities

and spelt out essential functions in each area. Most charts today follow similar lines although they are usually adapted towards the special needs of particular groups, for example geriatric or quadriplegic patients.

The charts start with listing independence in bed activities and self care and proceed to listing activities involving mobility and special needs. The usual activities listed are:

1. Feeding
   a. Eating
   b. Drinking
2. Hygiene
   a. Toilet and bathing activities; oral hygiene
   b. Grooming – care of the hair and nails; make-up or shaving
   c. Dressing
3. Mobility
   a. Moving in bed, from bed to chair to standing
   b. Walking in and out of doors; use of a wheelchair
   c. Use of transport – car or public transport
4. Miscellaneous
   a. Communication – speech, use of telephone and radio, writing, opening letters, turning pages etc.
   b. Handling – money, switches, opening and closing doors and so on.

Grading

A useful grading is:

Grade 3 – The activity can be performed adequately at a reasonable speed
Grade 2 – The activity can be performed poorly at a slow speed
Grade 1 – The activity can be performed with one or two helpers
Grade 0 – The activity is impossible.

If the activity is not essential for the patient it can be cancelled out on the form. Once the activity can be achieved, the time taken to perform it is an important factor in testing achievements.[19]

This knowledge will help the physiotherapist to plan, with the patient, the most necessary activities that look possible and so provide goals. These goals may be far off but near goals should provide incentive.

THE USE OF A BODY CHART

A body chart is a helpful recording method (Fig. A.6). Its advantage is that it provides an inexpensive, compact visual record.

Some of the observations that can be mapped in this way include:

1. Painful areas
2. Areas of sensory disturbance
3. Damage to the skin – burns, scars, discoloration
4. Sites of abnormal tone
5. Deformity.

TRENDELENBURG, THOMAS', LEG LENGTH TESTS

A test for hip joint stability – the Trendelenburg sign[20,21]

The Trendelenburg test is a common test used to assess the ability of the hip abductors to stabilise the pelvis on the femur.

Normally in standing, each leg bears equal weight. When one leg is lifted, the other takes

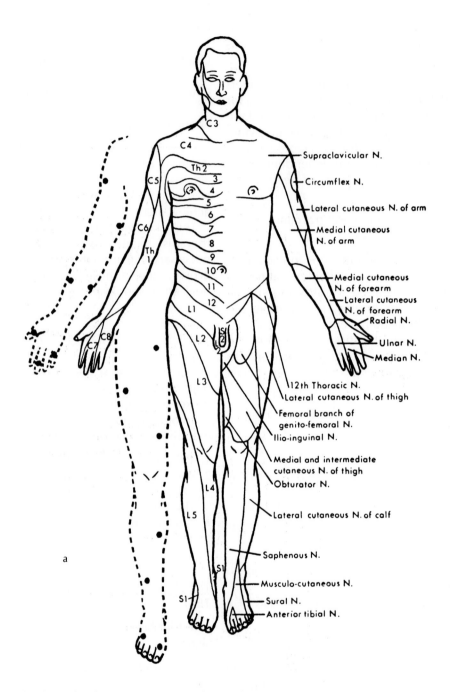

Fig. A.5 Segmental and peripheral nerve innervation and points for testing cutaneous sensation of limbs a. anterior, b. posterior. By applying stimuli at the points marked within the dotted outline, both the dermatomal and main peripheral nerve distribution are covered simultaneously. *Reproduced with kind permission from MacLeod, J. (1979) Clinical Examination, 5th edn. Edinburgh: Churchill Livingstone.*

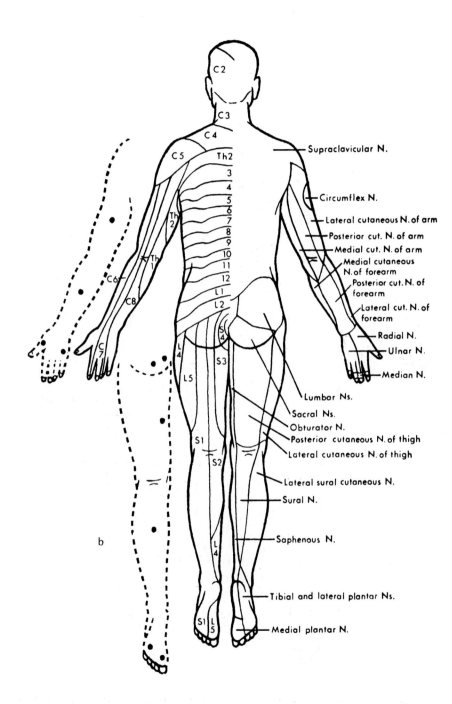

C 2

C 3

C 4

C 5

Th2
3
4
5
6
7
8
9
10
11
12

Th
2

Th
1

C6

C8

L 1
L 2

S
4

L
4

C
7

L 5

S 3

S1

S2

L
4

S1 L
5

Supraclavicular N.

Circumflex N.

Lateral cutaneous N. of arm

Posterior cut. N. of arm

Medial cut. N. of arm

Medial cutaneous
N. of forearm

Posterior cut. N. of
forearm

Lateral cut. N. of
forearm

Radial N.

Ulnar N.

Median N.

Lumbar Ns.

Sacral Ns.

Obturator N.

Posterior cutaneous N. of thigh

Lateral cutaneous N. of thigh

Lateral sural cutaneous N.

Sural N.

Saphenous N.

Tibial and lateral plantar Ns.

Medial plantar N.

b

BODY CHART

Surname :	First Names :	Age:	Date:
Physiotherapist :	Doctor :	Ward or Outpatients Clinic :	

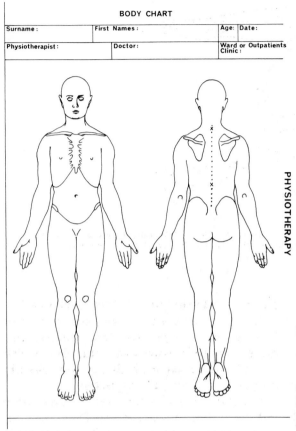

PHYSIOTHERAPY

Fig. A.6 Body chart.

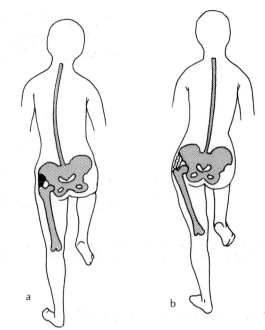

a   b

Fig. A.7 Trendelenburg test. a. Negative, b. Positive.

the full weight; the trunk tends to lean to the side of the supporting leg and the pelvis, through the action of the hip abductors of the supporting leg, rises on the unsupported side (Fig. A.7a).

If there is weakness of the hip abductors when weight is taken on the affected leg, the pelvis drops on the unsupported side. This is known as a positive Trendelenburg sign (Fig. A.7b).

Test for fixed flexion deformity of the hip – Thomas' test[20,21]

The Thomas' test is performed to determine whether there is a fixed flexion deformity of the hip.

When the patient is placed in supine lying, he compensates for his fixed hip flexion deformity by tilting his pelvis forwards so that his lumbar lordosis becomes more exaggerated (Fig. A.8a). This can be felt by the physiotherapist placing her hand between the patient's lumbar spine and the examination couch.

The unaffected hip is then flexed as far as possible thereby tilting the patient's pelvis backwards. This will produce a flattening of the lumbar curve provided there is no fixed lumbar lordosis as well.

As this manoeuvre is being completed, the affected limb, if it has a true fixed hip flexion deformity, will automatically lift from the supporting surface as the lumbar curve is reduced (Fig. A.8b). The angle through which the thigh of the affected side is lifted from the plinth is measured as the angle of the fixed flexion deformity.

Test for actual and apparent leg length[20,21]

In both tests the patient lies in a supine position with the trunk, pelvis and legs in straight alignment.

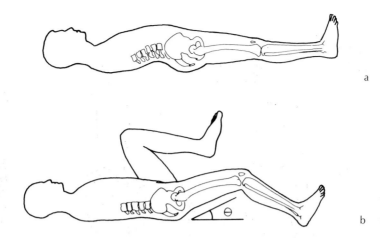

a

b

Fig. A.8 Thomas' test for fixed flexion deformity. In a. the fixed deformity is masked by an increased lumbar curve but becomes apparent when the sound hip is flexed as shown in b. θ is the angle of the fixed flexion deformity.

Measurement of actual leg length

The measurement is made from the anterior superior iliac spine to the medial malleolus.

Measurement of apparent leg length

The measurement is made from a fixed point in the middle of the trunk (such as the xiphisternum) to the medial malleolus.

TESTS OF RESPIRATORY FUNCTION[22]

The peak expiratory flow rate (PEFR) can be used to assess airways obstruction. It is a simple test to perform using a hand held peak flow meter. For this reason it can be readily performed at the bedside or in the patient's home.

The patient is asked to exhale as fast as he can into the mouthpiece attached to the flow meter. Care must be taken that the patient's mouth is firmly moulded around the mouthpiece as a seal, otherwise air can escape before passing through the meter.

It is advisable for the patient to be given a 'practice run' to familiarise him with the equipment and the procedure before readings are made. In some centres, the best of three attempts following the trial run is recorded.

The peak expiratory flow rate in normal healthy adults is 500–650 litres/minute. This measure correlates well with the FEV_1, which is the largest volume which can be expired in one second after a full inspiration.

A vitallograph can be used to give more detailed information than the PEFR. The apparatus used is a spirometer with an electronic recording device.

The patient is asked to inhale deeply and then exhale as much air as he possibly can into the mouthpiece. Care must be taken that the patient's lips are firmly sealed about the mouthpiece. The timing device is set in operation immediately he begins to exhale. Verbal encouragement by the physiotherapist to the patient to give of his best is essential.

Three readings are usually made, with adequate rest periods in between. The best response is the measurement used for further calculations.

Measurements which can be made using this test include:

1. Forced vital capcity (FVC) which is the greatest amount of air that can be expired after a maximal inspiration
2. Forced expiratory volume in one second (FEV_1) – already described.

The ratio of $\frac{FEV_1}{FVC}$ is usually expressed as a percentage. In healthy adults the FEV_1 is at least 80 per cent of the FVC.

Because in some obstructive airways diseases the FEV_1 is markedly reduced, the ratio $\frac{FEV_1}{FVC}$ is also reduced. However, in diseases which lead to rigidity of the chest wall or the lungs themselves, both the FEV_1 and the FVC will be reduced proportionally, so the normal ratio $\frac{FEV_1}{FVC}$ is preserved.

REFERENCES AND FURTHER READING

Manual muscle testing
1. Daniels, L. & Worthingham, C. (1980) *Muscle Testing*, 4th edn. Philadelphia: W. B. Saunders.
2. Kendall, F. P. & McCreary, E. K. (1983) *Muscles – Testing and Function*, 3rd edn. Baltimore: Williams & Wilkins.
3. Medical Research Council (1974) *War Memorandum No. 7 (1943) Aids to the Investigation of Peripheral Nerve Injuries*, 2nd edn. Her Majesty's Stationery Office.

Isometric (static) strength tests
4. International Committee for the Standardisation of Physical Fitness Tests, Larson, L. A. (Ed.) (1974) *Fitness, Health and Work Capacity: International Standards of Assessment*. New York: Macmillan.

Isokinetic testing
5. Moffroid, M., Whipple, E. A., Hofkosh, J., Lowman, E. & Thistle, H. (1969) A study of Isokinetic Exercise. *Physical Therapy*, Vol. 49, No. 7, pp. 735–746.
6. Molnar, G. E. & Alexander, J. (1974) Development of quantitative standards of muscle strength in children. *Archives of Physical Medicine and Rehabilitation*, Vol. 55, pp. 490–493.

Tests of muscle length
7. Janda, V. (1983) *Muscle Function Testing*. London: Butterworths.
8. Kendall, F. P. & McCreary, E. K. (1983) *Muscles – Testing and Function*, 3rd edn. Baltimore: Williams and Wilkins.

Measurement and recording of joint range
9. American Academy of Orthopaedic Surgeons. (1966) *Joint Measurement*. Edinburgh: Churchill Livingstone.
10. Moore, M. L. (1949) The measurement of joint motion Part 1 – Introductory review of literature. *Physical Therapy Review*, Vol. 29, pp. 195–205.
11. Moore, M. L. (1949) The measurement of joint motion Part 2 – the Technic of Goniometry. *Physical Therapy Review*, Vol. 29, pp. 256–264.
12. Moore, M. L. (1984) Clinical assessment of joint motion. In Basmajian, J. V. (Ed.) *Therapeutic Exercise*, 4th edn. Baltimore: Williams & Wilkins.

Sensory Testing
13. Macleod, J. (Ed.) (1979) *Clinical Examination*, 5th edn. Edinburgh: Churchill Livingstone.
14. Wood Jones, F. (1941) *The function of Anatomy as seen in the hand*. London: Baillière Tindall & Cox.
15. Wynn Parry, C. B. (1981) *Rehabilitation of the Hand*, 4th edn. London: Butterworths.

A test of the activities of daily living
16. Bromley, I. (1977) *Tetraplegia and Paraplegia*. Edinburgh: Churchill Livingstone.
17. Buchwald, E. (1952) *Physical Rehabilitation for Daily Living*. New York: McGraw-Hill.
18. Buchwald Lawton, E. (1963) *Activities of Daily Living for Physical Rehabilitation*. New York: McGraw-Hill.
19. Veteran's Administration Medical Rehabilitation Service (1946) *What's My Score? Handbook for patients with disabilities resulting from spinal cord injuries*. V. A. Pamphlet 10–10.

Trendelenburg sign: Thomas' test: test for actual and apparent leg length
20. Adams, J. C. (1981) *Outline of Orthopaedics*, 9th edn. Edinburgh: Churchill Livingstone.
21. Apley, A. G. (1977) *System of Orthopaedics and Fractures*, 5th edn. London: Butterworths.

Tests of respiratory function
22. Macleod, J. (Ed.) (1979) *Clinical Examination*, 5th edn. Edinburgh: Churchill Livingstone.

Appendix 2

Basic guidelines for the analysis, planning and teaching of a functional activity

Three major factors need to be considered when planning the teaching of a functional activity to a patient. These are:

1. The analysis of the activity
2. The demands placed on the patient by the activity and his ability to meet them safely
3. An effective teaching programme.

THE ANALYSIS OF THE ACTIVITY

The activity can be divided into several distinct phases which go to form the movement sequence. The movements in one phase flow smoothly into the next and so on until the activity is completed. Once each phase has been clearly defined it can be subdivided into its basic motions.

Further analysis is necessary in respect of:

1. The specific joint movements involved, i.e. which joints are moved through what range and which are stabilised
2. The muscles involved and the role each plays as well as the type of contraction occurring
3. The varying needs for postural stability at all stages of the activity
4. The sensory demands of the activity
5. The overall speed necessary for an economical performance.
6. Any mechanical considerations
7. Any physical or environmental hazards

8. The selection of any necessary equipment and its placement
9. Help needed by the patient from the physiotherapist for any particular phase of the movement sequence.

The demands on the patient

In planning for any activity a careful examination of the patient is necessary so that the therapist has a knowledge of his physical condition, his abilities, his need and desire to perform the activity, his fears and any special precautions necessary. The therapist must determine if the activity is within the patient's present capabilities and that he has the potential to succeed within a reasonable time period.

The teaching of the activity

A clear preliminary explanation and demonstration are given by the physiotherapist. She uses those words of instruction which will be repeated during the training programme. This should help the patient gain a knowledge of:

1. The movement as a whole, the sequence to be followed and the areas of potential difficulty
2. Any help needed to give him confidence and preserve his safety
3. Preliminary training of a specific part of the movement sequence as well as any supplementary help that may be given by the therapist at the point of need so that the total movement sequence may be achieved.

Following testing the training pattern should remain constant if possible and be practised regularly.

An example of the analysis of an activity

The activity to be briefly analysed here is 'standing to sitting on a straight chair'. As with most activities there are several ways of performing this task depending on such factors as the body proportions and abilities of the patient and the dimensions of the chair. Other factors such as the patient's initial position in relation to the chair will influence the movement sequence.

During the movement the arms may hang loosely by the side or if necessary, help control the rate of the final stage of the descent onto the chair.

Only the basic essentials will be analysed here but it is stressed that an analysis can be made as detailed as required by the circumstances. This analysis focuses on patient education rather than a full kinematic statement. The use of simple instructions which remain constant during the training period is highlighted.

Preparation for the activity

Action	Instruction
1. Check chair position for safety. Look at chair, gauge its height, place self with back to chair.	1. 'See that your chair is in a safe position.'
2. Check foot placement. There are two basic ways of placing the feet:	2. 'Check that your feet are firmly placed on the floor.'
a. feet parallel and slightly apart; or	
b. one foot placed slightly in front of the other (walk standing) – thus increasing the stability provided by the shape and size of the base. Both these positions influence the later movements at the ankles, knees, hips and trunk.	
3. Standing with back to the chair, feel the edge of the chair with either the back of one or both legs.	3. 'Feel the edge of the seat of the chair.'

Movement sequence

Action	Instruction
1. Slowly bend the knees, ankles and hips while simultaneously inclining the trunk forwards over the base.	1. 'Slowly lower your body on to the chair, keeping your trunk forward.'
2. Place the buttocks well back over the seat to ensure stability. This will also avoid the unnecessary friction from clothes on the seat occurring when pushing back on the chair.	2. 'Sit well back on to the seat.'
3. Once contact is made with the seat, raise and straighten the trunk to sit erect. Ensure that the legs are slightly apart and the feet are in a good position, parallel to each other and slightly apart with the soles firmly placed on the floor.	3. 'Sit up tall. Check to see that your legs are slightly apart and the soles of your feet are firmly on the floor.'

Postural stability

1. The head is held in alignment with the body throughout the movement sequence. Small 'righting' movements occur.
2. Body weight should be well balanced over both feet.
3. Trunk stability is maintained during the lowering action.
4. The arms may be used if necessary to help control and supplement the latter part of the lowering movement and thus provide an even flow of the movement and aid recovery.

Specific joint movements

The major joints involved are the hips, knees and ankles as well as the joints of the lumbar spine. The range of joint motion and angular velocity will vary from joint to joint according to the relative lengths of the body segments and the height of the chair. If one joint is restricted, any other joint or joints in the movement sequence may act at least temporarily in an increased range to allow the activity to be performed, though the pattern of the movement will change and be more awkward. The amount of pelvic rotation will vary.

Muscle activity

1. There will be active lengthening (eccentric contraction) primarily by the extensors of the ankles, knees and hips to brake gravity's action of pulling the body down onto the chair.
2. Bilateral extensor muscle activity of the trunk and neck will prevent the trunk and head from collapsing forward during the lowering movement. Active shortening (concentric contraction) of these same muscles as well as the extensors of the hip acting through the pelvis aid in pulling the body into an erect sitting position at the end of the sequence.
3. The depressors of the shoulder girdle and extensors of the elbow may be activated if the arms are used as props during part of the descent.

Sensory control of the movement sequence

The patient needs to be able to:

1. See the chair at the start of the action
2. Feel the chair and the floor
3. Hear the familiar words of instruction that the therapist uses when training the movement sequence
4. Appreciate his own movements, the effect of gravity on his body and the rate of his descent into the chair.

Mechanical factors involved

1. Gravity pulls the body downwards. This is controlled by forces produced through muscle activity.
2. Leverage alters due to the changing relationship of the line of gravity to the joint axes during the movement.

3. The line of gravity alters its projection in relation to the base.
4. Friction between the feet and the floor helps provide stability.
5. Friction can occur between the patient's clothing and the surface of the chair if he has to pull back on the seat of the chair.

This friction acts as a resistance to the movement.
6. Pressure between the buttocks, thighs and the seat can lead to discomfort if there is a poor match between the size and shape of the chair and the patient.

REFERENCES AND FURTHER READING

1. Bromley, I. (1976) *Tetraplegia and Paraplegia.* Edinburgh: Churchill Livingstone.
2. Broer, M. R. & Zernicke, R. F. (1979) *Efficiency of Human Movement*, 4th edn. Philadelphia: W. B. Saunders.
3. Buchwald, E. (1952) *Physical Rehabilitation for Daily Living.* New York: McGraw-Hill.
4. Buchwald Lawton, E. (1963) *Activities of Daily Living for Physical Rehabilitation.* New York: McGraw-Hill.
5. Carr, J. H. & Shepherd, R. B. (1982) *A Motor Relearning Programme for Stroke.* London: Heinemann Medical.
6. Hobson, E. P. G. (1956) *Physiotherapy in Paraplegia.* London: J. & A. Churchill.
7. Rasch, P. J. & Burke, R. K. (1978) *Kinesiology and Applied Anatomy*, 6th edn. Philadelphia: Lea & Febiger.
8. Rusk, H. A. & Taylor, E. J. (1953) *Living with a Disability.* New York: The Blakiston Company.
9. Veteran's Administration Medical Rehabilitation Service (1946) *What's My Score? Handbook for patients with disabilities resulting from spinal cord injuries.* V. A. Pamphlet 10–10.

Index